D0712614

Cerebral Reorganization of Function After Brain Damage

CEREBRAL REORGANIZATION OF FUNCTION AFTER BRAIN DAMAGE

Edited by

Harvey S. Levin
Departments of Physical Medicine and Rehabilitation,
Psychiatry, Neurosurgery, and Pediatrics
Baylor College of Medicine

Jordan Grafman
Cognitive Neuroscience Section
National Institute of Neurological Disorders and Stroke
National Institutes of Health

OXFORD
UNIVERSITY PRESS

2000

Oxford   New York
Athens   Auckland   Bangkok   Bogotá   Buenos Aires   Calcutta
Cape Town   Chennai   Dar es Salaam   Delhi   Florence   Hong Kong   Istanbul
Karachi   Kuala Lumpur   Madrid   Melbourne   Mexico City   Mumbai
Nairobi   Paris   São Paulo   Singapore   Taipei   Tokyo   Toronto   Warsaw

and associated companies in
Berlin   Ibadan

Published by Oxford University Press, Inc.,
198 Madison Avenue, New York, New York, 10016
http://www.oup-usa.org
1-800-334-4249

Library of Congress Cataloging-in-Publication Data
Cerebral reorganization of function after brain damage / edited by Harvey S. Levin, Jordan Grafman.
p.; cm.
Includes bibliographical references.
ISBN 0-19-512026-4
1. Neuroplasticity.   2. Brain damage—Patients—Rehabilitation.   I. Levin, Harvey S.
II. Grafman, Jordan.
[DNLM: 1. Brain Injuries—rehabilitation.   2. Brain Injuries—complications.
3. Cognition Disorders—rehabilitation.   4. Neuronal Plasticity. WL 354 C4146 2000]
QP363.3 .C47 2000
616.8—dc21   99-047749

9 8 7 6 5 4 3 2 1
Printed in the United States of America
on acid-free paper

I dedicate this book to Arthur Benton for the training I received under his leadership at the University of Iowa and for his mentorship throughout my career, to Robert Grossman and Howard Eisenberg for their encouragement during my transition to becoming an independent investigator, to Angela Williams for her support and understanding, and to Keisha S. Johnson for coordination with the authors and Oxford University Press.

H.S.L.

This book, like all my other research, is supported by the intellectual stimulation and care I receive from my wife Irene Litvan. To my mother, Phyllis, whose courage provided me the foundation that my career is built upon. Finally, I owe a great deal to all the staff and fellows who have passed through the Cognitive Neuroscience Section whose thoughts and creativity force me to continually challenge my own beliefs and methods.

J.G.

Foreword

Twenty years ago, a graduate student delving into the mysteries of nervous system injury or neurodegeneration understood the term *neuroplasticity* to refer to the developmental process and believed that after birth, it was downhill all the way. Today, a graduate student of neuroscience hardly knows where to begin to tackle the many processes that are involved in the dynamic, changing, responsive, "plastic" brain. Levin and Grafman have highlighted an exciting area of neuroscience from the important perspective of rehabilitation of the injured brain. The contents of this volume will lead the interested reader through the background, significance, practical applications, and potential future of neuroplasticity as a natural part of the living nervous system and as a tool to use in the treatment of neurological conditions.

The book has four well-rounded parts: a history and introduction, a perspective on the types of research relevant to brain plasticity, techniques to evaluate changes in the brain, and the possible applications of concepts of neuroplasticity to rehabilitation practice.

Parts I and II present a comprehensive and thought-provoking overview of the concepts of plasticity, or the capacity for change within the nervous system. Important theories in neuroscience and psychology are discussed in light of recent findings. The chapters in these two parts of the volume point out the usefulness of animal models, from rodents to primates, in the study of brain development, circuitry, plasticity, and injury. In addition to the existing paradigms, new technologies to produce knockout or transgenic animals will allow genetic dissection of the mechanisms that underlie the establishment of and changes seen in the brain's circuitry. These chapters present a wide variety of basic research that highlights important advances in neuroplasticity theory. Studies of primates show that alterations can occur in limbic cortical areas that control emotion, executive function, and reasoning capacities; it is intriguing to relate these observations to the sequelae of human traumatic brain injury. The intense connectivity among brain regions and the implications of these associations are clearly presented. Primate models certainly provide brain maps that can be closely related to human maps, and rodent models provide the opportunity for fairly rapid assessment of the numerous intrinsic chemical alterations that occur after injury. These factors change after injury, and such alterations may contribute to the molecular and synaptic plasticity that are part of regeneration and fiber sprouting in damaged systems. The observations of changes in cortical maps can be put into the context of changes in neurotransmitters, growth-stimulating proteins, and hormones. Several chapters present the robust responses of neurons and glial cells in a way that encourages further inquiry and adds important information to the knowledge base of any reader interested in neural plasticity, brain injury, or rehabilitation.

The authors do not shy away from the complexities of interpreting the findings from animal models of stroke and traumatic brain injury (TBI) that include attempts at treatment. Seemingly contradictory results from different models are reconciled by introducing important concepts relating to the possible cascades of secondary injury that result from ischemia and trauma and the timing of interventions meant to overcome deficits. For rehabilitation strategies, there may be periods of increased tissue vulnerability. Very early or aggressive programs of therapy may actually promote maladaptive plastic changes, leading to more severe lesions and deficits. The same cautionary note is applied to drug therapies, and agents that may appear efficacious when given soon after injury may do harm if therapy is delayed. These observations are important to both researchers and clinicians in the field who wish to design therapies for TBI.

The second half of the book provides both an excellent overview and detailed studies of plasticity in the human brain, both in the developing child and in the injured adult. These chapters present numerous methods of studying brain function that include neuropsychological tests and medical imaging. As one author states, "The developing brain is a dynamic, responsive, and self-organizing system. Early injury constitutes a perturbation of normal development" (Stiles, Chapter 10, p. 201). The effects of TBI, especially a mild injury, may not be immediately apparent, but emerge later during development when language, reading, or social interactions are usually acquired. The complexities of development and damage are often difficult to dissect. Again, the authors present the difficulties as well as the possible interpretations and caveats of using a particular parameter to assess function. Such methods as functional magnetic resonance imaging, electroencephalography, dichotic listening, and position emission tomography, scanning, to name only a few, are presented along with case studies of a variety of developmental disorders, TBI, and stroke. Results are interpreted carefully, with an understanding of the techniques used, the disorders under study, and the developmental processes that may impinge on results. Such a careful overview presents the reader with an idea of the combination of assessment tools that are necessary when tackling a study of brain plasticity. The discussion of future directions for research and practice presented in Chapter 19 provides an exciting conclusion to the volume.

The book leads the reader through the complexities and promise of neuroplasticity, and presents insights into current and future research and clinical practice. It is a valuable overview for anyone interested in how the brain works, develops and creates, responds to injury, and forms itself in response to the environment.

Mary Ellen Cheung, Ph.D.
Repair and Plasticity, National Institute of Neurological Disorders and Stroke

Preface

It is compelling to watch a young child learn the meaning of a new word or how to play a computer game. Children learn through trial and error and at times demonstrate a remarkably rapid learning curve. Fortunately, learning is not restricted to children; we retain the capacity to learn throughout life. This capacity can even be seen when children and adults suffer brain damage and need to relearn knowledge or skills that they had previously acquired or need to learn new knowledge and skills. That the brain mediates this learning and is the storehouse of new knowledge and skills has been known for centuries. What has been less certain is how the brain manages to change to accommodate new learning under normal conditions or following damage at various stages in development. Within the last 30 years, there has been considerable progress in forming an understanding of the genetic, cellular, assembly, system, and psychological factors that contribute to learning and plasticity. The purpose of this volume is to provide an update of much of that work and to suggest ways in which the knowledge gained in the laboratory can be translated into practical gains in helping people recover from brain damage.

Although it is clear that plasticity can be reflected at various levels in the nervous system, it is by no means obvious which level is most important or appropriate for an understanding of different forms of learning. The dominant theme in this volume is that changes at the network level are crucial for an understanding of how new learning is accomplished. For example, some researchers believe that the capacity to learn is reflected in the density of connectivity (and neurons) in a network. There is also evidence that as a network is activated and used during learning, the boundaries of the network expand to reflect its growing participation in a functional activity. The idea of a flexible boundary is appealing because it suggests that while the brain has regional functional networks that become firmly established at maturity, their boundaries can be extremely flexible in childhood and even in adulthood. It is not known whether this functional map expansion comes at a cost to the functional capabilities of neighboring networks.

One of the goals of this volume is to understand whether the basic principles of neuronal plasticity such as those described above can be used to develop treatments that can facilitate recovery of function after brain injury. There appear to be at least four major forms of neuroplasticity that can occur after brain damage. One form was alluded to above and is indicated by an expansion in the size of the cortical map of a sensorimotor or cognitive function with use. Another form of plasticity concerns the apparent transfer of function from one region of cortex to another—usually to the contralateral cortex. This phenomenon is generally known as *homologous region adaptation*. It suggests that the transferred function was at least partially latent (and perhaps inhibited or masked) in the homologous region and could not emerge without concomitant brain damage in the contralateral hemisphere. A most dramatic form of functional plasticity, known as *sensory substitution*, indicates that a cortical region previously devoted to accepting the sensory input of one modality (e.g., vision) is now capable of processing a new kind of sensory input (e.g., tactile information). This form of sensory substitution has been documented in subjects who were blind from birth and whose visual cortices, area V1, now serve as a relay station for the tactile information used in Braille reading. The fourth form of neuroplasticity is compensatory and can complicate the interpretation of observed learning and plasticity in people recovering from brain injury. In this case, an alternative mode of processing is now used to accomplish a task that was previously performed by the damaged area of the brain. For example, many people rely on spatial cues to navigate a route. If they incur brain damage to the nondominant parietal cortex, they may be left with persistent spatial-cognitive deficits. In order to navigate routes, they may have to learn to rely on verbal instructions. Using verbal instructions, they still may be able to achieve their goal (to reach a location), but it will be via an alternative cognitive strategy. No doubt the use of this compensatory strategy results in an altered distributed neural network, but rather than the emergence of a new function, it is the reordering of weights in the previously established distributed network that accomplishes the task. These four kinds of functional and neural adaptation (of the brain) can be explored with a variety of tools ranging from single-cell and cell assembly recordings to functional neuroimaging techniques in humans. The advantages of any research effort are that the research at various levels of the nervous system proceeds in parallel and that the results obtained across levels can be integrated to achieve new insights.

Our desire to address these broad issues led to the organization of a workshop on neuroplasticity that was held at the National Institutes of Health in Bethesda, Maryland, and a series of lectures presented at Baylor College of Medicine in Houston, Texas. The chapters in this book are an outgrowth of the talks given at these two venues.

We want to thank Dr. Mary Ellen Cheung of the National Institute of Neurological Disorders and Stroke for her support and encouragement in organizing the workshop on neuroplasticity, which was held on the campus of the National Institutes of Health in Bethesda, Maryland. We also want to thank the late Dr. Sarah Broman for her critical comments on the organization of the workshop, as well as Jeffrey House and Fiona Stevens of Oxford University Press for their encouragement during the preparation of the book.

Houston, Texas   H. L.
Bethesda, Maryland   J. G.
August 1999

Contents

Contributors

JAROSLAW ARONOWSKI, PH.D.
Department of Neurology
University of Texas Health Science
  Center
Houston, Texas

JOCELYNE BACHEVALIER, PH.D.
Department of Neurobiology and Anatomy
University of Texas Health Science
  Center
Houston, Texas

PAUL BACH-Y-RITA, M.D.
Center for Neuroscience and Department
  of Rehabilitation Medicine and
  Department of Biomedical Engineering
University of Wisconsin
Madison, Wisconsin

HELEN BARBAS, PH.D.
Department of Health Sciences
Boston University and Department of
  Anatomy and Neurobiology
Boston University School of Medicine
  and New England Regional Primate
  Research Center
Harvard Medical School
Boston, Massachusetts

H. SCOTT BARBAY, PH.D.
Center on Aging and Department of
  Molecular and Integrative Physiology
University of Kansas Medical Center
Kansas City, Kansas

ARTHUR BENTON, PH.D.
Department of Neurology
Division of Cognitive Neuroscience
University of Iowa
College of Medicine
Iowa City, Iowa

SONDRA T. BLAND
Department of Psychology and Institute
  for Neuroscience
University of Texas
Austin, Texas

DEANNA L. BUCK, M.S.
Department of Psychology
Virginia Commonwealth University
Richmond, Virginia

RANDY L. BUCKNER, PH.D.
Department of Psychology
Washington University
St. Louis, Missouri

GÖRAN CARLSSON, PH.D.
Department of Pediatrics
Christian-Albrecht's University of Kiel
Kiel, Germany

LUCINDA J. CARR, M.D.
Great Ormond Street Hospital for
  Children
NHS Trust and The Institute of Child
  Health
London, England

SANDRA B. CHAPMAN, PH.D.
The Callier Center for Communication
  Disorders
University of Texas at Dallas
Dallas, Texas

LEONARDO G. COHEN, M.D.
Human Cortical Physiology Unit
National Institute of Neurological
  Disorders and Stroke
National Institutes of Health
Bethesda, Maryland

S. MICHELLE DeFORD, M.S.
Department of Psychology
Virginia Commonwealth University
Richmond, Virginia

EDWARD .R. ERGENZINGER, PH.D.
Department of Neurosurgery
Wake Forest University
School of Medicine
Winston-Salem, North Carolina

PAULINE A. FILIPEK, M.D.
Departments of Pediatrics and Neurology
University of California
Irvine Medical Center
Orange, California

CANDACE L. FLOYD, M.S.
Department of Psychology
Virginia Commonwealth University
Richmond, Virginia

RUEBEN GONZALES, PH.D.
Department of Pharmacology and
  Toxicology
Institute for Neuroscience
University of Texas
Austin, Texas

SHARON GOODALL, M.S.
Departments of Computer Science and
  Neurology
Institute for Advanced Computational
  Studies
University of Maryland
College Park, Maryland

JORDAN GRAFMAN, PH.D.
Cognitive Neuroscience Section
National Institute of Neurological
  Disorders and Stroke
National Institutes of Health
Bethesda, Maryland

JAMES GROTTA, M.D.
Department of Neurology
University of Texas School of Medicine
Houston, Texas

MARK HALLETT, M.D.
Human Motor Control Section
National Institute of Neurological
  Disorders and Stroke
National Institutes of Health
Bethesda, Maryland

ROBERT J. HAMM, PH.D.
Department of Psychology
Virginia Commonwealth University
Richmond, Virginia

HARRIET HARWARD, M.S., L.P.A.
The Callier Center for Communication
  Disorders
University of Texas at Dallas
Dallas, Texas

KENNETH HUGDAHL, PH.D.
Department of Biological and Medical
  Psychology
University of Bergen
Bergen, Norway

JEFFREY A. KLEIM, PH.D.
Center on Aging and Department
  of Molecular and Integrative
  Physiology
University of Kansas Medical Center
Kansas City, Kansas

BRYAN KOLB, PH.D.
Department of Psychology
University of Lethbridge
Lethbridge, Alberta
Canada

J. LEIGH LEASURE
Department of Psychology and Institute
   for Neuroscience
University of Texas
Austin, Texas

HARVEY S. LEVIN, PH.D.
Department of Physical Medicine and
   Rehabilitation
Department of Psychiatry and Behavioral
   Sciences
Department of Neurosurgery
Baylor College of Medicine
Houston, Texas

LUDISE MALKOVA, PH.D.
Laboratory of Neuropsychology
National Institute of Mental Health
National Institutes of Health
Bethesda, Maryland

RANDOLPH J. NUDO, PH.D.
Center on Aging and Department
   of Molecular and Integrative
   Physiology
University of Kansas Medical
   Center
Kansas City, Kansas

STEVEN E. PETERSEN, PH.D.
Department of Neurology
Washington University
School of Medicine
St. Louis, Missouri

TIM P. PONS, PH.D.
Department of Neurosurgery
Wake Forest University
School of Medicine
Winston-Salem, North Carolina

JAMES A. REGGIA, M.D., PH.D.
Departments of Computer Science and
   Neurology
Institute for Advanced Computational
   Studies
University of Maryland
College Park, Maryland

KEN REVETT, PH.D.
Departments of Computer Science
   and Neurology
Institute for Advanced Computational
   Studies
University of Maryland
College Park, Maryland

TIMOTHY C. RICKARD, PH.D.
Department of Psychology
University of California, San Diego
La Jolla, California

EYTAN RUPPIN, M.D., PH.D.
Departments of Computer Science
   and Physiology
Tel Aviv University
Tel-Aviv, Israel

TIMOTHY SCHALLERT, PH.D.
Department of Psychology
Institute for Neuroscience
University of Texas
Austin, Texas

JAMES SONG, M.S.
Department of Physical Medicine and
   Rehabilitation
Baylor College of Medicine
Houston, Texas

JOAN STILES, PH.D.
Department of Cognitive Science
University of California,
   San Diego
La Jolla, California

MEREDITH D. TEMPLE, PH.D.
Department of Psychology
Virginia Commonwealth
   University
Richmond, Virginia

JENNIFER TILLERSON
Department of Psychology and Institute
   for Neuroscience
University of Texas
Austin, Texas

DANIEL TRANEL, PH.D.
Department of Neurology
Division of Cognitive Neuroscience
University of Iowa
College of Medicine
Iowa City, Iowa

J.T. WALL, PH.D.
Department of Neurobiology and Anatomy
Medical College of Ohio
Toledo, Ohio

ERIC M. WASSERMAN, M.D.
Office of the Clinical Director
National Institute of Neurological
  Disorders and Stroke
National Institutes of Health
Bethesda, Maryland

IAN Q. WHISHAW, PH.D.
Department of Psychology
University of Lethbridge
Lethbridge, Alberta
Canada

LAWRENCE WILLIAMS, PH.D.
Guilford Pharmaceuticals
Baltimore, Maryland

J. XU, PH.D.
Department of Neurobiology and
  Anatomy
Medical College of Ohio
Toledo, Ohio

Cerebral Reorganization of Function After Brain Damage

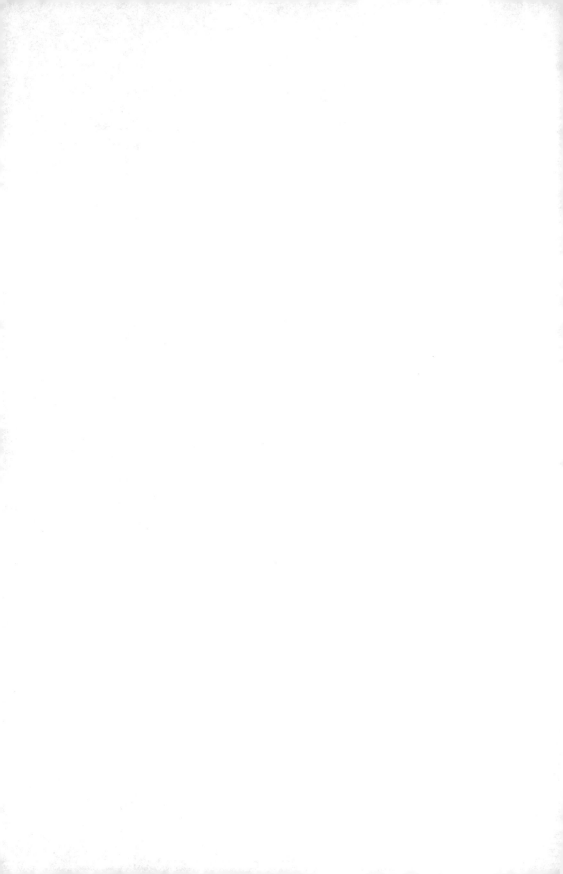

1

Historical Notes on Reorganization of Function and Neuroplasticity

ARTHUR BENTON AND DANIEL TRANEL

The Birth of Concepts

Spontaneous recovery of function after a disabling injury or illness must have been quite evident to observers since time immemorial. Early physicians and natural scientists had no great difficulty accounting for the phenomenon. Both natural and supernatural forces were considered to be quite capable of determining the course of disease, for better or for worse. Thus Hippocratic medicine generally ascribed unexpected recovery to the "healing power of nature" (*vis naturae medicatrix* in the Latin terminology). "Nature is the healer of disease. . . . It is nature itself that finds the way; though untaught and uninstructed, it does what is proper" (*Epidemics* VI, 5; cited by Neuburger, 1926, and Castiglione, 1958). Through the ages, the large element of truth in this doctrine has been amply confirmed. Neuburger (1926) provided a detailed account of its promulgation and interpretation by leading figures in medicine from antiquity to the middle of the 19th century. The recent rise of alternative medicine, which is striving in some cases for more or less equal footing with conventional medicine, is another testimonial to the power of this position.

Reliance on the efficacy of supernatural forces as a determinant of the outcome of illness dates back even earlier. And as the worldwide prevalence of faith healers and of prayers and supplications offered on behalf of the sick attests, this belief is still firmly held.

In the early 19th century a more specific factor was introduced by the French physiologist Pierre Flourens. This pioneer of the ablation experiment insisted that the cerebral lobes operated as a whole, without specialization of function in any particular region. All parts of the lobes (of the hen and the pigeon!) subserved all perceptual, intellectual, and volitional functions equally. When the lobes were completely removed, all of these capacities were completely lost. Ablations that were very large, but not complete, resulted in impairment, but not complete loss, of capacities. However, with smaller removals of tissue in any sector of the lobes there was complete return of function of all modalities. In short, Flourens argued for the equivalence, and against the localization, of function within the anterior lobes of his animals. His findings also supported the principle of *redundancy* to account for the restitution of functions after partial ablations. The assumption was that the anatomic substrate was more than enough to support the functions, so that tissue remaining after such ablations was quite sufficient to permit complete recovery after the initial surgical shock.

Finally, Flourens emphasized the importance of the *size of the lesion* as a determinant of whether or not restoration of function would occur. He was also a belligerent opponent and caustic critic of the localizationist system of Franz Joseph Gall, with its placement of some 27 abilities and personality traits in different regions of the human cerebral cortex. There ensued during the first half of the 19th century a rancorous controversy between the "localizationists" (not all of whom necessarily subscribed to Gall's scheme) and the "antilocalizationists," who insisted that the cerebral hemispheres operated as a unit. However, with Broca's correlation between speech disorder and focal left hemisphere disease in the 1860s, and the demonstration of the excitable motor cortex by Fritsch and Hitzig in 1870, the tide turned more or less irreversibly in favor of the doctrine of localization.

These momentous discoveries gave rise to remarkable advances in the identification of neuronal aggregates and pathways in the human cerebral cortex that formed the crucial anatomic substrates of sensation, perception, movement, and speech. Increasingly precise clinical and experimental studies established the concept of a system of stable connections involving afferent processes, central operating mechanisms, and efferent processes. This scheme proved to be notably successful in guiding clinical inference. A prime example is the progressive growth of knowledge of the visual system from the retina to the posterior and mesial occipital lobes, which accounted satisfactorily for the diverse visual field defects that were observed clinically (see Brouwer, 1936, and Polyak, 1955, for detailed accounts of this development). Similar advances in the delineation of the networks underlying audition, somesthesis, movement, and speech were achieved. Consequently, given that lower-level injury could be excluded, a physician who encountered a patient with a visual defect, a hemiparesis, a Broca (nonfluent) aphasia, or a Wernicke (fluent) aphasia could ascribe the disability with a reasonable degree of confidence to a focal lesion in a defined cortical area or its proximal connections with the rest of the brain.

However, this development, which established clinical neurology as a significant medical specialty and greatly enlarged the scope of neurological surgery, gave rise to a problem. It was commonly observed that many patients, after "stabilization" of their condition following stroke or trauma, i.e., after the global, nonspecific effects of the insult had disappeared, showed some degree of restitution of function; indeed, some patients showed complete recovery. For example, the condition of a patient with a Wernicke type of aphasia, with marked receptive speech defects, might evolve over months or even years into a less severe clinical picture more accurately characterized as *amnesic, conduction,* or *anomic* aphasia. Or a permanent visual field defect might no longer have the adverse effects on visual efficiency that it originally exerted. Severe anosognosia would evolve relatively quickly into a milder anosodiaphoria, in which a disability is acknowledged but its importance minimized. Severe hemineglect would resolve into a mild left-sided attentional defect. Or a dense hemiplegia might evolve over time into a mild hemiparesis.

The problem was that the concept of redundancy, dependent as it was on the principle of equivalence of function in all parts of the hemispheres, could not account adequately for these instances of recovery. When a lesion completely destroyed a neural region committed to the support of a behavioral capacity, such as Broca's area or Wernicke's area, one could hardly invoke redundancy as an explanation for the observed alleviation of the disability in speech following development of the lesion. In order for restitution of function, partial or complete, to occur, there had to be some alteration in the neural mechanism subserving the ability. In short, there had to be a *reorganization* of the neural substrate. The general idea of reorganization was often expressed more specifically as *vicarious functioning,* i.e., the mobilization of a region connected to the damaged substrate, such as the homologous area in the opposite hemisphere or the immediately surrounding area, to assume responsibility for mediating the lost or impaired function. (Current thinking regarding recovery from aphasia has focused on precisely these concepts, and new technology, e.g., positron emission tomography, may permit a definitive test of their validity.)

There was still another development in these early years. In 1868, only 3 years after Broca finally proclaimed that "one speaks with the left hemisphere," Jules Cotard reported that children with congenital or early acquired atrophy of the left hemisphere did not grow up to be aphasic. Thus, although the commitment of speech to the left hemisphere might be inborn, that commitment was not immutable; under some circumstances it was entirely circumvented. Evidently the neural substrate for the future development of speech in the infant or young child was sufficiently flexible to allow for alteration of the commitment. In short, some degree of *plasticity* was also a characteristic of the human brain. A few years later, the concept of plasticity received a measure of support from the observations of Otto Soltmann (1876) on the effects of hemispheric ablations in infant dogs and rabbits. Soltmann could not discern any abnormalities in the behavior of the animals after extirpation of cortical areas that presumably controlled movement, and he concluded that the region was not functional in the early postnatal period.

In the 1870s, Hughlings Jackson called attention to the significance of the *rate* of development of a lesion as a determinant of its symptomatology. A rapidly developing lesion (e.g., stroke) produced more severe disability than one that developed more slowly (e.g., tumor). "In all cases of nervous disease we must endeavor to estimate the element of rapidity of lesions, not only the quantity of nervous elements destroyed, but the rapidity of their destruction. We have to estimate the momentum of lesions" (Jackson, 1879, cited by Joynt, 1970). In a later study, Riese (1948) made the same point. The concept of *momentum* was concerned primarily with the issue of sparing of function. However, in its insistence that factors other than structural ones influenced the consequences of neuronal damage, it had a bearing on recovery as well.

As Joynt (1970) has pointed out, Jackson's "momentum" can be seen as a component of Von Monakow's (1911–1914) later concept of *diaschisis*. Distinguishing his concept from the global effects of traumatic or surgical shock, Von Monakow defined diaschisis as the selective disruptive effect of a focal lesion on the operations of areas with which it was structurally and functionally connected, such as the homologous region in the opposite hemisphere or an adjacent area. Diaschisis may be widespread if distant areas with neural connections to the lesioned area are affected. In contrast to shock, diaschisis is relatively longlasting, extending over months or even years. As its disruptive effects wane over time, recovery of function may occur.

Early Studies

Equivalence and Redundancy

Over the years, each of these early concepts regarding sparing and recovery of function after brain injury had its proponents. With respect to the concept of equivalence of function, the propositions of Flourens were supported a century later by Karl Lashley (1929) and also by his early collaborator, Shepherd Ivory Franz (1912). As is well known, Lashley concluded from his studies of the acquisition and retention of maze performances in rats that all areas of the cerebral cortex were equally important as the neural basis of these relatively complex learning and memory functions, and that the degree of behavioral impairment was simply proportional to the amount of tissue that had been removed.

Lashley also emphasized the extreme redundancy in the neural underpinnings of sensory and perceptual processes. For example, he reported that although complete removal of the visual cortical area did abolish pattern discrimination in rats, an *almost* complete removal that left only a small remnant of tissue sufficed to spare the capacity. In general, he argued against the assumption of sharply delimited cortical centers and for the concept of distributed neural circuits as the foundation for behavioral processes. In a number of studies he described recovery of motor function after focal ablations that, according to classical doctrine, should have produced permanent impairment.

In view of the steadily increasing evidence for the significance of regional cerebral differences in the determination of *human* cognitive performance, the doctrine of equivalence of function was viewed with extreme skepticism. Nevertheless, a large-scale investigation by Chapman and Wolff (1959) of patients with surgically excised lesions sought to support it. Based on the neurosurgeon's estimate of the amount of neural tissue lost, and utilizing a large battery of tests, the authors concluded that the size of the neural lesion was the sole determinant of the degree of impairment in the "highest integrative" cognitive functions. In general, moderate correlations between the mass of excised tissue and overall scores on neuropsycho-logical tests such as the Halstead-Reitan Battery were found. However, regional differences (e.g., frontal versus nonfrontal, right versus left hemisphere) were also evident. This massive study received very little attention.

The potential importance of *rehabilitation procedures* for restitution of func-tion was highlighted in a small study by Ogden and Franz (1917) that described almost complete recovery from paralysis after ablation of the cortical motor region in a monkey that was forced to use its hemiplegic arm. In contrast, there was little or no recovery in monkeys that were not subjected to the procedure. Decades later, Critchley (1949) and Furmanski (1950) reported that prolonged practice and cor-rection of errors significantly improved the performances of patients with parietal lobe lesions who showed extinction under the condition of double simultaneous stimulation.

Redundancy, in one form or another and explicitly or implicitly, was invoked by a host of other theorists, either in the context of discussions of cerebral localiza-tion or to account for recovery of function. For example, the physiologist Friedrich Goltz (1888) made the point that small lesions that presumably destroyed discrete cortical centers had absolutely no effect on the behavioral capacities of dogs, and that therefore the neural underpinnings of such capacities must be more extensive. Larger ablations (including hemispherectomy) produced surprisingly small defects in performance because the spared regions were capable of supporting the behav-ioral functions.

A rather different form of redundancy was postulated by Hughlings Jackson in his hierarchical conception of the organization of the nervous system. According to Jackson, sensory and motor functions are represented at each level, the more com-plex aspects (as well as the simpler aspects) being represented at the highest level. At the same time, the highest level includes the nerve fibers from the lower levels as well as its own, producing "multiple representation" of a function at that level. As a consequence, a lesion at the highest level leaves many fibers intact and pro-duces less (or no) impairment in some functions than the same lesion at a lower level. "Hence large destroying lesions in the hemisphere will result in no palsy, whereas palsy will follow lesions equally large in the corpus striatum. No fact is better recognized than that a large part of one cerebral hemisphere may be destroyed when there are no obvious symptoms of any kind," (Jackson 1870, 1873, reprinted in Clarke and O'Malley, 1968). Thus Jackson invoked a redundancy of neural el-ements to explain the sparing of at least elementary functions following brain in-jury. (However, it is clear that he would not have applied the principle to more complex mental functions, which, in his view, did require intact cortical function.)

Still another form of redundancy was implied by the dictum of Hughlings Jack-son that the behavioral capacities of a brain-lesioned patient were more an ex-pression of the properties of the spared regions of the brain than of the lesioned area. The idea, which was widely accepted, was applied primarily to account for differences in the extent of recovery from motor and speech impairments that were observed between younger and older patients. However, in principle it could apply to all individual differences in brain capacity.

Plasticity

The allied concept of plasticity also found broad support. Cotard's observation that presumed destruction of the cortical speech area in infants and young children did not result in lasting aphasia was repeatedly confirmed. For example, Henschen cited the case of a man with a paralyzed, atrophic right arm dating back to early infancy, whose speech had always been entirely normal. Autopsy after his death disclosed a massive lesion of the left hemisphere with deep cavitation in the posterior frontal, insular, and temporal regions. Henschen concluded that speech evidently had been mediated by the right hemisphere in this patient (cf. Henschen, 1920–1922, Vol. 7, p. 42).

Similarly, Nielsen (1946) described the sequelae of head injury in a 3-year-old girl. She exhibited a right hemiplegia and a right homonymous hemianopia and was unable to speak for a few days after the injury. The hemiplegia improved markedly, although the hemianopia persisted. Subsequently she showed a left-hand preference for writing. As she reached school age, speech, reading, writing, and school progress were completely normal despite the fact that at the age of 6 years she developed epileptic seizures that persisted until her death at the age of 43. Autopsy disclosed that the left temporal and occipital lobes, including the angular gyrus, had been replaced by a porencephalic cyst.

The notion of a systematic decline of plasticity with age was suggested by the case report of Hillier (1954) describing a 14-year-old boy who underwent a left hemispherectomy for removal of a tumor. Six months after surgery, the boy was still clearly aphasic. However, in contrast to the status of the hemispherectomized adult patients of Zollinger (1935) and Crockett and Estridge (1951), who were virtually without speech and language capabilities, Hillier's young patient showed considerable recovery in the understanding and expression of speech, as well as some return of reading ability. Hillier concluded that the right hemisphere must have taken over speech functions in the boy.

In the early decades of the twentieth century, another approach to the issue of reorganization of function in the immature brain arose in connection with the discovery of *congenital wordblindness* in intelligent schoolchildren. Following the model of classical aphasiology theory, it was assumed that the disability resulted from focal maldevelopment of the "visual word center" in the territory of the angular gyrus of the left hemisphere. James Hinshelwood (1900, 1904) considered it highly probable that such reading as the dyslexic child was capable of was mediated by the right angular gyrus. Given the plasticity of the immature brain, it should be possible to "educate" the right angular gyrus to assume the function of reading. Hence Hinshelwood (1904), Thomas (1905), and others recommended that the dyslexic child be trained to write with the left hand in order to strengthen the functional capacity of the right angular gyrus in this regard.

The scattered observations of Soltmann on the sparing of functions after cortical ablations in immature animals were refined and expanded years later in the influential studies of Margaret Kennard (1938, 1940, 1942). As is well known, Kennard found that excisions in the motor cortex of infant monkeys produced much less severe contralateral motor deficits than did comparable lesions in the adult monkey. She attributed this relative sparing to a reorganization of function involving a shift of the substrate to a neighboring cortical area. In addition, Kennard pointed out that some types of motor abnormality that were observed in mature monkeys that had been operated on such as deviation of the head and eyes, rigidity, and spasticity, also appeared in infant monkeys as permanent deficits after excisions. The *Kennard principle,* as it came to be known, was widely accepted: the earlier the brain damage, the better, insofar as recovery was concerned.

Momentum of the Lesion

The Jacksonian dictum about the importance of the *momentum* of the *lesion* was amply confirmed by the results of subsequent animal experimentation (cf. Finger, 1978). Ades and Raab (1946, 1949) and Travis and Woolsey (1956) demonstrated conclusively that successive partial ablations produced far less severe disruptive effects on the perceptual and motor abilities of monkeys than did a single total ablation. The differences were particularly striking in the Travis-Woolsey study, in which the successive ablations were made over the course of months.*

Other Developments

The neurological basis and essential nature of recovery of function after injury to the nervous system was the theme of the 1930 meeting of the Deutsche Neurologische Gesellschaft (see the valuable lengthy English-language abstract by Bernis, 1932).

Degeneration and regeneration following injury to the nervous system were described and discussed in detail by Boeke, Spatz, and Matthei, with emphasis on the uncertainties as well as the firm findings and on the problematic relationship of observed neural changes to recovery of the function. Two major presentations by Otfrid Foerster and Kurt Goldstein dealing with the fundamental nature of restitution of function in patients expressed their respective views on the topic.

Otfrid Foerster. Foerster (1930) interpreted recovery of function as the outcome of compensatory alterations in the structure of the nervous system that occur after injury, the two major changes being (*1*) direct regeneration of neural tissue and (*2*) reorganization, i.e., changes in the structure and operations of uninjured elements associated with the injured part. For example, in some cases, direct regeneration of injured peripheral nerves effectively reinnervates the concerned muscles, with

---

*A relevant human study in this context was reported by Anderson et al. (1990). They conducted a systematic comparison of lesions caused by stroke versus lesions caused by tumor and found striking differences in the neuropsychological profiles of patients whose lesions were virtually identical in location but different in pathogenesis. Specifically, patients with stroke-caused lesions had more predictable neuropsychological deficits (e.g., aphasia if the lesion was left perisylvian) and more severe impairment; patients with tumor-caused lesions had much less impairment than would have been predicted from the location and size of the lesion.

consequent recovery of function. In other cases, regeneration is fostered by surgical removal of obstacles to regeneration, by exercise, and by physical therapy. On the other hand, direct regeneration of injured pathways in the spinal cord, brain stem, and cortex, if it occurs at all, is practically of no importance for restitution of function. Reorganization, in which the operations of other neural mechanisms are brought into play, is the key to restitution. Thus the effects of injury to the pyramidal tracts are alleviated by the action of extrapyramidal motor tracts. Again, both surgical intervention and prolonged exercise are valuable means of promoting recovery of function.

Confining his attention to motor and sensory impairments, Foerster emphasized redundancy of the neural mechanisms subserving these capacities. Given this redundancy, various forms of reorganization of the operations of these mechanisms could lead to restitution of functions that had been lost after focal injury to the nervous system.

Because he was a neurosurgeon, Foerster's primary interest was in detailed analysis of the processes of reorganization, especially the role of surgical intervention in fostering reorganization. Nevertheless, his view of the problem of recovery of function was organismic, even teleological, as his concluding statements quoted from the translation of Bernis (1932), indicate:

> When the processes that take place in the restitution of motility and sensation in lesions within the nervous system are observed, one can note that in addition to restoration, that is, the restoration of lost nerve tissue, the principle of replacement of substance, there also takes place a considerable reorganization of the remaining part of the nervous system, which serves for the restoration of function. All conducting tracts that can be of assistance are engaged; whether they be concerned with afferent or efferent conduction is immaterial; unsuitable connections are omitted, of course; appropriate connections are opened, and forces are mobilized that do not depend directly on innervation, but are based on the fact that all parts of the organism, including the noninnervated, belong to the physical basic laws. All serve the organism in a remarkably spontaneous manner, even though they may here and there be assisted by medical art.
>
> An indefatigable, immovable striving for adjustment rules the organism. The same rule that governs superficial wounds obtains in destruction of nerve tissue. There is a tendency toward replacement of substance, and when this is not possible, at least a replacement of function is attempted. Every biologic happening in the organism and every happening in the nervous system, whether they are concerned with a voluntary movement, involuntary reflex movements or with afferent simuli from the body periphery to the central nervous system, has a definite usefulness. And when the nervous system becomes deranged through sickness, the organism possesses and finds ways and means to serve the purpose of the moment.
>
> Bernis, 1932, p. 736

Kurt Goldstein. Kurt Goldstein addressed the problem of restitution of function rather differently, with little concern about the specific anatomophysiologic factors that might be involved and, instead, with primary emphasis on the drive of the individual to achieve optimal adaptation to environmental demands and satisfaction of his or her own needs. According to Goldstein, there is never complete restitution of function in the brain-injured patient, at least not in the adult. The taking over of function by the opposite hemisphere in patients with unilateral injury is questionable, as is the assumption of redundancy ("reserve") in the anatomic substrate. Nor can one part of the brain take the place of another part in mediating a behavioral function. In patients whose lesions produce sensory or motor defects, improvement of performances takes place not through an amelioration of the defect but by a change in strategy in dealing with the environment. For example, a patient with a lasting hemianopia will shift the center of vision to encompass the entire (although reduced) visual field. When lesions lead to impairment of the higher mental processes, other mental processes are brought into play to compensate (but only partially) for the lost performances. Moreover, lesions that compromise the higher mental processes lead to profound changes in the overall behavior of the patient.

When restitution appears to have occurred, either there has been a regression of the pathologic anatomic process (or of diaschisis) or the symptom picture has been misinterpreted. This misinterpreted restitution reflects substituted performance, not restoration of the lost performance.

Goldstein emphasized that the diminished capacity of the brain-injured patient may lead to a number of characteristic reactions. The patient may fixate on a stimulus for an excessively long time, i.e., the patient is "stimulus-bound." Alternatively, the patient may become abnormally restless. Both reactions are expressions of a loss of "flexibility." Faced with demands that cannot be met, the patient becomes emotionally upset and incapable of performing even simple tasks, i.e., the patient has a "catastrophic reaction." The reduction in adaptive capacity is also reflected in a loss of spontaneity and a decided preference for an orderly, predictable personal environment.

According to Goldstein, rehabilitation should not be focused on specific impairments per se, but rather on establishing situations in which the patient may succeed in performing tasks through intact capacities and in which catastrophic reactions are avoided.

> If this is accomplished, the organism is indeed not normal but he is not really sick. He feels well subjectively and shows little overt disturbance. This condition appears to be the aim of nature and it must also be the goal of our therapeutic efforts. It follows that specific symptoms should not be attacked therapeutically since the organism will be more capable and "healthier" than if an attempt is made to eliminate symptoms.
>
> Goldstein, 1930, p. 26

The contributions of Foerster and Goldstein present an interesting study in contrasts. The neurosurgeon was primarily concerned with the identifiable neural mechanisms underlying normal and defective behavioral capacities. The neurologist advanced a radically new conception of brain–behavior relationships that his fellow neurologists found hard to accept. Both spoke of *reorganization,* but their use of the term was quite different. To Foerster it meant the establishment of a new neural network that led to a true restoration of function; to Goldstein it was the re-placement of a lost function by another, less appropriate function that alleviated but did not fully eliminate the behavioral disability.

Neuroanatomic redundancy and plasticity were key components of Foerster's conceptions; for Goldstein these factors simply did not exist. Foerster was quite optimistic about the possibility of fostering recovery of function through surgical intervention and special exercises. Goldstein was quite guarded about the prospects, although he did strongly recommend the creation of a therapeutic environment as a means of permitting the patient to reach maximum potential. In this connection, it should also be recalled that Goldstein was the director of a major rehabilitation institute for brain-injured war veterans that was renowned for its innovative ap-proaches to treatment. One point on which these giants of a past era did agree was in their recognition that the spontaneous striving of the organism toward an opti-mal adjustment, i.e., the "healing power of nature," was a potent (and in some cases the decisive) factor in recovery of function.

Post–World War II Developments

The carnage of World War I provided abundant case material on which the think-ing and rehabilitation efforts of Foerster, Goldstein, and other workers in the inter-war period were based. World War II performed the same grim service for a new generation of researchers and clinicians, who were able to address the same ques-tions concerning recovery of function with enhanced technical resources. Recent advances such as the modernization of the *lesion method* in humans (Damasio & Damasio, 1989) and the development of functional imaging techniques, such as positron emission tomography (PET) and functional magnetic resonance imaging (MRI) have fostered rapid growth in the field (as exemplified by some of the con-tributions in this volume.

Developmental Plasticity and Critical Periods

During the several decades following World War II, a dominant influence in the field of neural plasticity came from experiments such as those conducted by Hubel and Wiesel (e.g., 1970; Wiesel & Hubel, 1963). Specifically, investigators empha-sized the notion of a *critical period* and suggested that neural systems, and sensory systems in particular, were highly plastic only during a relatively brief develop-mental time.

The work of Hubel and Wiesel showed that monocular eye closure in kittens during the first few months of life produced a dramatic and permanent reduction in the number of striate cortex cells that could be influenced by the previously closed eye. This effect, however, disappeared almost entirely if eye closure was in-troduced after the third month of life; in fact, monocular deprivation in adult cats produced no detectable effect. The notion of critical periods continues to be em-phasized in recent studies, although the principle has not been without controversy.

Other aspects of developmental plasticity also received attention. For example, Woolsey (1978) pointed out that when a lesion occurs, many normal anatomic relationships can be highly distorted, and in general, the shifts are greater in the developing brain than in the mature one. This notion predicts quite accurately some recent findings indicating the importance of age of onset of seizures in predicting the cognitive effects of temporal lobectomy. Specifically, temporal lobectomies conducted in patients with an early age of seizure onset (before age 5 years) are associated with minimal disruption of the functions normally associated with the resected brain region; by contrast, operations in patients with a later age of onset are associated with more significant and "typical" defects, e.g., naming impairment with left temporal lobectomy (cf. Hermann et al., 1995; Jokeit et al., 1996; Saykin et al., 1989).

In a recent summary of morphometric studies of cerebral cortex in humans, Huttenlocher (1990) noted that developmental changes extend up to the time of adolescence. Dendrites and synaptic connections grow during infancy and early childhood, while excess synaptic connections are eliminated in later childhood. Huttenlocher proposed that the "exuberant connections" that occur during infancy may form the anatomic substrate for neural plasticity and for certain types of early learning in the young child.

Adult Plasticity of Sensory and Motor Representations

Beginning in the 1980s, clear evidence of *adult plasticity* began to emerge (see Kaas, 1991, for a review). Convincing changes in sensory and motor maps were demonstrated in a number of laboratories. In short, the evidence indicated that alterations in afferent input can induce plastic reorganizational changes in the adult nervous system resulting in a systematic change in the relationship between peripheral sensory (or motor) fields and their central representations. In many of these experiments, it was shown that removal of the afferent input from a cortical region results in "invasion" by a neighboring region whose innervation remains intact.

The Evidence. The elegant experiments of Merzenich (e.g., Wang et al., 1995) have shown that changes in the neuronal response specificity and maps of the hand surfaces in the primary somatosensory cortex occur in response to serial application of stimuli to the fingers, a phenomenon the authors termed *representational remodelling*. The investigators further showed that this representational plasticity is cortical in origin and does not occur at the level of the thalamus. In owl monkeys, prolonged increase in tactile stimulation to a particular region on one or two phalanges resulted in a greatly increased cortical representation specific to that portion of the phalanges (Jenkins et al., 1990).

In humans, Pascual-Leone et al. (1993) reported an increased cortical representation of the index finger used in reading by blind Braille readers. It was also shown that the cortical representation of the hand and fingers was altered within a few weeks in patients who underwent surgical separation of webbed fingers. Using magnetoencephalography, the authors compared cortical representations of the hand in two patients with congenital syndactyly (webbed fingers) before and after surgical separation of the digits. A somatotopic representation of individual digits with near-normal spacing emerged within a few weeks, providing compelling evidence that dynamic reorganization is possible in the cortical topography of adult humans (see O'Leary et al., 1994, for review and comment).

The finding that humans with limb (usually arm) amputation sometimes report that touches to the face are perceived as touches to the amputated arm also suggests remapping of somatosensory inputs (Halligan et al., 1993; Ramachandran, 1993; see also Flor et al., 1995). In the Halligan et al. study, the authors described a case in which the topographic representation of the phantom limb onto the face included sensations symptomatic of carpal tunnel syndrome; it turned out that the patient had developed this condition in the amputated hand several months before the operation. Also, a number of patients who underwent mastectomies reported phantom sensations evoked by stimulation of skin regions near the amputated breast; in some cases, the apparent remapping took place as soon as 6 days after surgery (Aglioti et al., 1994).

A recent study from Ungerleider's laboratory, using functional MRI, demonstrated cortical activation patterns congruent with practice on a motor task (Karni et al., 1995). The experiment showed that the extent of cortex in M1 activated by a practiced motor sequence enlarged compared to the extent of cortex activated by an unpracticed sequence and that this change persisted for several months. The authors suggested that the results indicate a slowly evolving, long-term, experience-dependent reorganization of the adult M1, which may underlie the acquisition and retention of a motor skill.

A related finding was reported by Elbert et al. (1995), who studied the cortical representation of the digits in string players and controls (nonstring players). Based on magnetic source imaging, the string players showed increased cortical representation of the digits of the left hand. The effect was smallest for the left thumb, and there was no such difference for representations of the right hand. The authors also found that the amount of cortical reorganization in the representation of the fingering digits was correlated with the age at which the person had begun to play. Another interesting finding of this type was reported by Schlaug et al. (1995), who found that musicians with perfect pitch had stronger leftward planum temporale asymmetry than nonmusicians or musicians without perfect pitch.

Conclusions. Kaas (1995) included the following points in summarizing recent findings in the area of adult plasticity.

1. There are clear, consistent reorganizations of sensory maps following manipulation of sensory and other neural activity. In general, more active inputs expand and substitute for less active inputs, while missing inputs may lose their sensory mapping.
2. The capacity for reorganization may be a fundamental property of the adult nervous system, not just the developing nervous system. Moreover, this

plasticity may be possible throughout various levels of the nervous system, from cortical to subcortical.

3. Both rapid (within minutes or hours) and slow (over days or weeks) changes in sensory representations have been demonstrated.

4. In an intriguing recapitulation of the early ideas of Hughlings Jackson, among others, recent evidence supports the notion that sensory maps at different levels of the nervous system differ in the way they represent a sensory surface. Local modifications at one level may have widespread ramifications for other levels, particularly higher ones. Maps at higher levels tend to express greater change as a result of accumulating the effects of changes at lower (earlier) levels.

Intermodal Plasticity

The question of whether an organism deprived of one sensory modality develops "suprasensitivity" or "hypersensitivity" in other sensory modalities has been the subject of debate for nearly a century. There is considerable anecdotal as well as experimental evidence in favor of such a view.

Rauschecker and colleagues have shown that cats whose eyelids were sutured from birth (the blind cat preparation introduced by Hubel and Wiesel) developed superior capacity to localize sounds in space. Similar findings have been reported in humans (Muchnik et al., 1991; see Rauschecker, 1995, for a review). In the Muchnik et al. study, blind subjects were superior to sighted subjects in their ability to localize sounds, and the blind subjects had superior auditory acuity. Rauschecker has argued that the mechanism for this intermodal plasticity is primarily or perhaps even entirely cortical. For example, in the anterior ectosylvian cortex of binocularly deprived cats, where different sensory modalities converge, the anterior ectosylvian visual area is completely taken over by auditory and somatosensory inputs. Rauschecker noted that intermodal plasticity might involve several neural mechanisms, alone or in various combinations: unmasking of silent inputs, stabilization of normally transient connections, axonal sprouting.

Intermodal plasticity in humans has been demonstrated in studies in which blind humans were shown to activate brain regions normally associated with vision during auditory stimulation (Kujala et al., 1992; Veraart et al., 1990), haptic mental rotation (Rosler et al., 1993), or Braille reading (Uhl et al., 1993). Also, surgical studies using transplants have shown that one sensory modality can take on capacities normally associated with a different modality (Schlaggar & O'Leary, 1991; Sur et al., 1988).

The concept of intermodal plasticity formed the basis of the extensive rehabilitation program developed by Paul Bach-y-Rita in the late 1960s (Bach-y-Rita, 1972). At the core of the program was the tactile vision substitution system (TVSS), whereby blind individuals could receive "visual" information from a portable television camera by means of mechanical vibrators or electric pulses. Although the specifics of the TVSS program were only partially accepted, the concept of intermodal plasticity has figured prominently in much of the work done in the past two decades (cf. Bach-y-Rita, 1990).

Recovery of Function

According to Rosner (1970), there are two devices for achieving recovery of function in the mammalian brain: (*1*) redundant representation of a psychological capacity within a specialized center or region and (*2*) a given psychological capacity placed under control by several centers, which may be bilaterally paired or lie at different levels of the nervous system. Rosner described the concepts of *reestablishment* and *reorganization* to explain recovery of function and compensation following brain injury, and pointed out that these ideas were fundamentally the same as those proposed by Jackson nearly a century earlier.

Recovery from Aphasia: Neuropsychological Studies. In aphasia caused by focal and nonprogressive disease processes, including stroke and head injury, maximal recovery generally occurs in the first 3 months following onset (Culton, 1969; Demeurisse et al., 1980; Kertesz & McCabe, 1977; Pickersgill & Lincoln, 1983; Sarno & Levita, 1971; Vignolo, 1964; Wade et al., 1986). Holland and her colleagues have suggested that this period of more or less maximal recovery may actually be as short as 2 months (Holland, 1989; Holland et al., 1989; Pashek & Holland, 1988).

In a 1993 review, Kertesz raised the question of the role of right hemisphere structures in recovery from aphasia. The idea that restitution of speech in these cases is due to activity of the opposite hemisphere has been referred to as *Henschen's axiom* (see Kertesz, 1993). Henschen (1920–1922) himself gave credit to Wernicke and other early aphasiologists for this notion. Nielsen (1946) advocated the idea that the variable extent of recovery from aphasia is related to the variable capacity of the right hemisphere to subserve language. Geschwind (1969) also supported such a hypothesis.

Rubens (1977) suggested that some spontaneous recovery from aphasia appeared to be due to reversals of physiologic changes that initially occurred as a result of a stroke. These included lessening of edema, reestablishment of premorbid neurotransmitter activity, reabsorption of blood collection in the case of hemorrhagic lesions, and recovery from diaschisis. Further potential factors were enumerated by Johnson and Almli (1978): (*1*) *substitution*, implying redundancy or multiple representation in the central nervous system, which permits a secondary neural system to take over the functions of a primary one; (*2*) *vicariation* or *equipotentiality*, in which nonspecialized brain areas assume the functions of damaged ones; (*3*) *regeneration*, i.e., new growth in damaged neurons; (*4*) *collateral sprouting*, i.e., new growth in areas adjacent to damaged tissue; and (*5*) *denervation sensitivity*, i.e., increased sensitivity to transmitter substances by neurons that have lost innervation due to brain damage.

Pieniadz et al. (1983) reported a study of computed tomography (CT) scan asymmetries and recovery from global aphasia. They found that the recovery of globally aphasic patients with atypical right occipital asymmetry, or no asymmetry, was better than the recovery of patients with typical left asymmetries (all patients were right-handed), and the right occipital asymmetry (or lack of asymmetry) was interpreted as a suggestion of weaker left hemisphere dominance for language. This applied to word comprehension, one-word repetition, and naming. These findings parallel the pattern of right hemisphere linguistic capabilities observed in commissurotomy cases (Gazzaniga & Hillyard, 1971; Sidtis et al., 1981; Zaidel, 1976). More recently, Kertesz and Naeser (1994) have summarized such findings as suggesting that in global aphasics who show somewhat better recovery and who have atypical cerebral asymmetries, the right hemisphere may aid in the recovery by "complementing or cooperating" with the few preserved areas of the left hemisphere in "some unique manner" not usually seen in other globally aphasic patients. These findings are generally consistent with studies of left-handed aphasic patients, which have indicated somewhat greater recovery of certain linguistic abilities. It has been suggested that such recovery may be due to a higher degree of "bilateral" language representation (e.g., Borod et al., 1990; Naeser & Borod, 1986). In summary, these studies have hinted at the possibility that some recovery from aphasia may be attributable to activity in the opposite hemisphere.

Naeser's (1994) most recent summary on recovery from aphasia, with a focus on two particular aspects of language (recovery of auditory comprehension and recovery of spontaneous speech), shows that (1) recovery of auditory comprehension is better when less of Wernicke's area is invaded by a lesion and (2) recovery of spontaneous speech is better when less of the frontal operculum and its surround are invaded by the lesion.

Recovery from Aphasia: Functional Imaging Studies. As alluded to above, there are few neuropsychological data concerning the factors that play a role in recovering from aphasia, and there are even fewer data on the physiologic correlates of spared or recovered function in the aphasis population. Metter et al. (1992), Price et al. (1993), and Karbe et al. (1995) are among the investigators who have evaluated the use of resting PET measurements as predictors of the long-term outcome of poststroke aphasia.

Damasio et al. (1986) reported an activation study in ten subjects with aphasia and six nonaphasic control subjects using single positron emission computed tomography (SPECT). In comparison with a resting condition, performance of a phonemic rhyme detection task resulted in asymmetric increases in blood flow in the anterior and posterior language areas of nonaphasics. In the aphasics, both the right hemisphere counterparts of these areas and areas in the vicinity of damaged language areas showed increased blood flow. These increases appeared to be larger in the right hemisphere.

Application of the [^{15}O]-water method to subjects with acquired brain lesions has been reported in only a few cases. Using a three-dimensional PET scanner, Price et al. (1993) reported that a recovered aphasic, who had suffered a large left middle cerebral artery infarct, activated several specific areas in the right hemisphere while reading aloud highly imageable words. These areas included the right sensorimotor cortex, the right inferior frontal gyrus, and the right supplementary motor area. The only left hemisphere activation was in the left lingual gyrus.

Engelien et al. (1995) studied six normal subjects and a patient who had bilateral perisylvian strokes and auditory agnosia but had recovered the ability to recognize environmental sounds. In a sound categorization experiment, the normal subjects activated both auditory regions. The patient activated spared auditory cortex and inferior parietal cortex on the right and regions adjacent to the lesion on the left (anterior insula, frontal operculum, middle temporal gyrus, and inferior parietal lobe).

Weiller et al. (1995) conducted a PET investigation of six normal control subjects and six subjects who had had strokes in the left posterior superior temporal gyrus and Wernicke's aphasia but who enjoyed a good recovery. These subjects were not aphasic at the time of the study. In the patients, two distinct tasks, silent verb generation and pseudo-word repetition, activated the right hemisphere homologs of left hemisphere regions activated in the normal subjects. The authors reported that no activation occurred in the surround of the lesions in the left hemisphere.

Closing Remarks

From a historical perspective, it is quite evident that many of the principal issues and questions in the field of neural plasticity and recovery of function have endured for more than a century. Inspection of early attempts to address these issues, both theoretical and empirical, reveals a remarkable degree of commonality in the main lines of thinking regarding neural plasticity between the classic writers and contemporary theorists. As our historical overview indicates, findings in this field have had a major influence on the development of rehabilitation programs throughout history, and this trend continues to the present. Also, as neuroscience has matured and as some of the classic demarcations between subspecialties have blurred, there has been increasing cross-fertilization between ideas from work at very different levels of the nervous system; for example, findings from cortical map reorganization may trigger new approaches to the study of the genetic and molecular bases of neural plasticity.

Perhaps the most dramatic change in the field is the nature of the tools available to study these questions. The advent of structural MRI, PET, and functional MRI has led to a number of pathbreaking discoveries. The field of neural plasticity has exploded in the past decade or so in a manner parallel to the exponential growth of neuroscience in general. As the chapters in this volume demonstrate, the cutting edge of the field has generated new insights that will help to provide answers to traditional questions. Our next challenge will be to apply these answers to the more effective treatment of individuals whose cognitive and behavioral capacities have been compromised by neurologic disease.

ACKNOWLEDGMENT

This work was supported by NINDS Program Project Grant NS 19632.

References

Ades, H.W., and Raab, D.H. (1946) Recovery of motor function after two stage extirpation of area 4 in monkeys (*Macaca mulatta*). *Journal of Neurophysiology,* 9:55–59.

Ades, H.W., and Raab, D.H. (1949) Effects of preeoccipital and temporal decortication on learned visual discrimination in monkeys. Journal of Neurophysiology, 12:101–108.

Agliotti, S., Cortese, F., and Franchini, C. (1994) Rapid sensory remapping in the adult human brain as inferred from phantom breast perception. Neuroreport, 5:473–476.

Anderson, S.W., Damasio, H., and Tranel, D. (1990) Neuropsychological impairments associated with lesions caused by tumor or stroke. Archives of Neurology, 47:397–405.

Bach-y-Rita, P. (1972) Brain Mechanisms in Sensory Substitution. New York: Academic Press.

Bach-y-Rita, P. (1990) Brain plasticity as a basis for recovery of function in humans. Neuropsychologia, 28:547–554.

Bernis, W.J. (1932) German Neurological Society, Twentieth Annual Congress, Sept. 18–20, 1930. Archives of Neurology and Psychiatry, 461–480:725–752.

Borod, J.C., Carper, J.M., and Naeser, M.A. (1990) Long-term language recovery in left-handed aphasic patients. Aphasiology, 4:561–572.

Brouwer, B. (1936) Chifasma, Tractus Opticus, Sehstrahlung und Sehrinde. In O. Bumke and O. Foerster (eds.), Handbuch der Neurologie, Vol. 6. Berlin: Springer, pp. 449–532.

Castiglione, A. (1958) A History of Medicine, New York: Alfred A. Knopf.

Chapman, L.L., and Wolff, H.G. (1959) The cerebral hemispheres and the highest integrative functions of man. Archives of Neurology, 1:357–424.

Clarke, E., and O'Malley, C.D. (1968) The Human Brain and Spinal Cord: A Historical Study. Berkeley: University of California Press.

Cohen, L.G., Brasil-Neto, J.P., Pascual-Leone, A., and Hallett, M. (1993) Plasticity of cortical motor output organization following deafferentation, cerebral lesions, and skill acquisition. In O. Devinsky, A. Beric, and M. Dogali (eds.), Electrical and Magnetic Stimulation of the Brain and Spinal Cord. New York: Raven Press, pp. 187–200.

Cotard, J. (1868) Etude sur l'atrophie cérébrale. Paris: Thèse.

Critchley, M. (1949) Phenomenon of tactile inattention with special reference to parietal lesions. Brain, 72:538–561.

Crockett, H.G., and Estridge, N.M. (1951) Cerebral hemispherectomy. Bulletin of the Los Angeles Neurological Society, 15:71–87.

Culton, G. (1969) Spontaneous recovery from aphasia. Journal of Speech and Hearing Disorders, 12:825–832.

Damasio, H., and Damasio, A.R. (1989) Lesion Analysis in Neuropsychology. New York: Oxford University Press.

Damasio, H., Rezai, K., Eslinger, P., Kirchner, P., and VanGilder, J. (1986) SPECT patterns of activation in intact and focally damaged components of a language-related network. Neurology, 36:316.

Demeurisse, G., Demol, O., Derouck, M., deBeuckelaer, R., Coekaerts, M.J., and Capon, A. (1980) Quantitative study of the rate of recovery from aphasia due to ischemic stroke. Stroke, 11:455–460.

Elbert, T., Pantev, C., Wienbruch, C., Rockstroh, B., and Taub, E. (1995) Increased cortical representation of the fingers of the left hand in string players. Science, 270:305–307.

Engelien, A., Silbersweig, D., Stern, E., Huber, W., Doring, W., Frith, K., and Frackowiak, R.S.J. (1995) The functional anatomy of recovery from auditory agnosia: A PET study of sound categorization in a neurological patient and normal controls. Brain, 118:1395–1409.

Finger, S. (1978) Lesion momentum and behavior. In S. Finger (ed.), Recovery from Brain Damage: Research and Theory. New York: Plenum Press, pp. 135–164.

Flor, H., Elbert, T., Knecht, S., Wienbruch, C., Pantev, C., Birbaumer, N., Larbig, W., and Taub, E. (1995) Phantom-limb pain as a perceptual correlate of cortical reorganization following arm amputation. Nature, 375:482–484.

Foerster, O. (1930) Restitution der motilitat: Restitution der sensibilitat. *Deutsche Zeitschrift für Nervenheilkunde,* 115:248–314.

Fox, K. (1992) A critical period for experience-dependent synaptic plasticity in rat barrel cortex, Journal of Neuroscience, 12:1826–1838.

Franz, S.I. (1912) New phrenology. *Science,* 35:321–328.

Furmanski, A.R. (1950) The phenomenon of sensory suppression. *Archives of Neurology and Psychiatry,* 63:205–217.

Galaburda, A.M. (1990) Introduction to Special Issue: Developmental plasticity and recovery of function. *Neuropsychologia,* 28:515–516.

Gazzaniga, M.S., and Hillyard, S.A. (1971) Language and speech capacity of the right hemisphere. *Neuropsychologia,* 9:272.

Geschwind, N. (1969) Problems in the anatomical understanding of the aphasias. In A. Benton (ed.), *Contributions to Clinical Neuropsychology.* Chicago: Aldine, pp. 107–128.

Goldstein, K. (1930) Die Restitution bei Schädigungen der Hernrinde. *Deutsche Zeitschrift für Nervenheilkunde,* 116:2–26.

Goltz, F. (1888) Uber die Verrichtungen des Grosshirns (On the functions of the hemispheres). *Pfüger's Archiv für die gesamte Physiologie,* 42:419–467.

Halligan, P.W., Marshall, J.C., Wade, D.T., Davey, J., and Morrison, D. (1993) Thumb in cheek? Sensory reorganization and perceptual plasticity after limb amputation. *Neuroreport,* 4:233–236.

Henschen, S.E. (1920–1922) *Klinische und anatomische Beiträge zur Pathologie des Gehirns,* Vols. 6–7. Stockholm: Nordiske Bokhandeln.

Hermann, B.P., Seidenberg, M., Haltiner, A., and Wyler, A.R. (1995) Relationship of age at onset, chronologic age, and adequacy of preoperative performance to verbal memory change after anterior temporal lobectomy. *Epilepsia,* 36:137–145.

Hillier, W.F. (1954) Total left hemispherectomy for malignant glioma. *Neurology,* 4:718–722.

Hinshelwood, J. (1900) Congenital wordblindness. *Lancet,* 1:1506–1508.

Hinshelwood, J. (1904) A case of congenital wordblindness. *Ophthalmoscope,* 2:399–404.

Holland, A.L. (1989) Recovery in aphasia. In F. Boller and J. Grafman (eds.), *Handbook of Neuropsychology,* Vol. 2. Amsterdam: Elsevier, pp. 83–90.

Holland, A.L., Fromm, D., Greenhouse, J.B., and Swindell, C.S. (1989) Predictors of language restitution following stroke: A multivariate analysis. *Journal of Speech and Hearing Research,* 32:232–238.

Hubel, D.H., and Wiesel, T.N. (1970) The period of susceptibility to the physiological effects of unilateral eye closure in kittens. *Journal of Physiology,* 206:419–436.

Huttenlocher, P.R. (1990) Morphometric study of human cerebral cortex development. *Neuropsychologia,* 28:517–527.

Jackson, J.H. (1870) A study of convulsions. *Transactions, St. Andrews Medical Graduate Association,* 3:162–204 (excerpted in Clarke and O'Malley, 1968).

Jackson, J.H. (1873) On the anatomical and physiological localisation of movement in the brain. *Lancet,* 1:84–85, 162–164, 232–234 (excerpted in Clarke and O'Malley, 1968).

Jackson, J.H. (1879) On affections of speech from disease of the brain. *Brain* 2:323–356.

Jenkins, W.J., Merzenich, M.M., and Recanzone, G. (1990) Neocortical representational dynamics in adult primates: Implications for neuropsychology. *Neuropsychologia,* 28:573–584.

Johnson, D., and Almli, C.R. (1978) Age, brain damage, and performance. In S. Finger (ed.), *Recovery from Brain Damage.* New York: Plenum Press, pp. 115–134.

Jokeit, H., Ebner, A., Holthausen, H., Markowitsch, H.J., and Tuxhorn, I. (1996) Reorganization of memory function after human temporal lobe damage. *NeuroReport,* 7:1627–1630.

Joynt, R.J. (1970) Anatomical determinants of behavioral change. In A.L. Benton (ed.), *Behavioral Changes in Cerebrovascular Disease.* New York: Harper and Row, pp. 37–39.

Kaas, J.H. (1991) Plasticity of sensory and motor maps in adult mammals. *Annual Review of Neuroscience,* 14:137–167.

Kaas, J.H. (1995) The reorganization of sensory and motor maps in adult mammals. In M.S. Gazzaniga (ed.), *The Cognitive Neurosciences.* Cambridge, MA: MIT Press, pp. 51–71.

Karbe, H., Kessler, J., Herholz, K., Fink, G.R., and Heiss, W.D. (1995) Long-term prognosis of poststroke aphasia studied with positron emission tomography. *Archives of Neurology,* 52:186–190.

Karni, A., Meyer, G., Jezzard, P., Adams, M.M., Turner, R., and Ungerleider, L.G. (1995) Functional MRI evidence for adult motor cortex plasticity during motor skill learning. *Nature,* 377:155–158.

Kennard, M.A. (1938) Reorganization of motor function in the cerebral cortex of monkeys deprived of motor and premotor areas in infancy. *Journal of Neurophysiology,* 1:477–497.

Kennard, M.A. (1940) Relation of age to motor impairment in man and subhuman primates. *Archives of Neurology and Psychiatry,* 44:377–397.

Kennard, M.A. (1942) Cortical reorganization of motor function. Studies on series of monkeys of various ages from infancy to maturity. *Archives of Neurology and Psychiatry,* 48:227–240.

Kertesz, A. (1993) Recovery and treatment. In K.M. Heilman and E. Valenstein (eds.), *Clinical Neuropsychology,* 3rd ed. New York: Oxford University Press, pp. 647–674.

Kertesz, A., and McCabe, P. (1977) Recovery patterns and prognosis in aphasia. *Brain,* 100: 1–18.

Kertesz, A., and Naeser, M.A. (1994) Anatomical asymmetries and cerebral lateralization. In A. Kertesz (ed.), *Localization and Neuroimaging in Neuropsychology.* New York: Academic Press, pp. 213–244.

Kujala, T. Alho, K. Paavilainen, P. Summala, H., and Naatanen, R. (1992) Neural plasticity in processing of sound localization by the early blind: an event-related potential study. *Electroencephalography and Clinical Neurophysiology,* 84:469–472.

Lashley, K. (1929) *Brain Mechanisms and Intelligence.* Chicago: University of Chicago Press.

Merzenich, M.M., and Jenkins, W.M. (1993) Reorganization of cortical representations of the hand following alterations of skin inputs induced by nerve injury, skin island transfers, and experience. *Journal of Hand Therapy,* 90:89–104.

Metter, E.J., Jackson, C.J., Kempler, D., and Hanson, W.R. (1992) Temporoparietal cortex and the recovery of language comprehension in aphasia. *Aphasiology,* 6:349–358.

Mogilner, A., Grossman, J.A.I., Ribari, U., Joliet, M., Volkmann, J., Rapaport, D., Beasley, R.W., and Llinas, R.R. (1993) Somatosensory cortical plasticity in adult humans revealed by magnetoencephalography, Proceedings of the National Academy of Sciences, 90:3593:3597.

Muchnik, C., Efrati, M., Nemeth, E., Malin, M., and Hildesheimer, M. (1991) Central auditory skills in blind and sighted subjects. *Scandinavian Audiology,* 20:19–23.

Naeser, M.A. (1994) Neuroimaging and recovery of auditory comprehension and spontaneous speech in aphasia with some implications for treatment in severe aphasia. In A. Kertesz (ed.), *Localization and Neuroimaging in Neuropsychology.* New York: Academic Press, pp. 245–295.

Naeser, M.A., and Borod, J.C. (1986) Aphasia in left-handers: CT lesion site, lesion site, and hemispheric asymmetries. *Neurology,* 36:471–489.

Neuburger, M. (1926) *Die Lehre von der Heilkraft der Natur im Wandel der Zeiten.* Stuttgart: F. Enke.

Nielsen, J.M. (1946) *Agnosia, Apraxia, Aphasia: Their Value in Cerebral Localization.* New York: Paul R. Hoeber.

Ogden, R., and Franz, S.I. (1917) On cerebral motor control: The recovery of function from experimentally produced hemiplegia. *Psychobiology,* 1:33–50.

O'Leary, D.D.M., Ruff, N.L., and Dyck, R.H. (1994) Development, critical period plasticity, and adult reorganizations of mammalian somatosensory systems. *Current Biology,* 4:535–544.

Pascual-Leone, A., Cammarota, A., Wasserman, E.M., Brasil-Neto, J.P., Cohen, L.C., and Wallace, M. (1993) Modulation of motor cortical outputs to the reading hand of Braille readers. *Annals of Neurology,* 34:33–37.

Pashek, G.V., and Holland, A.L. (1988) Evolution of aphasia in the first year post onset. *Cortex,* 24:411–423.

Pickersgill, M.N., and Lincoln, N.B. (1983) Prognostic indicators and the pattern of recovery of communication in aphasic stroke patients. *Journal of Neurology, Neurosurgery and Psychiatry,* 46:130–139.

Pieniadz, J.M., Naeser, M.A., Koff, E., and Levine, H.L. (1983) CT scan cerebral hemispheric asymmetry measurements in stroke cases with global aphasia: Atypical asymmetries associated with improved recovery. *Cortex,* 19:371–391.

Polyak, S. (1955) *The Vertebrate Visual System.* Chicago: University of Chicago Press.

Price, C., Wise, R., Howard, D., Warburton, E., and Frackowiak, R.S.J. (1993) The role of the right hemisphere in the recovery of language after stroke. *Journal of Cerebral Blood Flow and Metabolism,* 13:S520.

Ramachandran, V.S. (1993) Behavioral and magnetoencephalographic correlates of plasticity in the adult human brain. Proceedings of the National Academy of Sciences, 90: 10413–10420.

Rauschecker, J.P. (1995) Compensatory plasticity and sensory substitution in the cerebral cortex. *Trends in Neurosciences,* 18:36–43.

Recanzone, G.H. Merzenich, N.M., and Dinze, H.R. (1992) Expansion of the cortical representation of a specific skin field in primary somatosensory cortex by intracortical microstimulation. *Cerebral Cortex,* 2:181–196.

Riese, W. (1948) Aphasia in brain tumors. *Confinia Neurologica,* 9:64–79.

Rosler, F., Roder, B., Heil, M., and Hennighausen, E. (1993) Topographic differences of slow event-related brain potentials in blind and sighted adult human subjects during haptic mental rotation. *Cognitive Brain Research,* 1:145–159.

Rosner, B.S. (1970) Brain functions. *Annual Review of Psychology,* 21:555–594.

Rubens, A. (1977) The role of changes within the central nervous system during recovery from aphasia. In M.A. Sullivan and M.S. Kommers (eds.), *Rationale for Adult Aphasia Therapy.* Lincoln: University of Nebraska Medical Center, pp. 28–43.

Sarno, M.T. (1991) Recovery and rehabilitation in aphasia. In M.T. Sarno (ed.), *Acquired Aphasia,* 2nd ed. New York: Academic Press, pp. 521–582.

Sarno, M.T., and Levita, E. (1971) Natural courses of recovery in severe aphasia. *Archives of Physical Medicine Rehabilitation,* 52:175–178.

Saykin, A.J., Gur, R.C., Sussman, N.M., O'Connor, M.J., and Gur, R.E. (1989) Memory deficits before and after temporal lobectomy: Effect of laterality and age of onset. *Brain and Cognition,* 9:191–200.

Schlagger, B.L., and O'Leary, D.D.N. (1991) Potential of visual cortex to develop and array of functional units unique to somatosensory cortex. *Science,* 252:1556–1559.

Schlaug, G., Jancke, L., Huang, Y., and Steinmetz, H. (1995) In vivo evidence of structural brain asymmetry in musicians. *Science,* 267:699–701.

Sidtis, J.J., Volpe, B.T., Wilson, D.H., Rayport, M., and Gazzaniga, M.S. (1981) Variability in right hemisphere language function after callosal section: Evidence for a continuum of generative capacity. *Journal of Neuroscience,* 1:323–331.

Soltmann, O. (1876) Experimentelle studien uber die Functionen des Grosshirns der Neugeborenen. *Jahrbuch für Kinderheilkunde und physische Erziehung,* 9:106–148.

Sur, M., Garraghty, P.E., and Roe, A.W. (1988) Experimentally induced visual projections into auditory thalamus and cortex. *Science,* 242:1437–1441.

Thomas, C.J. (1905) Congenital "wordblindness" and its treatment. *Ophthalmoscope,* 3: 380–385.

Travis, A.M., and Woolsey, C.N. (1956) Motor performance of monkeys after bilateral partial and total cerebral decortications. *American Journal of Physical Medicine,* 35:273–310.

Uhl, F., Franzen, P., Podreka, I., Steiner, M., and Deecke, L. (1993) Increased cerebral blood flow in inferior occipital cortex and cerebellum of early blind humans. *Neuroscience Letters,* 150:62–164.

Veraart, C., De Volder, A.G., Wanet-Defalque, M.C. Bol, A., Michel, C., and Goffinet, A.M. (1990) Glucose utilization in human visual cortex is abnormally elevated in blindness of early onset but decreased in blindness of late onset. *Brain Research,* 510:115–121.

Vignolo, A. (1964) Evolution of aphasia and language rehabilitation: A retrospective exploratory study. *Cortex,* 1:344–367.

Von Monakow, C. (1911) Lokalisation der Hirnfunktionen. *Journal für Neurologie and Psychiatrie,* 17:185–200.

Wade, D.T., Hewer, R.L., David, R.M., and Enderby, P.M. (1986) Aphasia after stroke: Natural history and associated deficits. *Journal of Neurology, Neurosurgery and Psychiatry,* 49:11–16.

Wang, X., Merzenich, M.M., Sameshima, K., and Jenkins, W.M. (1995) Remodelling of hand representation in adult cortex determined by timing of tactile stimulation. *Nature,* 378:71–75.

Weiller, C., Isensee, C., Rjntjes, M., Huber, W., Muller, S., Bier, D., Dutschka, K., Woods, R.P., Noth, J., and Diener, H.C. (1995) Recovery from Wernicke's aphasia: A positron emission tomographic study. *Annals of Neurology,* 37:723–732.

Weiskrantz, L. (1986) *Blindsight: A Case Study and Implications.* New York: Oxford University Press.

Wiesel, T.N., and Hubel, D.H. (1963) Single-cell responses in striate cortex of kittens deprived of vision in one eye. *Journal of Neurophysiology,* 26:1003–1017.

Woolsey, T.J. (1978) Lesion experiments: Some anatomical considerations. In S. Finger (Ed.), *Recovery from Brain Damage: Research and Theory.* New York: Plenum Press, pp. 71–89.

Zaidel, E. (1976) Auditory vocabulary of the right hemisphere following brain bisection or hemidecortication. *Cortex,* 12:191–212.

Zihl, J., and von Cramon, D. (1980) Registration of light stimuli in the cortically blind hemifield and its effect on localization. *Behavioural Brain Research,* 1:287–298.

Zollinger, R. (1935) Removal of left cerebral hemisphere: Report of a case. *Archives of Neurology and Psychiatry,* 34:1055–1064.

I

Neuroscience Research on Neuroplasticity and Reorganization of Function

2

Neuropsychological Indices of Early Medial Temporal Lobe Dysfunction in Primates

JOCELYNE BACHEVALIER AND LUDISE MÁLKOVÁ

Neural plasticity and reorganization of brain functions have been clearly demonstrated in young animals and children after early insult to the brain. The pioneering work of Margaret Kennard (1936) in this domain has led to the proposal that early damage to the brain results in a greater sparing of brain functions than later injury. Although the Kennard principle has been substantiated by numerous studies in animals as well as humans (Bates, 1992; Goldman-Rakic et al., 1983; Kolb & Whishaw, 1989; and other chapters in this volume), other reports indicate that early brain lesions may produce different results, depending on which neural structures are removed, which brain functions are investigated, and at what age the damage occurs (Schneider, 1979). After investigating a number of human patients of early brain lesions, Teuber and colleagues (1962) suggested the existence of more than just quantitative differences in the degree of sparing or loss of function between early and late injury. For example, in some cases the early injury led to apparently anomalous functions that had never been observed in adult-injured patients (Rudel, et al., 1966; Rudel & Teuber 1971; Woods & Teuber, 1978). From the wide variety of early lesion effects, they formulated the tentative hypothesis that the earlier the lesion occurred, the greater the reorganization of neural mechanisms underlying behavior. In turn, this neural reorganization would lead to different outcomes: (1) in some aspects of behavior, the effects of early injury would appear only with a delay as development progresses; (2) in other aspects of behavior, the effects of early injury would emerge early and remain unchanged with maturation; and (3) in still other aspects of behavior, the effects of early injury would occur immediately but disappear as development proceeds.

Numerous neuropathological studies of humans and lesion studies of monkeys have shown that damage to the medial temporal lobe region, including the hippocampal formation and adjacent cortical areas, causes a severe global anterograde

27

amnesia. When the insult also involves the amygdaloid complex, additional disorders of emotional regulation and social interaction occur. There is little evidence to suggest that the same behavioral syndrome results from medial temporal damage in early infancy. This chapter will review the long-term behavioral consequences of early medial temporal lobe damage in primates and compare the effects of early lesions to those of late lesions. Not only will the results illustrate the three aspects of behavioral reorganization proposed by Teuber, but they will also provide support for the view advanced by Schneider (1979) that early insult to the structures in the medial temporal lobe may be the origin of developmental psychosis in humans.

Medial Temporal Lobe Functions

The medial temporal lobe comprises two subcortical structures, the hippocampal formation and the amygdaloid complex (Fig. 2-1, left hemisphere), as well as several cortical areas lying over and around these two structures (Fig. 2-1, right hemisphere). The cortical areas include area TG on the temporal pole; the entorhinal (area 28) and perirhinal (areas 35 and 36) cortices located in and around the rhinal sulcus; the parahippocampal cortical areas TH/TF, just posterior to the entorhinal and perirhinal areas; and, more laterally, the cortex on the inferior temporal gyrus (area TE). Studies over the last few decades have provided strong evidence that particular regions in the medial temporal lobe are specialized, by virtue of their connections and physiology, for subserving the cognitive processes of learning and memory, emotionality, and sociality.

Learning and Memory

Much of our knowledge about the role of the medial temporal lobe structures, particularly the hippocampus, in memory functions is derived from well-studied clinical patients who have either undergone selective medial temporal lobe ablations for relief of epilepsy or suffered neuropathology in this brain region secondary to anoxia or ischemia. Among these patients are the famous H.M., who underwent bilateral resection of the medial temporal lobe to alleviate his epileptic seizures (Scoville & Milner, 1957), and, more recently, a few patients with selective cell loss in the hippocampal formation due to ischemia (Damasio et al., 1985; Rempel-Clower et al., 1996; Zola-Morgan et al., 1986). All these patients suffer a profound inability to remember recent events and to learn many types of new information and thus display profound global anterograde amnesia. They can, however, recollect old events, and their intelligence, perception, and language are either unaffected or only minimally impaired. Paradoxically, despite their profound memory defects, amnesic patients demonstrate normal performance on certain kinds of learning tasks (Brooks & Baddeley, 1976; Cohen & Squire, 1980; Corkin, 1968; Milner, 1962; Squire et al., 1984; Warrington & Weiskrantz, 1968). For example, amnesic subjects show steady learning of mirror drawing, tactile mazes, and rotary pursuit,

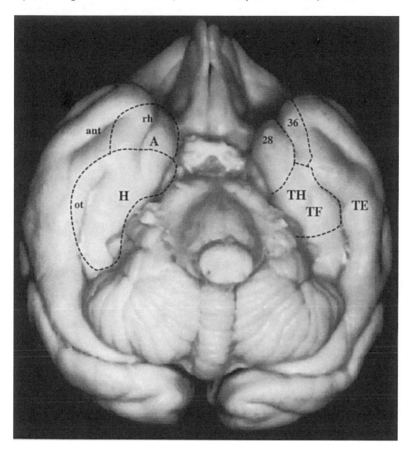

Figure 2-1. Ventral surface of a macaque brain illustrating the localization of the medial temporal cortical areas on the right and subcortical amygdala (A) and hippocampus (H) on the left. Abbreviations: amt: anterior medial temporal sulcus; ot: occipitotemporal sulcus; rh: rhinal sulcus; TE: inferior temporal cortical areas; TF/TH: parahippocampal cortical areas; area 36: perirhinal cortex; area 28: entorhinal cortex. Note that perirhinal area 35 is buried in the fundus of the rhinal sulcus.

and they can improve on other cognitive tasks, such as completing jigsaw puzzles or solving the Tower-of-Hanoi problem.

Subsequent studies conducted with nonhuman primates have converged on a similar dichotomy of spared learning abilities in the presence of profound amnesia (Mishkin & Petri, 1984; Mishkin et al., 1984; Zola-Morgan & Squire, 1985). For example, monkeys with bilateral damage to the medial temporal lobe, similar to that of H.M., are unable to recognize an object they saw just a minute or two earlier (Mishkin, 1982; Saunders et al., 1984; Zola-Morgan & Squire, 1985) or to remember for even a few seconds whether or not the object was previously associated with a food reward (Spiegler & Mishkin, 1979). In addition, as was the case in amnesic humans, the surgically operated monkeys display global memory impairment (Mishkin, 1978; Murray & Mishkin, 1984; Parkinson et al., 1988), although they have no difficulty mastering a multiple-trial concurrent-object discrimination task in which successive trials on a given pair are separated by 24-hour intertrial intervals (Malamut et al., 1984).

These clinical and experimental findings have led to the proposal that retaining the effects of experience depends on two fundamentally different neural systems (Hirsh, 1974; Mishkin & Appenzeller, 1987; Mishkin & Petri, 1984; Mishkin et al., 1984; Zola-Morgan & Squire, 1985), one of which is critically dependent on the integrity of structures in the medial temporal lobe.

Emotional States and Social Relationships

Behavioral and emotional changes following bilateral damage to the medial temporal lobe region in adult monkeys were first described by Brown and Schafer (1888). These changes, later described by Klüver and Bucy (1938, 1939), include (1) hypoemotionality, as reflected by a tendency to become unnaturally fearless and tame; (2) hyperexploratory behavior, as shown by excessive examination of objects, often with the mouth; (3) purposeless hyperactivity; and (4) impairment in social interaction. More recent studies have shown that many similar behavioral changes can be observed after restricted bilateral damage to either the amygdala (Aggleton & Mishkin, 1986; Aggleton & Passingham, 1981; Kling, 1972; Kling & Brothers, 1992; Rosvold et al., 1954; Weiskrantz, 1956; Zola-Morgan et al., 1991) or the inferior temporal cortex (Horel et al., 1975; Iwai et al., 1986). Interestingly, different emotional changes follow selective lesions of the ento- and perirhinal cortical. Thus, monkeys with such lesions exhibit an increased amount of freezing behavior and an absence of facial expressions in the presence of fear-inducing stimuli (Meunier et al., 1991).

The role of the medial temporal lobe structures in emotional behavior has also received support from clinical cases (see Aggleton, 1992, for a review). Hypoemotionality has been described both in patients suffering from viral encephalitis, a disease that can produce extensive damage to the medial temporal lobe structures and the neocortex in the temporal lobe (Friedman & Allen, 1969; Gascon & Gilles, 1973; Marlowe et al., 1975), and in patients who receive bilateral temporal lobectomy as a treatment either for psychosis (Obrador, 1947; Pool, 1952; Terzian & Delle Ore, 1955) or for otherwise untreatable epileptic seizures, such as H.M. (Hebben et al., 1981; Scoville & Milner, 1957). In addition to hypoemotionality, some of these patients have exhibited the complete pattern of behavioral disturbances seen in Klüver-Bucy syndrome. Involvement of the amygdala in social cognition and affect in humans was demonstrated by the studies of Gloor (1972, 1986), involving patients' reports of their subjective experiences on stimulation of different portions of the temporal lobe. These experiences tended to involve actions, attitudes, or intentions of others, perceived by the subjects to be directed at themselves. More recently, descriptions of a few patients with neuropathology in the amygdala provide additional information on the emotional changes that follow such brain damage. These patients demonstrate impairment in the recognition of facial expressions of fear and in the recognition of facial emotion in a single facial expression (Adolphs et al., 1994, 1995), as well as in the identification of facial expressions of emotion (Young et al., 1996). Finally, neuroimaging studies in normal human subjects have shown increased neuronal activity in the amygdala in response to facial expressions (Irwin et al., 1996; Morris et al., 1996), indicating that the amygdala is a key structure for extracting affective significance from external stimuli.

Neonatal Medial Temporal Lobe Lesions

To study the long-term behavioral consequences of early medial temporal lobe damage, we prepared newborn monkeys by removing the medial temporal lobe structures. Then we followed in some detail the development of their cognitive and socioemotional behavior from infancy to adulthood.

Medial Temporal Lobe Lesions

Eight newborn monkeys sustained two-stage bilateral aspiration of the medial temporal lobe structures, and eight were age-matched, unoperated controls. Surgery was performed aseptically when the animals were about 1 week of age for the removal in the left hemisphere and at about 3 weeks of age for the removal in the right hemisphere. The surgical removals included the amygdaloid complex and the adjacent entorhinal cortex, plus the hippocampal formation and the adjacent parahippocampal gyrus. All details of the surgical procedures, as well as pre- and postoperative care, are given elsewhere (Bachevalier et al., 1990). Lesions were verified histologically for all operated animals, and one representative case (AH-5) is presented in Figure 2-2. In all cases, the extent of the medial temporal lobe removal was largely as intended. The only deviations from the intended removal were encroachment on the fundus of the rhinal sulcus along its entire length, damaging area 35 of the perirhinal cortex. In addition, at the caudal tip of the rhinal sulcus, the lesion included a small amount of damage to perirhinal cortical area 36. Finally, there was minor unintended damage to the inferior temporal cortex, along the medial border of areas TE and TEO, presumably due to a combination of mechanical and ischemic damage.

Rearing Conditions

All newborn monkeys were laboratory raised. On arrival in the primate nursery (National Institute of Mental Health, Bethesda, Maryland), they were assigned to social groups consisting of one normal animal and one or two operated animals. All infant monkeys were reared in individual wire cages that allowed visual, auditory, and some somatosensory contact between a pair of animals. They were

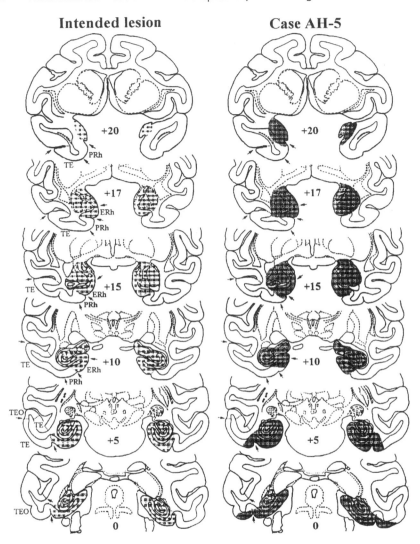

Figure 2-2. Coronal sections through the medial temporal lesions illustrating the intended lesions (left) and the extent of lesion in one representative case, AH-5 (right). Abbreviations: ERh: entorhinal area 28; PRh: perirhinal areas 35 and 36; TE, anterior two-thirds of the inferior temporal cortex; TEO, posterior one-third of the inferior temporal cortex.

handled several times each day by the experimenters. In addition, the animals forming each dyad or triad were placed for up to 4 hours daily in a playpen containing toys and towels located in the nursery. These rearing conditions have proven to be optimal for the establishment of normal social relationships in infant primates reared with peers (Ruppenthal et al., 1991).

Learning and Memory Abilities

To determine whether neonatal removal of the medial temporal lobe structures would yield an amnesic syndrome similar to the one described in adult monkeys with equivalent lesions, visual, tactile, and spatial memory were measured in monkeys with early medial temporal lobe lesion and their age-matched controls at different time points from infancy through adulthood.

Visual Memory Abilities

At 1 month of age (i.e., almost immediately after the surgical removals), object recognition was investigated using a paired-comparison task. In this task, for each trial, a pair of identical objects was shown on a screen for a 30 second familiarization period, followed after a 10 second delay by two preference tests in which one of the familiar stimuli was presented together with a new one for 5 seconds. The two preference tests were separated by a 10 second interval, and between these tests the left-right position of the objects was reversed. An interval of 20 seconds separated the trials, each involving a different pair of objects, and a total of ten trials was used. The direction of a subject's visual fixation was recorded, and the percentage of time spent fixating the new object on each trial was calculated. Preference for novelty was investigated in infant monkeys with early medial temporal lobe lesions and their controls and was compared to the preference of adult monkeys that had received the same lesions in adulthood (Bachevalier et al., 1993). At 30 days of age, normal infant monkeys showed a strong preference for viewing novel objects, indicating the presence of some recognition memory processes at this early age. This object memory was absent both in monkeys that had received medial temporal lobe ablations in infancy and in those that had received the same lesion in adulthood (Fig. 2-3A, parts a and b), suggesting that the medial temporal lobe structures make a critical contribution to this form of object memory even at this early age.

This impairment in object recognition was still evident later on when the infant monkeys were tested on another recognition task, the delayed nonmatching-to-sample (DNMS) task, at 10 months of age (Bachevalier & Mishkin, 1994). In this task, monkeys first had to learn the rule of avoiding a familiar object and to displace the novel object in an object pair. On each trial, a single object was presented first and then, after a delay of 10 seconds, the familiar object was presented together with a new one for choice. New objects were used for each trial until the animal reached a criterion of 90 correct choices in 100 trials. Monkeys' recognition memory was then taxed further by either increasing the delay between the first and second appearances of the sample object (delays of 30, 60, and 120 seconds) or by increasing the number of objects to be remembered (lists of three, five, and ten objects). Under these conditions, monkeys with early medial temporal lesions were severely impaired compared to age-matched controls; their average performance across the six conditions dropping 23% below that of normal controls. Thus, early damage to the medial temporal lobe in monkeys results in a visual recognition loss

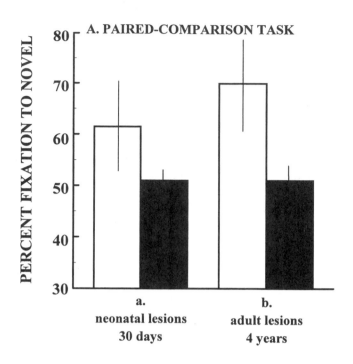

A. PAIRED-COMPARISON TASK

PERCENT FIXATION TO NOVEL

a.
neonatal lesions
30 days

b.
adult lesions
4 years

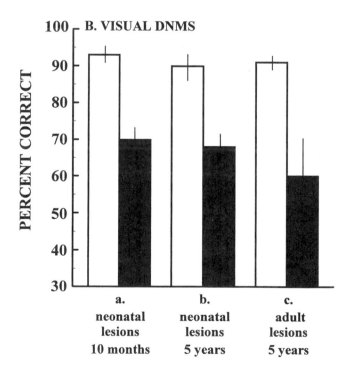

B. VISUAL DNMS

PERCENT CORRECT

a.
neonatal
lesions
10 months

b.
neonatal
lesions
5 years

c.
adult
lesions
5 years

nearly as severe as that found after late damage (Fig. 2-3B; compare parts a and c) to the same region (Bachevalier & Mishkin, 1994). In addition, like monkeys with late damage to the medial temporal lobe, those with early damage showed unimpaired abilities in mastering concurrent object discriminations with 24 hour, intertrial intervals at 3 months of age (Bachevalier et al., 1990). Hence, the good performance on the object discrimination task indicated that the impairment in visual recognition tasks reflects a genuine memory loss rather than a deficiency in such processes as perception, attention, or motivation or in the performance of instrumental responses.

Thus, the data indicate that the medial temporal lobe structures appear to operate early to sustain visual recognition memory, that other regions cannot assume this function even when the damage occurs neonatally, and that recovery from early damage to this region is therefore limited at best. Nevertheless, whether functions are permanently lost or spared after early brain damage depends on several factors besides the locus of injury, including the age at testing and the precise function measured (Goldman, 1971, 1974; Schneider, 1979). Thus, it remains possible that the evidence for loss of visual recognition observed after early medial temporal lesions when the monkeys were still infants might change with further maturation of the animals. For example, operated monkeys showing early visual recognition impairment initially may show eventual recovery (Goldman, 1971, 1974). To examine this possibility, monkeys with early medial temporal lobe lesions and their normal controls were retrained in adulthood on the same visual DNMS and concurrent object discrimination tasks they were trained on as infants (Málková et al., 1995). The results on both visual memory tasks were the same as those obtained when the monkeys were less than 1 year of age. Specifically, early medial temporal lesions, similar to late lesions, left visual discrimination intact but severely impaired recognition memory (Fig 2-3B; compare parts b and c).

Global Memory Loss

In addition to their severe visual recognition impairment, monkeys given medial temporal lobe lesions in adulthood are profoundly impaired in recognizing objects by touch as well as in recalling spatial locations, indicating that their amnesia is global (Angeli et al., 1993; Murray & Mishkin, 1984; Parkinson et al., 1988). To determine whether the same global amnesia holds for the effects of neonatal lesions, the monkeys with early medial temporal lobe lesions were tested on tactile DNMS and spatial DNMS tasks.

Training on tactile DNMS proceeded in the same way as for visual DNMS, except that the animals were trained in complete darkness, so that they had to feel

Figure 2-3. Percentage of fixation to novel objects in the paired-comparison task (A) and average scores across the six conditions of the visual DNMS performance task (B) in infant and adult monkeys (operated on neonatally) and adult monkeys (operated on in adulthood). White bars give the scores of normal controls, and black bars give the scores of animals with medial temporal lobe lesion.

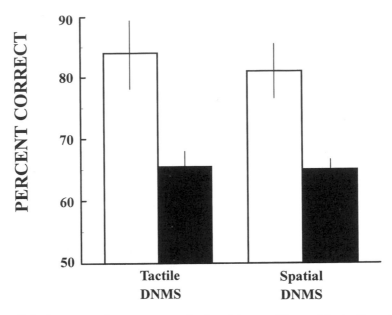

Figure 2-4. Average performance across the four delay conditions of the tactile and spatial DNMS in monkeys with neonatal damage to the medial temporal lobe (black bars) and their normal controls (white bars).

the objects presented on the tray to make their choice and displace them to retrieve the reward. For the spatial DNMS, the tray contained three rows of three wells, and two identical plaques served as stimuli. For each trial, one of the wells was covered with a plaque and the animal had to displace it to retrieve the reward. After a delay of 10 seconds, the same well was recovered but unbaited, and a new baited well was covered with the second plaque. The animal had to displace the new covered well to receive a reward. In these two versions of the DNMS, monkeys were first trained to learn the tasks to a criterion of 90 correct responses in 100 trials; their memory was then taxed further by increasing the delay from the original 10 seconds during learning to 30, 60, and 120 seconds. As shown in Figure 2-4, the loss of visual recognition memory following early medial temporal lesions was accompanied by a severe loss of tactile and spatial memory formation. Thus, neonatal medial temporal lesions, like those sustained in adulthood, cause enduring and global amnesia (Málková et al., 1995; see also Mahut & Moss, 1986).

Critical Neural Substrate Responsible for Severe Global Memory Loss

The severe global and long-lasting memory loss observed after early medial temporal lobe lesions demonstrates that the medial temporal lobe structures operate early in life to sustain memory processes and that recovery from early damage does not occur. These findings also raise the question of whether a specific structure, namely the hippocampus, is responsible for the global amnesia or whether different structures within the medial temporal lobe might underlie the specific memory losses described. Recent studies in adult monkeys, as well as preliminary findings on memory loss following early damage to selective structures within the medial temporal lobe, offer some evidence that specific areas within the medial temporal lobe are responsible for specific memory loss.

During the last decade, it has become apparent that the medial temporal lobe tissue that is critical for visual recognition memory, as measured by visual DNMS, is the cortex located in and around the rhinal sulcus. Thus, in adult monkeys, severe visual recognition deficits were found after combined damage to the entorhinal and perirhinal cortices (Buckley et al., 1997; Eacott et al., 1994; Meunier et al., 1993; Zola-Morgan et al., 1989), but not after combined excitotoxic lesions of the amygdala and hippocampus that spared the underlying rhinal and parahippocampal cortices (Murray & Mishkin, 1998). Severe deficits in tactile as well as visual recognition were also found after bilateral damage restricted to the perirhinal and parahippocampal cortices (Suzuki et al., 1993). It is thus likely that the enduring loss of visual and tactile recognition memory sustained by the animals with early medial temporal lobe lesions in the present study is also attributable mainly to damage to the cortex in and around the rhinal sulcus and not to damage of the subcortical medial temporal lobe structures themselves. This proposal is strengthened by recent findings indicating that neonatal ablations of the hippocampal formation that include much of the parahippocampal gyrus but do not encroach on the perirhinal or entorhinal areas appear to leave visual recognition memory intact (Beauregard & Bachevalier, 1993). Nevertheless, the proposal regarding the locus of the critical tissue for recognition memory may not extend to relational memory, in view of the evidence that severe impairment in the latter function can be produced by hippocampal ablations that largely spare the rhinal cortex, whether the lesions occur in early infancy (Alvarado et al., 1996) or in adulthood (Alvarado et al., 1998). Thus, additional studies are clearly needed to identify the effects of damaging each component of the medial temporal lobe on specific memory processes.

Emotional Reactions and Social Interactions

To investigate the emotional and social development of infant monkeys with neonatal medial temporal lobe lesions, the social interactions between operated monkeys and their age-matched normal controls were analyzed at different points in their maturation and compared to those of normal infants raised together.

At the ages of 2 months, 6 months, and 5 years, operated infant monkeys and their age-matched controls were placed in a play cage containing toys and towels. The behavior of each pair was videotaped for two periods of 5 minutes each, separated by a 5 minute interval, for 6 consecutive days. The frequency and duration of behaviors for each animal on the videotapes were scored independently by two observers, who assigned the behaviors to one of eight different behavioral categories. These behavioral categories included *Approach*—social contact initiated by the observed monkey; *Acceptance of approach*—acceptance of social contact initiated by the other monkey; *Dominant approach*—immature forms of aggression, such as snapping at the other monkey, taking toys away from the other monkey, or pushing the other monkey away; *Active withdrawal*—active withdrawal from a social approach initiated by the other monkey; *Inactivity*—passive behavior; *Manipulation*—manipulations of toys or parts of the cage with the limbs or mouth; *Locomotor stereotypies*—abnormal motor behaviors, such as circling or doing somersaults; and *Self-directed activities*—self-administered actions such as pressing the head with hands or sucking part of the body.

At both 2 and 6 months of age, pairs of normal animals spent most of their time in social interactions, locomotion, or manipulation. They exhibited virtually no behaviors considered to be abnormal, such as active withdrawal, locomotor stereotypies, or self-directed activities, and almost no inactivity. Between 2 and 6 months, however, the nature of social interactions between the normal animals did change. Whereas at 2 months social behavior consisted primarily of following the other monkey and clinging to it, at 6 months these immature behaviors were replaced primarily by rough-and-tumble play and chasing. As adults, normal monkeys remain mainly in close proximity to or physical contact with each other, with few episodes of locomotor behaviors and no stereotypies.

Unlike normal infant monkeys, those with neonatal medial temporal lobe lesions began to show numerous socioemotional abnormalities as they matured (Bachevalier, 1994). At 2 months of age, these infant monkeys showed more inactivity and manipulated objects less than the controls. The analysis of their social interactions revealed that these animals did not initiate social contact as much as did their unoperated controls, but they did have a normal amount of accepting approach from their controls, indicating that the normal animal in the pair initiated most of the social interactions (Fig. 2-5A, part a). Interestingly, at 6 months of age, the operated monkeys displayed even more striking pathology. The amount of social interaction between the operated animals and their controls decreased dramatically compared with that of animals in the normal dyads (Fig. 2-5A, part b). These results indicate that not only did the animals with medial temporal lobe lesions display less initiation of social approach, they also displayed less acceptance of social contacts. In addition, the normal controls adapted to the social unresponsiveness of the operated animals by reducing the amount of social contact attempted. There were also qualitative differences in appearance and social interactions between the animals with early medial temporal lobe lesions and their controls at 6 months of age. They had blank, unexpressive faces and poor body expression (i.e., a lack of normal playful posturing), and they displayed very few eye contacts.

Social dominance was measured by analyzing dominant approach and active withdrawal. At 2 months of age, there was virtually no dominant approach or active withdrawal by any animals. At 6 months of age, however, there was more dominant approach in the control animals paired with the operated monkeys—even more than in animals from dyads with two normal controls—and more active withdrawal in animals with early medial temporal lobe lesions. This is of particular interest because the increase in active withdrawal, which occurs in response to an

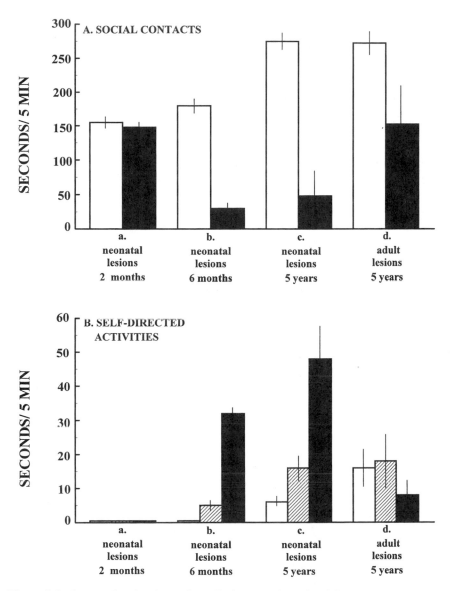

Figure 2-5. Average duration (seconds per 5 minute session) of social contacts (A) and self-directed activities (B) in animals with neonatal medial temporal lobe damage and their age-matched controls at 2 months, 6 months, 4–5 years, and 4- to 5-years-old animals with the same damage in adulthood and their age-matched normal controls. Total social contacts included Approach and Accepts Approach across both members of each dyad at 2 and 6 months and Proximity and Contact across both members of each dyads at 4–5 years. Conventions: for social behavior, white bars represent social contacts measured in dyads comprising two age-matched normal animals; black bars represent social contacts in dyads comprising one animal with a medial temporal lobe lesion and its age-matched, unoperated controls; for self-directed activities, white bars are scores of normal animals in the normal dyads, hatched bars are scores of normal controls in dyads including an animal with a medial temporal lobe lesion, and black bars are scores of animals with medial temporal lobe lesions.

initiation of social contact by the other animal, suggests that animals with early medial temporal lobe lesions were not only uninterested in social contact and socially inept, but also that they actively avoided social contact. Perhaps as a result of the drastic reduction in the amount of social contact, both animals with early medial temporal lobe lesions and their controls exhibited an increase in manipulation. In addition to these social disturbances, animals with early medial temporal lobe lesions developed stereotypies (Fig. 2-5B; compare parts a and b).

Finally, all of the socioemotional disturbances in infants with medial temporal lobe lesions were still present when these animals reached adulthood (Fig. 2-5A and B, part c). At adult age, compared to the normal dyads, dyads containing an operated and a normal animal engaged in dramatically less social interaction and more object manipulation. In addition, compared to normal controls, the monkeys with early medial temporal lobe lesions displayed more self-directed activities and more locomotion. The results therefore indicate that the socioemotional effects of early damage of the medial temporal lobe are long-lasting and probably permanent, and appear even to increase in magnitude over time.

The effects of early medial temporal lobe lesions on socioemotional development were then compared to those of late lesions (Málková, et al., 1997). Adult monkeys were raised in conditions similar to those of infant monkeys but were given similar bilateral medial temporal lobe lesions in adulthood. Two and 6 months after their surgery, they were paired with normal controls with which they had had social interactions in their infancy and early adulthood. Their behavior was videotaped in the large enclosure in the same way as that of the monkeys with early lesions. Although the dyads containing one operated animal displayed less social contact than the normal dyads, this reduction in social interactions was milder than the severe drop in social contact seen in the dyads containing animals with lesions. As shown in Figure 2-5A and 2-5B (compare parts c and d), social interactions were substantially and significantly less after lesions in infancy than after lesions in adulthood. In addition, monkeys operated on in adulthood displayed none of the other behavioral abnormalities observed in those operated on in infancy. The finding of more profound socioemotional disturbances after early lesions suggests that the monkeys given lesions in adulthood retained at least some aspects of the socioemotional repertoire they had acquired during maturation, whereas the neonatally lesioned animals never succeeded in acquiring them. Supporting this suggestion is the finding that the original dyads containing animals with early medial temporal lobe lesions did not show the increase in social interaction from infancy to adulthood that was observed in the normal dyads.

Thus, our findings confirm those of earlier studies demonstrating that damage to the medial temporal lobe impairs socioemotional behavior in rhesus monkeys. Interestingly, our findings also demonstrate that such damage in infancy yields more profound socioemotional effects than does damage in adulthood, the reverse of the pattern commonly reported for other types of behavioral effect after early versus late cerebral damage. These experimental findings may therefore have important implications for socioemotional development, as distinct from other types of behavioral and cognitive development, after medial temporal lobe damage in children.

Concluding Remarks

In sum, this developmental study in nonhuman primates has shown that early damage to the medial temporal lobe results in a severe, global, and long-lasting anterograde amnesia strikingly similar to the anterograde amnesia observed in adult monkeys with the same neural damage. This finding clearly indicates that compensatory mechanisms do not always operate to ensure recovery of functions after early brain damage. In addition, the severe anterograde amnesia was accompanied by profound changes in the formation of social bonds and emotionality. Not only did the early lesions cause a loss of social bonds that was greater in magnitude than that found after late lesions, but they also resulted in the development of abnormal behaviors that had never been reported in adult monkeys with the same lesions. Thus, in the case of the socioemotional behavior, the results suggest that, as proposed earlier by Teuber and Rudel (1962), the early medial temporal lobe damage may have caused a reorganization in other neural systems, and this reorganization may have been functionally debilitating rather than beneficial. This has recently been confirmed by our neurobiological studies on the same monkeys (Bertolino et al., 1997, Saunders et al., 1998).

These results in infant monkeys are consistent with the clinical observation that children who sustain medial temporal lobe damage in infancy develop significant anterograde amnesia and, in some cases, changes in socioemotional behaviors. As shown in Table 2-1, there are anecdotal reports of severe memory loss in children who developed a Klüver-Bucy syndrome resulting either from hypoxic insults affecting the medial temporal lobe (Tongstard et al., 1987) or from bitemporal arachnoid cysts (Rossitch & Oakes, 1989). Detailed neuropsychological evaluation of a few cases has also indicated the presence of childhood anterograde amnesia following either encephalopathy (Ostergaard, 1987), herpes simplex encephalitis (Wood et al., 1989), anoxia (Broman et al., 1990), or medial temporal sclerosis and hippocampal atrophy (Levick, 1992; Vargha-Khadem et al., 1992). In all these amnesic cases, the damage was sustained some years after birth, with the youngest patients being 4 and 5 years old and all the others being between 9 and 15 years of age. There are also reports of amnesic syndrome in children with congenital insult to the medial temporal lobe (Maurer, 1991), indicating that the same anterograde amnesia might well develop no matter how early postnatally such damage occurs. Conversely, the apparent absence of memory disorders in children with agenesis of the temporal lobe (Karvounis et al., 1970; Lang et al., 1981; Nathan & Smith, 1950; Tuyman et al., 1974;) suggests that there could well be a critical period in fetal development before which medial temporal damage may still be fully compensated for.

Finally, recent reports demonstrate that neonatal damage to restricted portions of the medial temporal lobe in monkeys has different impacst on the development of memory functions and socioemotional behavior, causing different patterns of functional recovery or dysfunction. Indeed, such restricted neonatal damage cause specific behavioral syndromes in monkeys that share similarities with developmental behavioral disorders in humans, resembling autism (Bachevalier, 1994) and

Table 2-1. Cognitive and Behavioral Deficits After Early Medial Temporal Lobe Insult in Humans

Authors	Cases	Neuropathology	Symptoms
Nathan & Smith (1950)	34-year-old man	Agenesis of the temporal lobes	No behavioral changes, no memory loss
Karvounis et al. (1970)	48-year-old woman	Agenesis of the temporal lobes	No behavioral changes, no memory loss
Chutorian & Antunes (1981)	13-year-old girl	Biopsy-proven herpes encephalitis of the temporal lobe	Klüver-Bucy symptoms
Lang et al. (1981)	76-year-old man	Agenesis of the temporal lobes	No behavioral changes, no memory loss
Martinius (1983)	14-year-old boy	Cystic defect of left amygdala	Aggressive behavior, lags in cognitive development
Tonsgard et al. (19i87)	4-year-old boy 11-year-old boy 14-year-old girl	Hyposix insult	Klüver-Bucy symptoms, memory loss
Ostergaard (1987)	10-year-old boy	Left hippocampus, parahippocampal gyrus, and right orbitofrontal region	Memory losses
Wood et al. (1989)	9-year-old girl	Herpes simplex encephalitis	Dense amnesia
Rossitch & Oakes (1989)	11-year-old boy	Bilateral temporal arachnoid cysts	Klüver-Bucy symptoms, poor memory
Broman et al. (1990)	27-year-old man	Anoxic encephalopathy at age 7 years	Severe anterograde amnesia
DeRenzi & Lucchelli (1990)	22-year-old man	Not known	Dyslexia and poor memory from childhood
Vargha-Khadem et al. (1992)	10-year-old boy	Right temporal lobectomy	Impaired memory
Levick (1992)	11-year-old boy	Not known	Amnesic syndrome
Lanska & Lanska (1993)	11-year-old boy	Neuronal ceroid lipofuscinosis	Klüver-Bucy syndrome

schizophrenia (Beauregard & Bachevalier, 1996; Bertolino et al., 1997). Thus, the developmental studies of early medial temporal lobe lesions in monkeys substantiate an earlier proposal from Schneider (1979) that early dysfunction of the medial temporal lobe is the origin of developmental psychosis in humans and provides insights into the neural substrates of these debilitating disorders of human neurodevelopment.

References

Adolphs, R., Tranel, D., Damasio, H., and Damasio, A.R. (1994) Impaired recognition of emotion in facial expressions following bilateral damage to the human amygdala. *Nature*, 372:669–672.

Adolphs, R., Tranel, D., Damasio, H., and Damasio, A.R. (1995) Fear and the human amygdala. *Journal of Neuroscience*, 15:5880–5891.

Aggleton, J.P. (1992) The functional effects of amygdala lesions in humans: A comparison with findings from monkeys. In J.P. Aggleton (ed.), *The Amygdala: Neurobiological Aspects of Emotion, Memory, and Mental Dysfunction*. New York: Wiley-Liss, pp. 485–504.

Aggleton, J.P., and Mishkin, M. (1986) The amygdala: Sensory gateway to the emotions. In R. Plutchik and H. Kellerman (eds.), *Emotion: Theory, Research, and Experience*, Vol. 3 of *Biological Foundations of Emotion*. New York: Academic Press, pp. 281–299.

Aggleton, J.P., and Passingham, R.E. (1981) Syndrome produced by lesions of the amygdala in monkeys (*Macaca mulatta*). *Journal of Comparative and Physiological Psychology*, 95:961–977.

Alvarado, M.C., Barnhill, J.W., and Bachevalier, J. (1996) Long-term effects of neonatal hippocampal lesions on spatial recognition memory in rhesus monkeys. *Society for Neuroscience Abstracts*, 22:1120.

Angeli, S.J., Murray E.A., and Mishkin, M. (1993) Hippocampectomized monkeys can remember one place but not two. *Neuropsychologia*, 31:1021–1030.

Bachevalier, J. (1994) Medial temporal lobe structures and autism: A review of clinical and experimental findings. *Neuropsychologia*, 32:627–648.

Bachevalier, J., Brickson, M., and Hagger, C. (1993) Limbic-dependent recognition memory in monkeys develops early in infancy. *NeuroReport*, 4:77–80.

Bachevalier, J., Brickson, M., Hagger, C., and Mishkin, M. (1990) Age and sex differences in the effects of selective temporal lobe lesions on the formation of visual discrimination habits in rhesus monkeys (*Macaca mulatta*). *Behavioral Neuroscience*, 104:885–899.

Bachevalier, J., and Mishkin, M. (1994) Effects of selective neonatal temporal lobe lesions on visual recognition memory in rhesus monkeys. *Journal of Neuroscience*, 14:2128–2139.

Bates, E. (1992) Language development. *Current Opinion in Neurobiology*, 2:180–185.

Beauregard, M., and Bachevalier, J. (1993) Long-term effects of neonatal hippocampal lesions on visual recognition memory. *Society for Neuroscience Abstracts*, 19:1004.

Beauregard, M., and Bachevalier, J. (1996) Neonatal insult to the hippocampal region and schizophrenia: A review and a putative animal model. Canadian Journal of Psychiatry, 41:446–456.

Bertolino, A., Saunders, R.C., Mattay, V.S., Bachevalier, J., Frank, J.A., and Weinberger, D.R. (1997) Altered development of prefrontal neurons in rhesus monkeys with neonatal mesial temporo-limbic lesions: A proton magnetic resonance spectroscopic imaging study. *Cerebral Cortex,* 7:740–768.

Broman, M., Kriengkrairut, S., McCarthy, C. and Rose, A. (1990) A case of severe antero-grade amnesia in an adult with onset at seven years of age as a result of presumed anoxic encephalopathy. Presented at the 11th annual conference of the New York Neuropsychology Group, New York.

Brooks, D.N., and Baddeley, A.D. 1976. What can amnesic patients learn? *Neuropsychologia,* 14:111–122.

Brown, S., and Schafer, E.A. (1888) An investigation into the functions of the occipital and temporal lobes of the monkey's brain. *Philosophical Transactions of the Royal Society of London,* 179B:303–327.

Buckley, M.B., Gaffan, D., and Murray, E.A. (1997) A functional double-dissociation between two inferior temporal cortical areas: Perirhinal cortex vs. middle temporal gyrus. *Journal of Neurophysiology,* 77:587–598.

Chutorian, A.B., and Antunes, J.L. (1981) Klüver-Bucy syndrome and herpes encephalitis: Case report. Neurosurgery, 8:388–390.

Cohen, N.J., and Squire, L.R. (1980) Preserved learning and retention of pattern-analyzing skill in amnesia: Dissociation of "knowing how" and "knowing that". *Science,* 210:207–209.

Corkin, S. (1968) Acquisition of motor skill after bilateral medial temporal-lobe excision. *Neuropsychologia,* 6:255–266.

Damasio, A.R., Eslinger, P.J., Damasio, H., Van Hoesen, G.W., and Cornell, S. (1985) Multimodal amnesic syndrome following bilateral temporal and basal forebrain damage. *Archives of Neurology,* 42:252–259.

De Renzi, E., and Lucchelli, F. (1990) Developmental dysmnesia in a poor reader, Brain, 113:1337–1345.

Eacott, M.J., Gaffan, D., and Murray, E.A. (1994) Preserved recognition memory for small sets, and impaired stimulus identification for large sets, following rhinal cortex ablations in monkeys. *European Journal of Neuroscience,* 6:1466–1478.

Friedman, H.M., and Allen, N. (1969) Chronic effects of complete limbic lobe destruction in man. *Neurology,* 19:679–690.

Gascon, G.G., and Gilles. F. 1973. Limbic dementia. *Journal of Neurology, Neurosurgery, and Psychiatry,* 36:421–450.

Gloor, P. (1972) Temporal epilepsy: Its possible contribution to the understanding of the functional significance of the amygdala and its interaction with neocortical-temporal mechanisms. In B.E. Eleftheriou (ed.), *The Neurobiology of the Amygdala.* New York: Plenum Press, pp. 423–457.

Gloor, P. (1986) The role of human limbic system in perception, memory, and affect: Lessons from temporal epilepsy. In B.K. Doane and K.E. Livingston (eds.), *The Limbic System: Functional Organization and Clinical Disorders.* New York: Raven Press, pp. 159–169.

Goldman, P.S. (1971) Functional development of the prefrontal cortex in early life and the problem of neuronal plasticity. *Experimental Neurology,* 32:366–387.

Goldman, P.S. (1974) An alternative to development plasticity: Heterology of CNS structures in infants and adults. In D.G. Stein, J. Rosen, and N. Butters (eds.), *Plasticity and Recovery of Function in the Central Nervous System.* New York: Academic Press, pp. 149–174.

Goldman-Rakic, P.S., Isseroff, A., Schwartz, M.L., and Bugbee, N.M. (1983) The neurobiology of cognitive development. In P. Mussen (ed.), *Handbook of Cognitive Development: Biology and Infancy Development,* New York: Wiley, pp. 281–344.

Hebben, N., Shedlack, K., Eichenbaum, H., and Corkin, S. (1981) The amnesic patient H.M.: Diminished ability to interpret and report internal states. *Society for Neurosciences Abstracts,* 7:235.

Hirsh, R. (1974) The hippocampus and contextual retrieval of information from memory: A theory. *Behavioral Biology,* 12:421–445.

Horel, J.A., Keating, E.G., and Misantone, L.J. (1975) Partial Klüver-Bucy syndrome produced by destroying temporal neocortex or amygdala. *Brain Research,* 94:347–359.

Irwin, W., Davidson, R.J., Lowe, M.J., Mock, B.J., Sorenson, J.A., and Turski, P.A. (1996) Human amygdala activation detected with echo-planar functional magnetic resonance imaging. *NeuroReport,* 7:1765–1769.

Iwai, E., Nishio, T., and Yamaguchi, K. (1986) Neuropsychological basis of a K-B sign in Klüver-Bucy syndrome produced following total removal of inferotemporal cortex of macaque monkeys. In Y. Oomura (ed.), *Emotion: Neural and Chemical Control.* Tokyo: Japan Scientific Society Press, pp. 299–311.

Karvounis, P.C., Chiu, J.C., Parsa, K., and Gilbert, S. (1970) Agenesis of temporal lobe and arachnoid cyst. *New York State Journal of Medicine,* 70:2349–2353.

Kennard, M.A. (1936) Age and other factors in motor recovery from presentral lesions in monkey. *American Journal of Physiology,* 115:138–146.

Kling, A. (1972) Effects of amygdalectomy on social-affective behavior in nonhuman primates. In B.E. Eleftheriou (ed.), *The Neurobiology of the Amygdala.* New York: Plenum Press, pp. 511–536.

Kling, A., and Brothers, L.A. (1992) The amygdala and social behavior. In J.P. Aggleton (ed.), *The Amygdala: Neurobiological Aspects of Emotion, Memory, and Mental Dysfunction.* New York: Wiley-Liss, pp. 353–377.

Klüver, H., and Bucy, P.C. (1938) An analysis of certain effects of bilateral temporal lobectomy in the rhesus monkey, with special reference to "psychic blindness." *Journal of Psychology,* 5:33–54.

Klüver, H., and Bucy, P.C. (1939) Preliminary analysis of function of the temporal lobe in monkeys. *Archives of Neurology,* 42:979–1000.

Kolb, B., and Whishaw, I.Q. (1989) Plasticity in the neocortex: Mechanisms underlying selective neonatal temporal lobe lesions on learning and memory in monkeys. *Progress in Neurobiology,* 32:235–276.

Lang, C., Lehrl, S., and Huk, W. (1981) A case of bilateral temporal lobe agenesis. *Journal of Neurology, Neurosurgery and Psychiatry,* 44:626–630.

Landska, D.J., and Landska, M.J. (1996) Klüver-Bucy syndrome in juvenile neuronal ceroid lipofuscinosis, Journal of Child Neurology, 9:67–69.

Levick, W. (1992) A developmental amnesic syndrome? The life cycle: Development, maturation, senescence. Proceedings of the 16th Annual Brain Impairment Conference, Sydney, Australia, pp. 1–5.

Mahut, H., and Moss, M. (1986) The monkey and the sea horse. In R.L. Isaacson and K.L. Pribram (eds.), *The Hippocampus,* Vol. 4. New York: Plenum Press, pp. 241–279.

Malamut, B.L., Saunders, R.C., and Mishkin, M. (1984) Monkeys with combined amygdalo-hippocampal lesions succeed in object discrimination learning despite 24-hour intertrial intervals. *Behavioral Neuroscience,* 98:759–769.

Málková, L., Mishkin, M., and Bachevalier, J. (1995). Long-term effects of selective neonatal temporal lobe lesions on learning and memory in monkeys. *Behavioral Neuroscience,* 109:1–15.

Málková, L., Mishkin, M., Suomi, S.J., and Bachevalier, J. (1997) Socioemotional behavior in adult rhesus monkeys after early versus late lesions of the medial temporal lobe. *Annals of the New York Academy of Sciences,* 807:538–540.

Marlowe, W.B., Mancall, E.L., and Thomas, J.J. (1975) Complete Klüver-Bucy syndrome in man. *Cortex,* 11:53–59.

Martinius, J. (1983) Homicide of an aggressive adolescent boy with right temporal lesion: A case report. Neuroscience and Biobehavioral Review, 7:419–422.

Maurer, R.G. (1991) Disorders of memory and learning. In S.J. Segalowitz and I. Rapin (vol. eds.) and F. Boller and J. Grafman (series eds.), *Handbook of Neuropsychology: Child Neuropsychology,* Vol. 7. Amsterdan Elsevier, pp. 241–260.

Meunier, M., Bachevalier, J., Mishkin, M., and Murray, E.A. (1993) Effects on visual recognition memory of combined and separate ablations of the entorhinal and perirhinal cortex in rhesus monkeys. *Journal of Neuroscience,* 13:5418–5432.

Meunier, M., Bachevalier, J., Murray, E.A., Merjanian, P.M., and Richardson, R. (1991) Effects of rhinal cortical or limbic lesions on fear reactions in rhesus monkeys. *Society for Neuroscience Abstracts,* 17:337.

Milner, B. (1962) Les troubles de la mémoire accompagnant des lésions hippocampiques bilatérales. In P. Passouant (Ed.), *Physiologie de l'hippocampe.* Paris: Centre de la Recherche Scientifique, pp. 257–272.

Mishkin, M. (1978) Memory in monkeys severely impaired by combined but not separate removal of amygdala and hippocampus. *Nature,* 273:297–298.

Mishkin, M. (1982) A memory system in the monkey. *Philosophical Transactions of the Royal Society of London,* B298:85–95.

Mishkin, M., and Appenzeller, T. (1987) The anatomy of memory. *Scientific American,* 256:80–89.

Mishkin, M., Malamut, B.L., and Bachevalier, J. (1984) Memories and habits: Two neural systems. In G. Lynch, L. McGaugh, and N.M. Weinberger (eds.), *Neurobiology of Learning and Memory.* New York: Guildford Press, pp. 65–77.

Mishkin, M., and Petri, H.L. (1984) Memories and habits: Some implications for the analysis of learning and retention. In N. Butters and L. Squire (eds.), *Neuropsychology of Memory.* New York: Guildford Press, pp. 287–296.

Morris, J.S., Frith, C.D., Perrett, D.I., Rowland, D., Young, A.W., Calder, A.J., and Dolan, R.J. (1996) A differential neural response in the human amygdala to fearful and happy facial expressions. *Nature,* 383:812–815.

Murray, E.A., and Mishkin, M. (1984). Severe tactual as well as visual memory deficits follow combined removal of the amygdala and hippocampus in monkeys. *Journal of Neuroscience,* 4:2565–2580.

Murray, E.A., and Mishkin, M. (1998). Object recognition and Location in monkeys with excitotoxic lesions of the amygdala and hippocampus. Journal of Neuroscience, 18:6568–6582.

Nathan, P.W., and Smith, M.C. (1950) Normal mentality associated with a maldeveloped rhinencephalon. *Journal of Neurology, Neurosurgery and Psychiatry,* 13:191–197.

Obrador, S. (1947) Temporal lobotomy. *Journal of Experimental Neurology,* 6:185–193.

Ostergaard, A.L. (1987) Episodic, semantic, and procedural memory in a case of amnesia at an early age. *Neuropsychologia,* 25:341–357.

Parkinson, J.K., Murray, E.A., and Mishkin, M. (1988) A selective mnemonic role for the hippocampus in monkeys: Memory for the location of objects. *Journal of Neuroscience,* 8:4159–4167.

Pool, J.L. (1952) The visceral brain of man. *Journal of Neurosurgery,* 96:209–248.

Rempel-Clower, N.L., Zola, S.M., Squire, L.R., and Amaral, D.G. (1996) Three cases of enduring memory impairment after bilateral damage limited to the hippocampal formation. *Journal of Neuroscience,* 16:5233–5255.

Rossitch, E., and Oakes, W.J. (1989) Klüver-Bucy syndrome in a child with bilateral arachnoid cysts: Report of a case. *Neurosurgery,* 24:110–112.

Rosvold, H.E., Mirsky, A.F., and Pribram, K. (1954) Influence of amygdalectomy on social behavior in monkeys. *Journal of Comparative and Physiological Psychology,* 47:173–178.

Rudel, R.C., and Teuber, H.L. (1971) Spatial orientation in normal children and in children with early brain injury. *Neuropsychologia,* 9:401–407.

Rudel, R.C., Teuber, H.L., and Twitchell, T.E. (1966) A note on hyperesthesia in children with early brain damage. *Neuropsychologia,* 4:351–356.

Ruppenthal, G.C., Walker, C.G., and Sackett, G.P. (1991) Rearing infant monkeys (*Macaca nemestrina*) in pairs produces deficient social development compared with rearing in single cages. *American Journal of Primatology,* 25:103–113.

Saunders, R.C., Kolachana, B.S., Bachevalier, J., and Weinberger, D.R. (1998) Neonatal lesions of the medial temporal lobe disrupt prefrontal cortical regulation of striatal dopamine, *Nature,* 393:169–171.

Saunders, R.C., Murray, E.A., and Mishkin, M. (1984) Further evidence that amygdala and hippocampus contribute equally to recognition memory. *Neuropsychologia,* 22:785–796.

Schneider, G.E. (1979). Is it really better to have your brain lesion early? A revision of the "Kennard Principle." *Neuropsychologia,* 17:557–583.

Scoville, W.B., and Milner, B. (1957) Loss of recent memory after bilateral hippocampal lesions. *Journal of Neurology, Neurosurgery and Psychiatry,* 20:11–21.

Spiegler, B.J., and Mishkin, M. (1979) Associative memory severely impaired by combined amygdalo-hippocampal removals. *Society for Neuroscience Abstracts,* 5:323.

Squire, L.R., Cohen, N.J., and Zouzounis, J.A. (1984) Preserved memory in anterograde amnesia: Sparing of a recently acquired skill. *Neuropsychologia,* 22:145–152.

Suzuki, W.A., Zola-Morgan, S., Squire, L.R., and Amaral, D.G. (1993) Lesions of the perirhinal and parahippocampal cortices in the monkey produce long-lasting memory impairments in the visual and tactual modalities. *Journal of Neuroscience,* 13:2430–2451.

Teuber, H.L., and Rudel, R.G. (1962) Behaviour after cerebral lesions in children and adults. *Developmental Medicine and Child Neurology,* 4:3–20.

Tonsgard, J.H., Harwicke, N., and Levine, S.C. (1987) Kluver-Bucy syndrome in children. *Pediatric Neurology,* 3:162–165.

Tuynman, F.H.B., Hekster, R.E.M., and Pauwels, E.K.J. (1974) Intracranial arachnoid cyst of the middle fossa demonstrated by positive 99m Tc brain scintigraphy. *Neuroradiology,* 7:41–44.

Vargha-Khadem, F., Isaacs, E.B., and Watkins, K.E. (1992) Medial temporal lobe versus diencephalic amnesia in childhood. *Journal of Clinical and Experimental Neuropsychology,* 14:371–372.

Warrington, E.K., and Weiskrantz, L. (1968). New method of testing long-term retention with special reference to amnesic patients. *Nature (Lond.),* 217:972–974.

Weiskrantz, L. (1956) Behavioral changes associated with ablations of the amygdaloid complex in monkeys. *Journal of Comparative and Physiological Psychology,* 49:381–391.

Wood, F.B., Brown, I.S., and Felton, R.H. (1989) Long-term follow-up of a childhood amnesic syndrome. *Brain and Cognition,* 10:76–86.

Woods, B.T., and Teuber, H.L. (1978) Mirror movements after childhood hemiparesis. *Neurology,* 28:1152–1158.

Young, A.W., Hellawell, D.J., Van de Wakl, C., and Johnston, M. (1996) Facial expression processing after amygdalectomy. *Neuropsychologia,* 34:31–39.

Zola-Morgan, S., and Squire, L.R. (1985). Complementary approaches to the study of memory: Human amnesia and animal models. In N.W. Weinberger, J.L. McGaugh, and L. Lynch (eds.), *Memory Systems of the Brain: Animal and Human Cognitive Processes.* New York: Guildford Press, pp. 463–477.

Zola-Morgan, S., Squire, L.R., Alvarez-Royo, P., and Clower, R.P. (1991) Independence of memory functions and emotional behavior: Separate contributions of the hippocampal formation and the amygdala. *Hippocampus,* 1:207–220.

Zola-Morgan, S., Squire, L.R., and Amaral. D.G. (1986) Human amnesia and the medial temporal region: Enduring memory impairment following a bilateral lesion limited to field CA1 of the hippocampus. *Journal of Neuroscience,* 6:2950–2967.

Zola-Morgan, S., Squire, L.R., Amaral, D.G., and Suzuki, W. (1989) Lesions of perirhinal and parahippocampal cortex that spare the amygdala and hippocampal formation produce severe memory impairment. *Journal of Neuroscience,* 9:4355–4370.

3

Cognitive Recovery from Traumatic Brain Injury: Results of Posttraumatic Experimental Interventions

ROBERT J. HAMM, MEREDITH D. TEMPLE, DEANNE L. BUCK,
S. MICHELLE DEFORD, AND CANDACE L. FLOYD

This chapter reviews experimental work on posttraumatic interventions aimed at improving cognitive recovery.[*] Its scope is limited to animate models of traumatic brain injury (TBI) in which injury is mechanically induced to the whole brain and is nonpenetrating. Also, the interventions tested must have been initiated after the injury and continued for a period of time following the injury (usually several days). To provide a context for these experimental studies, we give a brief summary of some the features of human head injury.

Human Head Injury

Epidemiology

Head injury is a major cause of disability and is the leading source of brain damage in previously healthy adults (Kraus, 1987). Data from the largest study of head-injured patients, the Major Trauma Outcome Study, indicate the occurance of head injury is the single most significant factor contributing to morbidity and mortality in hospital admissions (Gennarelli et al., 1994). In the United States alone, there are approximately 500,000 hospital admissions due to head injury each year (Frankowski, 1986).

---

[*]The term *recovery* is used here to describe a reduction in cognitive deficits. No reference is implied to the issue of restorative versus compensatory processes.

Disability Following Head Injury

Traumatic brain injury is a multifactorial and often diffuse injury process. There-fore, traumatically induced impairments encompass a wide range of disabilities. The most frequently reported complaint by patients following head injury is cognitive impairment (Brooks et al., 1987; Gronwall & Wrightson, 1974; Oddy et al., 1985: van Zomeren & van den Burg, 1985). Two features of posttraumatic cognitive im-pairment are particularly important for experimental studies. First, there is usually a graded retrograde memory deficit. For example, most mildly injured patients can recall remote memories but cannot remember events that occurred just before the trauma (Levin, 1992). Second, anterograde amnesia, or loss of memory for events occurring after the injury, is also prominent following head injury. For example, head-injured patients consistently perform poorly on free recall tasks in which a list of words is presented and the patient is required to learn the words and recall them later (Levin & Goldstein, 1986).

Experimental Traumatic Brain Injury

While a comprehensive review of the physiological changes produced by TBI is beyond the scope of this chapter, a brief review of selected features is necessary because many of the experimental interventions target these changes.

Acute Physiological Alterations

Over the past few years, numerous findings have supported the hypothesis that TBI initiates a cascade of events that lead to a period of abnormally excessive neuronal excitation (for more extensive reviews, see Hayes et al., 1992; McIntosh et al., 1994). For example, TBI causes neuronal depolarization, as measured by large increases in extracellular potassium, which leads to massive, indiscriminate neurotrans-mitter release and further depolarization (Faden et al., 1989; Gorman et al., 1989; Katayama et al., 1990). The resulting excessive activation of receptors may produce changes in intracellular signaling mechanisms that result in long-lasting alteration in cell function.

In addition to abnormal neurotransmitter receptor-effector function, the con-sequences of necrotic and apoptotic processes initiated by TBI may combine with diffuse axonal injury to contribute to the chronic impairment of cognitive function observed after injury.

Chronic Physiological Alterations

The mechanisms that mediate chronic[†] disability after TBI have been less inten-sively investigated and are not fully understood. However, as early as 1905, von Monakow (1969) hypothesized that the central nervous system (CNS) enters a

---

[†] The word *chronic* refers to a postinjury time period in rats that begins approximately 24 hours after injury and continues for weeks. In humans, the time scale would probably be much longer.

state of "functional depression" following insult. This theory of diaschisis has recently been revised by Feeney (1991) as *remote functional depression (RFD)*. The theory of RFD posits that the behavioral deficits observed after neurological insult are due, in part, to functional depression of normal neuronal activity. Thus, according to theories of diaschisis and RFD, behavioral recovery should be associated with the dissipation of this neuronal depression.

A Biphasic Hypothesis

A comparison of the pathobiology of the acute and chronic phases of TBI suggests there is a dramatic reversal in a number of physiological processes. As predicted by the acute phase of excessive neuronal excitation after TBI, antagonists of excitatory neurotransmitters improved outcome when administered shortly (generally <30 minutes) after injury (Hamm et al., 1993; Hayes et al., 1992; Lyeth et al., 1992; McIntosh et al., 1994). When the same excitatory antagonists are administered several days after TBI, behavioral deficits are exacerbated (Dixon et al., 1994c; Hamm et al., 1994). Microdialysis studies have documented that glutamate and acetylcholine (ACh) levels are elevated shortly after TBI (Faden et al., 1989; Gorman et al., 1989), and many features of cholinergic function are depressed chronically after TBI (Dixon et al., 1994a, 1994b, 1996, 1997; Grady et al., 1992; Leonard et al., 1994; Schmidt & Grady, 1995). A similar biphasic change is observed when cerebral metabolism is measured: acutely (<6 hours), metabolism is elevated; chronically after TBI, metabolism is depressed (Yoshino et al., 1991). Other physiological processes have been examined in both the acute and chronic injury phases. In each case there is a reversal in the measured variable between the acute and chronic phases. Moreover, the alterations are consistent with an acute phase characterized by excessive neuronal activation and a chronic phase typified by neuronal depression or hypofunction. These changes in neuronal function can be represented graphically. In Figure 3-1, neuronal activity is represented on the ordinate. A normal level of neuronal activity necessary for optimal neuronal communication and function is assumed to take place within the horizontal dotted lines. Time after injury is represented on the abscissa (in a nonlinear fashion). The graph shows that immediately following TBI there is an abnormal increase in neuronal activity that resolves within a relatively short period of time. In rats, the period of excessive activity may end within a period of time ranging from minutes to a few hours after injury (Hamm et al., 1993; Hayes et al., 1992; Lyeth et al., 1992). Following, and perhaps in response to, the period of excessive activation, neuronal activity becomes suppressed. The degree and duration of the chronic hypofunctional phase depend on the severity of the injury.

If neuronal function is depressed chronically after TBI, as predicted by the biphasic model, then interventions initiated during the chronic phase should be designed to increase neuronal activity in order to return neuronal function to the normal range. In the following sections, the various types of posttraumatic interventions are reviewed. For convenience, they are divided on the basis of the targeted receptor system.

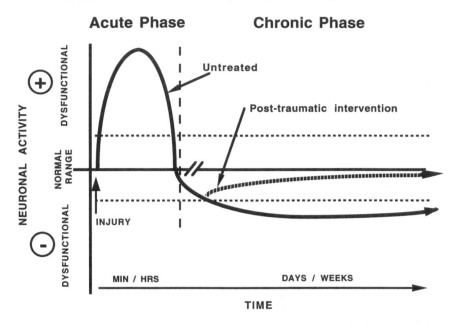

Figure 3–1. A hypothetical biphasic model of the changes in neuronal activity after injury. Normal neuronal function is assumed to be restricted to the area within the dashed lines. The graph shows that after TBI there is an abnormal, excessive increase in neuronal activity. This acute activation phase resolves fairly quickly and is followed by a period of depressed neuronal activity. If this model is correct, treatments initiated during the chronic phase of the injury process should be designed to increase neuronal function to the normal range.

Posttraumatic Neurotransmitter-Based Interventions

Monoamine System

L-deprenyl. Because manipulations of the monoamine system enhance motor recovery following non-TBI neuronal injury (Feeney et al., 1982, 1987), it seems reasonable to examine its role in posttraumatic recovery of cognitive function. The drug chosen for this experiment (L.L. Phillips, personal communication) was L-deprenyl, a monoamine oxidase-B (MAO-B) inhibitor. L-deprenyl has been shown to protect neurons from excitotoxic and ischemic damage (Semkova et al., 1996), as well as to improve the cognitive performance of aged rats (Yavich et al., 1996).

Rats were subjected to a moderate level of central fluid percussion injury. Twenty-four hours after injury, rats were injected (intraperitoneally [i.p.]) with either saline or 1 mg/kg of L-deprenyl. Drug treatments were continued daily for 7 days after injury and then terminated. On days 11–15 after TBI, rats were tested in the Morris water maze (MWM, four trials per day). Results indicated that injured animals previously treated with L-deprenyl performed significantly better in the MWM (i.e., reached the goal more quickly) than injured animals treated with saline. While the enhancement of monoamine activity is correlated with improved cognitive performance, there are a number of additional effects of L-deprenyl treatment that may have contributed to the improved cognitive outcome. For example, recent studies suggest that L-deprenyl has neurotrophic effects that are independent of its inhibition of MAO-B (Finnegan et al., 1990).

Cholinergic System

Research indicates that a decline in central cholinergic neurotransmission contributes to memory impairment following TBI (Dixon et al., 1994c, 1995; Hayes et al., 1992; Leonard et al., 1994; O'Dell & Hamm, 1995; Pike & Hamm, 1995; Schmidt & Grady, 1995). Therefore, increasing cholinergic transmission may attenuate cognitive deficits following TBI (Bartus et al., 1986). Pharmacotherapeutic interventions directed at enhancing cholinergic function include inhibition of the enzyme that catabolizes ACh, increased ACh availability and/or release, direct stimulation of the M1 muscarinic receptor subtype, or the addition of a cholinergic precursor. Additionally, antagonism of the presynaptic M2 autoreceptor (Doods, 1995; Sarter et al., 1990) could facilitate ACh release.

CDP-Choline. Dixon et al. (1997) investigated the ability of cytidine-5'-diphosphate choline (CDP-choline) to increase cholinergic transmission following TBI. The mechanism of action for CDP-choline is unknown; however, when administered exogenously, it is hydrolyzed to choline and cytidine. When applied to the cholinergic hypofunction hypothesis of TBI, CDP-choline should improve postinjury cognitive performance by enhancing ACh availability. Dixon et al. (1996) administered CDP-choline and examined the cognitive effect, as well as the drug's ability to increase ACh release in the dorsal hippocampus and neocortex.

Rats were prepared surgically and then injured (or sham injured) via the controlled cortical impact (CCI) injury device. Injured animals were administered (i.p.) either 100 mg/kg CDP-choline or saline for 18 days, beginning on day 1 postinjury. Cognitive performance was evaluated by the MWM on days 14 through 18 postinjury. CDP-choline–treated injured rats had significantly improved cognitive performance compared to saline-treated injured rats.

To assess the effect of CDP-choline on ACh levels, microdialysis was performed in a separate study. Rats were given (i.p.) a 100 mg/kg dose of CDP-choline. Microdialysis probes were implanted stereotaxically in the right dorsal hippocampus and the right neocortex. Baseline samples were collected; then CDP-choline or saline was injected. Samples were collected continuously over the next 3 hours. Extracellular ACH levels were assayed using high-performance liquid chromatography—(HPLC). The exogenous administration of CDP-choline resulted in significant increases in ACh levels in the dorsal hippocampus and neocortex. The results of this study support the hypothesis that a hypofunctional cholinergic system contributes to cognitive deficits following TBI, as exogenous activation of the cholinergic system with CDP-choline reduced these deficits. However, it is possible that CDP-choline's beneficial effects are the result of other mechanisms. For example, CDP-choline increases brain phospholipid metabolism, may account for the neuroprotective effects evidenced in this study.

BIBN-99. Another pharmacotherapeutic strategy involves antagonism of the ACh autoreceptor. Activation of the M2 muscarinic acetylcholine receptor (mAChR) regulates the release of ACh from the presynaptic terminal. Blockade of the M2 mAChR has been shown to increase release of ACh in the hippocampus and neocortex (Hoss et al., 1990; Lapchak et al., 1989; Richards, 1990; Richard et al., 1991). Thus, antagonism of M2 mAChR mitigated cholinergic hypofunction and potentially could provide a mechanism for chronic therapy following TBI. BIBN-99 is a highly selective M2 antagonist hypothesized to reduce cognitive deficits after TBI (Pike & Hamm, 1995).

Rats were prepared surgically and then administered a central injury (or sham injury) via the fluid percussion device. Injured rats were injected subcutanousely (s.c.) with either saline, 0.5 mg/kg, or 1.0 mg/kg BIBN-99. Two time courses of chronic BIBN-99 administration were tested. The early postinjury administration group was injected daily on days 1–15 postinjury. The delayed postinjury administration group was injected on days 11–15 postinjury. All injections were given 1 hour prior to cognitive assessment with the MWM on days 11–15 postinjury.

In the early postinjury administration injured group, animals treated with 0.5 or 1.0 mg/kg of BIBN-99 had significantly improved MWM performance compared to injured saline-treated animals. However, injured animals in the delayed postinjury administration group treated with either dose of BIBN-99 did not have improved MWM performance. These results show that selective antagonism of the M2 autoreceptor is an effective chronic therapy for attenuating cognitive deficits following TBI if the intervention is initiated early after the injury.

Tacrine. Tetrahydroaminoacridine (THA, Tacrine) is a reversible acetylcholinesterase (AChE) inhibitor that has been approved for clinical treatment in patients with mild to moderate Alzheimer's disease (Enz et al., 1993, Knapp et al., 1994). Acetylcholinesterase inhibitors inhibit enzymatic catabolism of ACh, thus maintaining synaptic levels of ACh. Consequently, Pike et al. (1997) tested the hypothesis that administration of THA would improve MWM performance following TBI.

Rats were prepared surgically and then centrally injured (or sham injured) via the fluid percussion device. Injured rats were injected (i.p.) either with saline, 1, 3, or 9 mg/kg THA on days 1–15 postinjury. Cognitive performance following TBI was assessed with the MWM on days 11–15 postinjury; rats were injected 30 minutes prior to MWM assessment. Injured rats treated with either 1 or 3 mg/kg of THA did not perform significantly differently on the MWM than injured saline-treated rats. However, injured rats treated with 9 mg/kg THA had significantly poorer performance than injured animals treated with saline.

These results suggest that THA is not an effective cholinomimetic therapy for treatment of cognitive deficits following TBI. The negative behavioral effect of THA observed in this study is consistent with reports indicating that repeated cholinesterase inhibition may reduce ACh synthesis by competing for choline up-take sites (Becker et al., 1988). Similarly, because presynaptic M2 autoreceptors regulate ACh release (Doods, 1995; Potter et al., 1984), THA-induced increase in extracellular ACh levels may inhibit presynaptic ACh release.

LU 25-109. As shown in the THA study, a nonselective mAChR agonist can have opposing effects on cellular function by stimulating postsynaptic M1 receptors (pos-itive modulation) as well as M2 presynaptic autoreceptors (negative modulation), producing a net zero effect on ACh activity. Consequently, a potentially more physiologically effective approach to increasing cholinergic function would involve partial agonism of the M1 mAChR combined with antagonism of the presynaptic M2 mAChR autoreceptor (Moltzen & Bjornholm, 1995; Sarter et al., 1990). The compound LU 25-109 has the binding profile of a partial M1 mAChR agonist and a M2 and M3 antagonist (Meier et al., 1995).

Pike and Hamm (1997a) investigated the effect of LU 25-109 in reducing cog-nitive deficits after TBI. Rats were prepared surgically and then centrally injured (or sham injured) via the fluid percussion device. Injured rats were injected (s.c.) with either saline or 3.6 or 15.0 μmol/kg LU 25-109 on days 1–15 postinjury. Cognitive deficits were assessed on days 11–15 via the MWM. There was no significant difference between injured saline-treated and injured 3.6 μmol/kg LU 25-109-treated rats. However, treatment with 15.0 μmol/kg LU 25-109 signifi-cantly improved MWM performance. In a separate experiment testing the effect of delayed postinjury administration of LU 25-109, rats were injured and drug treatment was initiated on days 11–15 postinjury 10 minutes prior to MWM assess-ment. This delayed treatment did not improve cognitive performance. Thus, as was observed with BIBN-99, delaying the initiation of drug treatment for 10 days af-ter injury eliminated the drug's beneficial effects.

A follow-up experiment assessed whether it was necessary for LU 25-109 to be pharmacologically active at the time of MWM assessment to be effective. Rats were injured and 15 μmol/kg LU 25-109 was administered on days 1–15 post-injury, with the drug administered 4 hours after MWM testing on days 11–15. The results demonstrated that LU 25-109 treatment was effective in reducing cognitive deficits. These experiments demonstrate that early chronic postinjury administration of LU 25-109 is effective in reducing cognitive deficits after TBI. Additionally, the drug does not need to be pharmacologically active at the time of cognitive testing.

To examine the relationship between chronic drug treatment and an index of cholinergic function, choline acetyltransferase (ChAT) immunoreactivity in the basal forebrain was examined in rats administered 15 μmol/kg LU 25-109 on post-injury days 1–15 (Pike et al., 1997). In the analysis of ChAT immunoreactivity, TBI caused a significant reduction in the number of ChAT-positive neurons in basal forebrain nuclei on day 15 postinjury. Chronic treatment with 15 μmol/kg LU 25-109 attenuated the injury-induced reductions in ChAT-positive neurons. Thus, the LU 25-109 treatment that was cognitively enhancing also normalized a neurochemical index of cholinergic function.

Gamma-aminobutyric Acid System

Much brain injury research has concentrated on the contribution of excitatory neurotransmitter systems such as ACh and N-methyl-D-aspartate (NMDA) to trauma-induced pathophysiology. However, recent behavioral and anatomical evidence indicates that the gamma-aminobutyric acid (GABA) system also plays a significant role in the mechanisms of neuronal injury (Schwartz et al., 1994).

Pentylenetetrazol. Hamm et al. (1995) investigated the influence of posttraumatic seizures on cognitive outcome. Pentylenetetrazol (PTZ), a $GABA_A$ receptor antagonist, was used to kindle rats chemically. Beginning 24 hours after central fluid percussion injury, injured (and sham-injured) rats were injected (i.p.) once daily with either saline or 25 mg/kg PTZ on days 1–24 postinjury. In both the injured and sham-injured groups, daily administration of PTZ resulted in an increase in behavioral seizure severity over days 1–24.

On days 25–29 postinjury, cognitive function was assessed using the MWM. Analysis of maze performance indicated that PTZ had a deleterious effect on sham-injured rats. In contrast, PTZ enhanced cognitive performance of injured rats. These results indicate that posttraumatic kindled seizures do not increase behavioral impairment. Chronic postinjury antagonism of an inhibitory neurotransmitter system can improve the cognitive outcome. This finding is consistent with the biphasic hypothesis indicating that blocking an inhibitory neurotransmitter system during the chronic phase results in a net excitatory effect, possibly normalizing neuronal activity.

MDL 26,479 (Suritozole). O'Dell and Hamm (1995) examined the indirect enhancement of cholinergic function via suppression of GABA activity on postinjury cognitive performance. The $GABA_A$ inverse agonist MDL 26,479 was tested. This experiment tested both early and delayed postinjury dosing protocols of MDL 26,479 following central fluid percussion injury or sham injury. In the delayed dosing procedure, animals received (i.p.) either vehicle, 5 mg/kg, or 10 mg/kg MDL 26,479 on days 11–15 postinjury. In the early dosing procedure, animals received either vehicle, 5 mg/kg, or 10 mg/kg MDL 26,479 on days 1–15 postinjury. Results indicated that both doses of MDL 26,479 were effective in reducing cognitive impairment following injury. However, improved MWM performance was observed only with the early dosing procedure. If drug treatment was delayed until days 11–15 after injury, no beneficial effects of MDL 26,479 were observed.

These results suggest that indirect enhancement of cholinergic function by negative modulation of the $GABA_A$ receptor during the chronic phase of TBI is also an effective strategy to attenuate TBI-induced cognitive deficits. In addition, this study provides additional evidence of the importance of timing a chronic posttraumatic intervention.

Glutamatergic System

D-Cycloserine. The NMDA receptor system is a major contributor not only to learning and memory function (Morris et al., 1986) but also to the pathophysiological mechanisms of TBI (Faden et al., 1989; Hamm et al., 1993; Katayama et al., 1990; Miller et al., 1991). Most of what is documented about the role of NMDA in TBI involves acute postinjury mechanisms (McIntosh, 1993). In contrast, little is known about NMDA involvement in the chronic phase of TBI.

Temple and Hamm (1996) evaluated the NMDA receptor's contribution to chronic cognitive dysfunction. Specifically, chronic postinjury administration of D-cycloserine (DCS), an NMDA partial agonist, was evaluated to determine its effects on cognitive performance. D-cycloserine modulates the glycine site associated with the NMDA receptor (Hood et al., 1989; Johnson & Ascher, 1987). It has been well documented to produce cognitive enhancement in multiple models of memory impairment, including aging, scopolamine challenge, and quinolinic acid lesions (Baxter et al., 1994; Fishkin et al., 1993; Schuster & Schmidt, 1992; Sirvio et al., 1992).

The effect of DCS was tested with the use of an early postinjury dosing procedure. After lateral fluid percussion injury or sham injury, rats received either vehicle, 10 mg/kg, or 30 mg/kg DCS (i.p.) on days 1–15 postinjury. Cognitive performance was assessed on days 11–15 postinjury using the MWM task; injections were given 30 minutes prior to testing. Results indicated that early chronic administration of 30 mg/kg of DCS was highly effective in reducing TBI-associated cognitive impairment. In fact, MWM performance of injured, DCS-treated (30 mg/kg) rats was not statistically different from sham-vehicle performance.

The effectiveness of a delayed post-TBI administration of DCS was also tested. In the delayed administration procedure, 30 mg/kg DCS was given on days 11–15 postinjury 30 minutes prior to assessment with the MWM. Results illustrated that DCS lost its cognitive-enhancing effects when administration was delayed for 10 days, a finding observed with chronic cholinergic therapies as well.

This study demonstrates that the NMDA receptor does contribute to chronic postinjury cognitive disruption. It also shows that therapies designed to chronically enhance NMDA receptor activity after injury are particularly effective in reducing TBI-induced deficits. Because this drug has been approved by the Food and Drug Administration (FDA) as an antibiotic, it may be a strong candidate for testing in clinical trials.

Nonselective Neurotransmitter Intervention

BMY-21502. Although the specific neurotransmitters affected by the nootropic drug BMY-21502 are not known, this drug has been shown to improve cognitive performance of rats. To determine whether BMY-21502 improved posttraumatic cognitive performance, Pierce and colleagues (1993) subjected rats to a lateral fluid percussion injury or a sham injury. Thirty minutes before MWM testing, on days

7–8 postinjury, animals were injected (s.c.) with either vehicle or BMY-21502 (10 mg/kg). Injured animals treated with BMY-21502 reached the goal platform with a shorter latency than injured vehicle-treated animals. Results also indicated that the drug treatment increased swimming speed of injured rats. This raises the possibility that the shorter goal latencies were the result of an increase in swim speed rather than a consequence of improved cognitive function. In addition, drug treatment had a tendency to impair the performance of uninjured animals.

Posttraumatic Neurotrophic Interventions

Endogenous trophic factors are typically increased following neurological insults and alter pathophysiological consequences of TBI (for a review, see Mattson & Scheff, 1994). Various trophic factors administered after CNS injury provide neuronal protection (Korsching, 1993; Maness et al., 1994).

Nerve Growth Factor

Sinson and colleagues (1995) investigated the chronic effects of nerve growth factor (NGF) infusion on cognitive deficits following lateral fluid percussion brain injury in rats. Prior to TBI, rats were trained on the MWM task. Twenty-four hours after injury, animals received intracerebral infusion (0.5 µl/h) of vehicle or NGF until 3, 7, or 14 days after injury, at which time animals were assessed for retrograde memory deficits on the MWM. Nerve growth factor infusion significantly attenuated cognitive deficits in injured animals at 7 and 14 days following injury. Following assessment, brains were fixed for Nissl staining with toluidine blue to examine hippocampal CA3 cell loss. However, no significant differences in cell loss were found between the NGF-treated and control groups. Also, Sinson et al. (1996) found that cognitive deficits after TBI were reduced with the combined treatment of NGF infusion and fetal tissue transplant.

Basic Fibroblast Growth Factor

McDermott et al. (1997) investigated the chronic posttraumatic effects of basic fibroblast growth factor (bFGF) infusion on histopathological damage and cognitive deficits following lateral fluid percussion brain injury. Rats were first trained in the MWM, then were prepared for and received lateral or sham fluid percussion injury. Twenty-four hours after injury, they received an intracerebral infusion of vehicle or bFGF (2 g) in vehicle for 7 days. On day 8, rats were assessed for memory of the MWM task and then were sacrificed. Their brains were fixed and stained with toluidine blue or glial fibrillary acidic protein (GFAP) antibody to evaluate CA3 hippocampal cell loss or gliosis, respectively. Treatment with bFGF was found to significantly reduced retrograde memory deficits in injured animals. Basic FGF did not significantly decrease CA3 cell loss. Immunohistochemical analysis revealed increased astrocytosis in the injured cortex of bFGF-treated animals compared to injured-vehicle animals.

Posttraumatic Environmental Interventions

Several studies utilizing different models of neurological damage, such as lesions, ischemia, and neurotoxins, illustrate the effectiveness of postinsult exposure to an enriched environment (EE) on recovery (Brenner et al., 1983; Johansson, 1996; Kolb & Gibb, 1991; Murtha et al., 1990; Rose et al., 1993). Since the chronic phase of TBI is characterized by suppression of neuronal signaling, increasing environmental complexity could enhance recovery from TBI. Hamm et al. (1996) studied the effect of EE on TBI-induced cognitive deficits.

Rats received a central fluid percussion injury or a sham injury. On regaining consciousness, they were either returned to the standard vivarium environment or placed in the EE for 15 days. Their cognitive performance was assessed on days 11–15 postinjury using the MWM task. Results indicated that exposure to the EE significantly enhanced recovery of postinjury cognitive deficits. This study illustrates the value of postinjury EE for cognitive performance.

The physiological mechanisms of EE on cognition have not been elucidated. However, trophic factors have been studied as a possible mechanism (Falkenberg et al., 1992; Mohammed et al., 1990). Falkenberg et al. found a significant increase in brain-derived neurotrophic factor (BDNF) mRNA following EE and MWM assessment. A current study in this laboratory examined the interaction between TBI and EE on BDNF at 2 and 15 days postinjury. Histopathological analysis revealed an interaction between EE and TBI on levels of BDNF in the hippocampus; levels of BDNF were increased in injured animals exposed to an EE (Buck et al., 1997).

Summary and Speculations

As discussed above, many different posttraumatic interventions have been found to improve cognitive performance after TBI. To facilitate the comparison of the relative effectiveness of the different manipulations, a *percent improvement* score was estimated for each intervention. The percent improvement measure was approximated by first calculating the difference between the performances of the injured-untreated and injured-treated groups (as a measure of the improvement produced by the treatment). Second, as an estimate of the total injury-induced deficit, the difference between the sham-injured and injured-untreated groups was calculated. The ratio of these two numbers was computed (i.e., treatment improvement / total deficit) and was expressed as a percentage. While the percent improvement score can be influenced by a number of factors (e.g., experiments not determining the maximally effective dose, differences in method and time of behavioral assessment, type and severity of injury), it provides at least a crude means of comparing

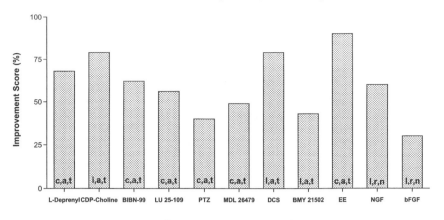

Post-traumatic Interventions

Figure 3–2. The improvement score was calculated as described in the text and was based on estimates from the published graphs. A score of 100% indicates that the treatment completely eliminated the injury-induced deficit (i.e., the injured-treated group's performance was equivalent to the uninjured group's performance). A score of 0% indicates that the treatment had no effect on the injury-induced deficits. Abbreviations: c, central fluid percussion injury; l, lateral fluid percussion injury; i, cortical impact; a, an anterograde amnesia paradigm was used; r, a retrograde amnesia paradigm was used; t, the behavioral measure of maze performance was based on the time needed to reach the goal platform; n, the behavioral measure was based on a "neuroscore," which is an indirect measure of the rat swimming near the goal platform.

the efficacy of the different interventions. Figure 3-2 presents the results of this calculation for each of the experimental interventions reviewed in this chapter. The improvements in cognitive performance range from 90% (EE) to 30% (bFGF).

It should also be noted that the vast majority of posttraumatic interventions were begun shortly after the injury (usually within 24 hours). Experiments examining the effect of delay in initiating treatment have found that postponing the start of treatment for several days after TBI turns an effective treatment into an ineffective one (O'Dell & Hamm, 1995; Pike & Hamm, 1995, 1997; Temple & Hamm, 1996). Similarly, in the case of L-deprenyl, treatment was given on days 1–7 after TBI and then terminated. The L-deprenyl-treated group demonstrated improved performance when tested 4 days after the termination of drug treatment. Treatment with LU 25-109 was also found to improve maze performance when it was administered 4 hours after maze testing. These findings strongly suggest that the effectiveness of neurotransmitter-based pharmacological interventions is not simply the result of receptor activation at the time of behavioral testing. Posttraumatic neurotransmitter-based interventions must be operating through some other mechanism. In the case of the cholinergic drug LU 25-109, treatment reduces the loss of ChAT-positive cells observed after TBI. Similarly, the partial NMDA agonist DCS appears to normalize NMDAR1 immunoreactivity after injury (unpublished data).

Thus, chronic posttraumatic neurotransmitter treatments that enhance behavioral performance also ameliorate (or normalize) aspects of altered receptor function after injury.

While each of the posttraumatic interventions has its own rationale for improving recovery after TBI (whether the modulation of a specific neurotransmitter system or a neurotrophic factor), there may be a common mechanism of action for all beneficial interventions. As discussed at the beginning of the chapter, the biphasic model of posttraumatic neuronal activity assumes that the chronic postinjury period is characterized by suppression of normal neuronal function. Thus, any therapy that enhances neuronal activity would be predicted to improve cognitive function after TBI. In the case of treatments that are neurotransmitter agonists, it is clear that these treatments increase neuronal activity. These treatments also result in the release of neurotrophic factors. For example, L-deprenyl has been shown to enhance NGF synthesis (Semkova et al., 1996). Similarly, excitatory neurotransmitter agonists (cholinergic and NMDA) and inhibitory (GABA) antagonists increase neurotrophic factors (Gwag et al., 1993; Hughes et al., 1993; Metsis et al., 1993; Zafra et al., 1990). Exposure to an EE has also been shown to increase both neurotransmitter and neurotrophic activity (Falkenberg et al., 1992). In the case of neurotrophic treatment, neurotrophins result in the release of neurotransmitters. For example, BDNF treatment increases serotonin, dopamine, and/or norepinephrine, as well as ChAT activity and NMDA release (Alderson et al., 1990; Siuciak et al., 1996; Takei et al., 1997). Thus, treatments based on neurotransmitter modulation or neurotrophic factors activate a biochemical cascade that share many features. At this initial stage of research in posttraumatic interventions, it is not clear what mechanism(s) are responsible for the improved cognitive outcome. The most likely global conclusions are that the interventions stimulate neuronal repair mechanisms and/or optimize the performance of the surviving neuronal systems. Obviously, additional research will be required to explicate the biochemical processes involved in the recovery of cognitive function following TBI.

Implications for Rehabilitation of Human Head Injury

Although experimental research on posttraumatic interventions is quite limited, the data do support several tentative conclusions that are relevant to rehabilitation of human head injury. First, animal model research clearly indicates that initiating therapy as soon as possible after the injury will increase the probability that the treatment will be effective. Second, the results of the EE experiment strengthen the argument for placing patients in an invigorating and active rehabilitation program after injury. The experimental work has also identified several promising pharmacological treatments for head injury. D-Cycloserine, an FDA-approved antibiotic, produced a large improvement in the cognitive performance of rats after experimental TBI. It is an attractive candidate for clinical testing for improving the cognitive outcome in patients. Cytidine-5'-diphosphate choline and L-deprenyl are also reasonable candidates for clinical testing. Levin (1996) found that a small sample of head-injured patients had a beneficial response to treatment with CDP-choline. L-deprenyl has produced clinical benefits in patients with neurodegenerative conditions (Brannan & Yahr, 1995; Martignoni et al., 1991). Administration of neurotrophic factors is also a possible treatment for head injury. However, neurotrophic factors do not normally cross the blood-brain barrier. Consequently, they must be centrally administered, which makes the clinical delivery of these drugs more problematic. In any case, the positive results obtained thus far provide hope that further progress will be made in developing interventions that can be used to treat posttraumatic cognitive impairment effectively.

ACKNOWLEDGMENTS
We would like to acknowledge the support of NIH Grant NS12857. We also would like to acknowledge the valuable contributions of Dianne O'Dell, Bruce Lyeth, Brian Pike, Linda Phillips, Thomas Reeves, and Jiepei Zhu.

References

Alderson, R.F., Alterman, A.L., Barde, Y.-A., and Lindsay, R.M. (1990) Brain-derived neurotrophic factor increases survival and differentiated functions of rat septal cholinergic neurons in culture. *Neuron,* 5:297–306.

Bartus, R.T., Dean, R.L., Pontecorvo, M.J., and Flicket, C. (1986) The cholinergic hypothesis: A historical overview, current perspective, and future directions. *Annals of the New York Academy of Sciences,* 444:332–358.

Baxter, M.G., Lanthorn, T.H., Frick, K.M., Golski, S., Wan, R.-Q., and Olton, D.S. (1994) D-Cycloserine, a novel cognitive enhancer, improves spatial memory in aged rats. *Neurobiology of Aging,* 15:207–213.

Becker, R.E., and Giacobini, E. (1988) Mechanisms of cholinesterase inhibition in senile dementia of the Alzheimer's type: Clinical, pharmacological, and therapeutic aspects. *Drug Development Research,* 12:163–195.

Brannan, T., and Yahr, M.D. (1995) Comparative study of selegiline plus L-dopa-carbidopa versus L-dopa-carbidopa alone in the treatment of Parkinson's disease. *Annals of Neurology,* 37:95–98.

Brenner, E., Mirmiran, M., Uylings, H.B.M., and Van der Gugten, J. (1983) Impaired growth of cerebral cortex of rats treated neonatally with 6-hydroxydopamine under different environmental conditions. *Neuroscience Letters,* 42:13–17.

Brooks, N., McKinlay, W., Simington, C., Beattie, A., and Campsie, L. (1987) Return to work within the first seven years of severe head injury. *Brain Injury,* 1:5–19.

Buck, D.L., Hamm, R.J., Zhu, J.P., Phillips, L.L., Giebel, M.L., and Floyd, C.L. (1997) Changes in brain-derived neurotrophic factor immunoreactivity in the hippocampus after 2 and 15 days of enriched environment following traumatic brain injury. *Journal of Neurotrauma,* 14:802.

Dixon, C.E., Bao, J., Bergmann, J.S., and Johnson, K.M. (1994a) Traumatic brain injury reduces hippocampal high-affinity [^{3}H]choline uptake but not extracellular choline levels in rats. *Neuroscience Letters,* 180:127–130.

Dixon, C.E., Bao, J., Liu, S., Johnson, K., and Hayes, R.L. (1994b) Cortical impact produces chronic cholinergic deficits that are associated with reduced ACh release and can be attenuated behaviorally by CDP-choline. *Journal of Neurotrauma,* 11:107 (abstract).

Dixon, C.E., Bao, J., Long, D.A., and Hayes, R.L. (1996) Reduced evoked release of acetyl-choline in the rodent hippocampus following traumatic brain injury. *Pharmacology, Biochemistry, and Behavior,* 53:679–686.

Dixon, C.E., Hamm, R.J., Clifton, G.L., and Hayes, R.L. (1994c) Increased anticholinergic sensitivity following closed skull impact and controlled cortical impact traumatic brain injury in the rat. *Journal of Neurotrauma,* 11:275–287.

Dixon, C.E., Liu, S.J., Jenkins, L.W., Bhattachargee, M., Whitson, J.S., Yang, K., and Hayes, R.L. (1995) Time course of increased vulnerability of cholinergic neurotrans-mission following traumatic brain injury in the rat. *Behavioural Brain Research,* 70: 125–131.

Dixon, C.E., Ma, X., and Marion, D.W. (1997) Effects of CDP-choline treatment on neuro-behavioral deficits after TBI and on hippocampal and neocortical acetylcholine release. *Journal of Neurotrauma,* 14:159–166.

Doods, H.N. (1995) Lipophilic muscarinic M_2 antagonists as potential drugs for cognitive disorders. *Drugs of the Future,* 20:157–164.

Enz, A., Amstutz, R., Boddeke, H., Gmelin, G., and Malanowski, J. (1993) Brain selective inhibition of acetylcholinesterase: A novel approach to therapy for Alzheimer's disease. *Progress in Brain Research,* 98:431–438.

Faden, A.I., Demediuk, P., Panter, S.S., and Vink, R. (1989) The role of excitatory amino acids and NMDA receptors in traumatic brain injury. *Science,* 244:798–800.

Falkenberg, T., Mohammed, A.K., Henriksson, B., Persson, H., Winblad, B., and Linde-fors, N. (1992) Increased expression of brain-derived neurotrophic factor mRNA in rat hippocampus is associated with improved spatial memory and enriched environment. *Neuroscience Letters,* 138:153–156.

Feeney, D.M. (1991) Pharmacologic modulation of recovery after brain injury: A recon-sideration of diaschisis. *Journal of Neurologic Rehabilitation,* 5:113–128.

Feeney, D.M., Gonzalez, A., and Law, W.A. (1982) Amphetamine, haloperidol and ex-perience interact to affect rate of recovery after motor cortex injury. *Science,* 217: 855–857.

Feeney, D.M., and Sutton, R.L. (1987) Pharmacotherapy for recovery of function after brain injury. *CRC Critical Review Neurobiology,* 3:135–197.

Finnegan, K.T., Skrattt, J.S., Irwin, I., DeLanney, L.E., and Langston, J.W. (1990) Protec-tion against DSP-4-induced neurotoxicity by deprenyl is not related to its inhibition of MAO-B. *European Journal of Pharmacology,* 184:119–126.

Fishkin, R.J., Ince, E.S., Carlezon, W.A., Jr., and Dunn, R.W. (1993) D-Cycloserine atten-uates scopolamine-induced learning and memory deficits in rats. *Behavioral and Neural Biology,* 59:150–157.

Frankowski, R.F. (1986) Descriptive epidemiologic studies of head injury in the United States 1974–1984. *Advances in Psychometrics and Medicine,* 16:153.

Gennarelli, T.A., Champion, H.R., Copes, W.S., and Sacco, W.J. (1994) Comparison of mortality, morbidity, and severity of 59,713 head injured patients with 114,447 patients with extracranial injuries. *Journal of Trauma,* 37:962–968.

Gorman, L.K., Fu, K., Hovda, D.A., Becker, D.P., and Katayama, Y. (1989) Analysis of acetylcholine release following concussive brain injury in the rate. *Journal of Neuro-trauma,* 6:203.

Grady, M.S., Leonard, J., and Maris, D.O. (1992) Lateral fluid percussion brain injury causes cholinergic forebrain neuron death. *Society for Neuroscience Abstracts,* 18:172.

Gronwall, E., and Wrightson, P. (1974) Delayed recovery of intellectual function after mi-nor head injury. *Lancet,* 2:605–609.

Gwag, B.J., Sessler, F.M., Waterhouse, B.D., and Springer, J.E. (1993) Regulation of NGF and mRNA in the hippocampal formation: Effects of N-methyl-D-aspartate receptor activation. *Experimental Neurology,* 121:160–171.

Hamm, R.J., O'Dell, D.M., Pike, B.R., and Lyeth, B.G. (1993) Cognitive impairment following traumatic brain injury: The effect of pre- and post-injury administration of scopolamine and MK-801. *Cognitive Brain Research,* 1:223–226.

Hamm, R.J., Pike, B.R., O'Dell, D.M., and Lyeth, B.G. (1994) Traumatic brain injury enhances the amnesic effect of NMDA antagonist. *Journal of Neurosurgery,* 81:267–271.

Hamm, R.J., Pike, B.R., Temple, M.D., O'Dell, D.M., and Lyeth, B.G. (1995) The effect of postinjury kindled seizures on cognitive performance of traumatically brain-injured rats. *Experimental Neurology,* 136:143–148.

Hamm, R.J., Temple, M.D., O'Dell, D.M., Pike, B.R., and Lyeth, B.G. (1996) Exposure to environmental complexity promotes recovery of cognitive function after traumatic brain injury. *Journal of Neurotrauma,* 13:41–47.

Hayes, R.L., Jenkins, L.W., and Lyeth, B.G. (1992) Neurotransmitter-mediated mechanisms of traumatic brain injury: Acetylcholine and excitatory amino acids. *Journal of Neurotrauma,* 9:S173–S187.

Hood, W.F., Compton, R.P., and Monahan, J.B. (1989) D-Cycloserine: A ligand for the N-methyl-D-aspartate coupled glycine receptor has partial agonist characteristics. *Neuroscience Letters,* 98:91–95.

Hoss, W., Messer, W.S., Monsma, F.J., Miller, M.D., Ellerborck, B.R., Scranton, T., Ghodsi-Hovsepian, S., Price, M.A., Balan, S., Mazloum, Z., and Bohmett, M. (1990) Biochemical and behavioral evidence for muscarinic autoreceptors in the CNS. *Brain Research,* 517:195–201.

Hughes, P., Beilharz, E., Gluckman, P., and Dragunow, M. (1993) Brain-derived neurotrophic factor is induced as an immediate early gene following N-methyl-D-aspartate receptor activation. *Neuroscience,* 57:319–328.

Johansson, B.B. (1996) Functional outcome in rats transferred to an enriched environment 15 days after focal brain ischemia. *Stroke,* 27:324–326.

Johnson, J.W., and Ascher, P. (1987) Glycine potentiates the NMDA response in the cultured mouse brain neurons. *Nature,* 325:529–531.

Katayama, Y., Becker, D.P., Tamura, T., and Hovda, D.A. (1990) Massive increases in extracellular potassium and the indiscriminate release of glutamate following concussive brain injury. *Journal of Neurosurgery,* 73:889–900.

Knapp, M.J., Knopman, D.S., Solomon, P.R., Pendlebury, W.W., Davis, C.S., and Gracon, S.I. (1994) A 30-week randomized controlled trial of high-dose Tacrine in patients with Alzheimer's disease. *Journal of the American Medical Association,* 271:985–991.

Kolb, B., and Gibb, R. (1991) Environmental enrichment and cortical injury: Behavioral and anatomical consequences of frontal cortex lesions. *Cerebral Cortex,* 1:189–198.

Korsching, S. (1993) The neurotrophic factor concept: A reexamination. *Journal of Neuroscience,* 13:2739–2748.

Kraus, J.F. (1987) Epidemiology of head injury. In P.R. Cooper (ed.), *Head Injury.* New York: Williams & Wilkins, pp. 1–19.

Lapchak, P.A., Araujo, D.M., Quirion, R., and Collier, B. (1989) Binding sites for [^{3}H]AF-DX 116 and effect of AF-DX 116 on endogenous acetylcholine release from rat brain slices. *Brain Research,* 496:285–294.

Leonard, J.R., Maris, D.O., and Grady, M.S. (1994) Fluid percussion injury causes loss of forebrain choline acetyltransferase and nerve growth factor receptor immunoreactive cells in the rat. *Journal of Neurotrauma,* 11:379–392.

Levin, H.S. (1992) Neurobehavioral recovery. *Journal of Neurotrauma,* 9(1):S359–S373.

Levin, H.S. (1996) Treatment of postconcussional symptoms with CDP-choline. *Journal of the Neurological Sciences,* 103:S39–S42.

Levin, H.S., and Goldstein, F.C. (1986) Organization of verbal memory after severe closed head injury. *Journal of Clinical and Experimental Neuropsychology,* 8:643–656.

Lyeth, B.G., Ray, M., Hamm, R.J., Schnabel, J., Saady, J.J., Poklis, A., Jenkins, L.W., Gudeman, S.K., and Hayes, R.L. (1992) Postinjury scopolamine administration in experimental traumatic brain injury. *Brain Research,* 569:281–286.

Maness, L.M., Kastin, A.J., Weber J.T., Banks, W.A., Beckman, B.S., and Zadina, J.E. (1994) The neurotrophins and their receptor: Structure, function, and neuropathology. *Neuroscience and Biobehavioral Reviews,* 18:143–159.

Martignoni, E., Bono, G., Blandini, F., Sinforiani, E., Merlo, P., and Nappi, G. (1991) Monoamines and related metabolite levels in the cerebrospinal fluid of patients with dementia of Alzheimer type: Influence of treatment with L-deprenyl. *Journal of Neural Transmission [PD Sect.],* 3:15–26.

Mattson, M.P., and Scheff, S.W. (1994) Endogenous neuroprotection factors and traumatic brain injury: Mechanisms of action and implications for therapy. *Journal of Neurotrauma,* 11:3–33.

McDermott, K.L., Raghupathi, R., Fernandez, S.C., Saatman, K.E., Protter, A.A., Finklestein, S.P., Smith, D.H., and McIntosh, T.K. (1997) Delayed administration of basic fibroblast growth factor attenuates cognitive dysfunction following parasagittal fluid percussion brain injury in the rat. *Journal of Neurotrauma,* 14:191–200.

McIntosh, T.K. (1993) Novel pharmacologic therapies in the treatment of experimental traumatic brain injury: A review. *Journal of Neurotrauma,* 10:215–261.

McIntosh, T.K. (1994) Neurochemical sequelae of traumatic brain injury: Therapeutic implications. *Cerebrovascular and Brain Metabolism Reviews,* 6:109–162.

Meier, E., Arnt, J., Frederidsen, K., Lembol, H.L., Sanchez, C., Skarsfeldt, T., Dragsted, N., Pederson, H., and Hyttel, H. (1995) Pharmacological characterization of LU 25-109-T, a compound with M_1-agonistic and M_2/M_3-antagonistic effects on muscarinic receptors. *Life Sciences,* 56:1006.

Metsis, M., Timmusk, T., Arenas, E., and Persson, H. (1993) Differential usage of multiple brain-derived neurotrophic factor promoters in the rat brain following neuronal activation. *Proceedings of the National Academy of Science of the USA,* 90:8802–8806.

Miller, L.P., Lyeth, B.G., Jenkins, L.W., Oleniak, L., Panchision, D., Hamm, R.J., Phillips, L.L., Dixon, C.E., Clifton, G.L., and Hayes, R.L. (1991) Excitatory amino acid receptor subtype binding following traumatic brain injury in the rat. *Brain Research,* 526:103–107.

Mohammed, A.K., Winblad, B., Ebendal., T., and Larkfors, L. (1990) Environmental influence on behavior and nerve growth factor in the brain. *Brain Research,* 528:62–72.

Moltzen, E.K., and Bjornholm, B. (1995) Medicinal chemistry of muscarinic agonists: Development since 1990. *Drugs of the Future,* 20:37–54.

Morris, R.G.M., Anderson, E., Lynch, G.S., and Baudry, M. (1986) Selective impairment of learning and blockade of long-term potentiation by an *N*-methyl-D-aspartate receptor antagonist, AP5. *Nature,* 319:774–776.

Murtha, S., Pappas, B.A., and Raman, S. (1990) Neonatal and adult forebrain norepinephrine depletion and the behavioral and cortical thickening effects of enriched/impoverished environment. *Behavioral Brain Research,* 39:249–261.

Oddy, M., Coughlan, T., Tyerman, A., and Jenkins, D. (1985) Social adjustment after closed head injury: A further follow-up seven years after injury. *Journal of Neurology, Neurosurgery, and Psychiatry,* 48:564–568.

O'Dell, D.M., and Hamm, R.J. (1995) Chronic postinjury administration of MDL 26,479 (Suritozole), a negative modulator at the $GABA_A$ receptor, and cognitive impairment in rats following traumatic brain injury. *Journal of Neurosurgery,* 83:878–883.

Pierce, J.E.S., Smith, D.H., Eison, M.S., and McIntosh, T.K. (1993) The nootropic compound BMY-21502 improves spatial learning ability in injured rats. *Brain Research,* 624: 199–208.

Pike, B.R., and Hamm, R.J. (1995) Post-injury administration of BIBN 99, a selective muscarinic M_2 receptor antagonist, improves cognitive performance following traumatic brain injury in rats. *Brain Research,* 686:37–43.

Pike, B.R., and Hamm, R.J. (1997a) Chronic administration of a partial muscarinic M_1 receptor agonist attenuates decreases in forebrain choline acetyltransferase immunoreactivity following experimental brain trauma. *Experimental Neurology,* 147:55–65.

Pike, B.R., and Hamm, R.J. (1997b) Activating the post-traumatic cholinergic system for the treatment of cognitive impairment following traumatic brain injury. *Pharmacology, Biochemistry and Behavior,* 57:785–791.

Pike, B.R., Hamm, R.J., Temple, M.D., Buck, D. L., and Lyeth, B.G. (1997) Effect of tetrahydroaminoacridine, a cholinesterase inhibitor, on cognitive performance following experimental brain injury. *Journal of Neurotrauma,* 14:897–905.

Potter, L.T., Flynn, D.D., Hanchett, H.E., Kalinoski, D.L., Luber-Narod, J., and Mash, D.C. (1984) Independent M_1 and M_2 receptors: Ligands, autoradiography and functions. *Trends in Pharmacological Science,* 5:22–31.

Richard, J.W., Wilson, A., and Quirion, R. (1991) Muscarinic M_2 negative autoreceptors regulate acetylcholine release in cortex and hippocampus: A microdialysis study in freely moving rats. *Society for Neuroscience Abstracts,* 17:781.

Richards, M.H. (1990) Rat hippocampal muscarinic autoreceptors are similar to the M_2 (cardiac) subtype: Comparison with hippocampal M_1, atrial M_2, and ileal M_3 receptors. *British Journal of Pharmacology,* 99:753–761.

Rose, F.D., Al-Khamees, K., Davey, M.J., and Attree, E.A. (1993) Environmental enrichment following brain damage: An aid to recovery or compensation? *Behavioural Brain Research,* 5:93–100.

Sarter, M., Bruno, J.P., and Dudchenko, P. (1990) Activating the damaged basal forebrain cholinergic system: Tonic stimulation versus signal amplification. *Psychopharmacology,* 101:1–17.

Schmidt, R.H., and Grady, M.S. (1995) Loss of forebrain cholinergic neurons following fluid-percussion injury: Implications for cognitive impairment in closed head injury. *Journal of Neurosurgery,* 83:496–502.

Schuster, G.M., and Schmidt, W.J. (1992) D-Cycloserine reverses the working memory impairment of hippocampal-lesioned rats in a spatial learning task. *European Journal of Pharmacology,* 224:97–98.

Schwartz, R.D., Huff, R.A., Xiao, Y., Carter, M.L., and Bishop, M. (1994) Postischemic diazepam is neuroprotective in the gerbil hippocampus. *Brain Research,* 647:153–160.

Semkova, I., Wolz, P., Schilling, M., and Krieglestein, J. (1996) Selegiline enhances NGF synthesis and protects central nervous system neurons from excitotoxic and ischemic damage. *European Journal of Pharmacology,* 315:19–30.

Sinson, G., Voddi, M., and McIntosh, T.K. (1995) Nerve growth factor administration attenuates cognitive but not neurobehavioral motor dysfunction or hippocampal cell loss following fluid-percussion brain injury in rats. *Journal of Neurochemistry,* 65:2209–2216.

Sinson, G., Voddi, M., and McIntosh, T.K. (1996) Combined fetal neural transplantation and nerve growth factor infusion: Effects on neurological outcome following fluid-percussion brain injury in the rat. *Journal of Neurosurgery,* 84:655–662.

Sirvio, J., Ekonsalo, T., Riekkinen, P., Jr., Lahtinen, H., and Riekkinen, P., Sr. (1992) D-Cycloserine, a modulator of the *N*-methyl-D-aspartate receptor, improves spatial learning in rats treated with muscarinic antagonist. *Neuroscience Letters,* 146:215–218.

Siuciak, J.A., Boylan, C., Fritsche, M., Altar, C.A., and Linsay, R.M. (1996) BDNF increases monoaminergic activity in rat brain following intracerebroventricular or intra-parenchymal administration. *Brain Research,* 710:11–20.

Takei, N., Sasaoka, K., Inoue, K., Takahshi, M., Endo, Y., and Hatanaka, H. (1997) Brain-derived neurotrophic factor increases the stimulation-evoked release of glutamate and the levels of exocytosis-associated proteins in cultured cortical neurons from embryonic rats. *Journal of Neurochemistry,* 68:370–375.

Temple, M.D., and Hamm, R.J. (1996) Chronic, post-injury administration of D-cycloserine, an NMDA partial agonist, enhances cognitive performance following experimental brain injury.*Brain Research,* 741:246–251.

van Zomeren, A.H., and van den Burg, W. (1985) Residual complaints of patients two years after severe head injury. *Journal of Neurology, Neurosurgery and Psychiatry,* 48:21–28.

von Monakow, C. (1969) Diaschisis, the localization in the cerebrum and functional impairment by cortical loci. In K. Pribram (ed.), *Brain and Behavior: Moods, States, and Mind,* Vol. 1 (trans. G. Harris). Baltimore: Penguin Books, pp. 27–36.

Yavich, L., Sirvio, J., Haapalinna, A., Puumala, T., Koivisto, E., Heinonen, E., and Riekkinen, P.J. (1996) The systemic administration of Tacrine or selegiline facilitate spatial learning in aged fisher 344 rats. *Journal of Neural Transmission,* 103:619–626.

Yoshino, A., Hovda, D.A., Kawamata, T., Katayama, Y., and Becker, D.P. (1991) Dynamic changes in local cerebral glucose utilization following cerebral concussion in rats: Evidence of hyper- and subsequent hypometabolic state. *Brain Research,* 561:106–119.

Zafra, F., Hengerer, B., Leibrock, J., Thoenen, H., and Lindhol, D. (1990) Activity dependent regulation of BDNF- and NGF-mRNAs in the rat hippocampus is mediated by non-NMDA glutamate receptors. *EMBO Journal,* 9:3545–3550.

4

Growth of New Connections and Adult Reorganizational Plasticity in the Somatosensory System

EDWARD R. ERGENZINGER AND TIM P. PONS

Over the past 15 years, the capacity of adult sensory systems to reorganize in response to injury has been unequivocally demonstrated (Pons et al., 1991; see Kaas, 1991, 1995 for reviews). Studies of the plasticity of sensory maps in the central nervous system have shown that adult sensory systems are dynamic and mutable, a discovery that has altered the static and hardwired view of the adult brain held by a generation of neuroscientists. That view was not unfounded and in fact was suggested by the classic demonstration of a critical period for plasticity early in visual development (Hubel & Wiesel, 1970). The realization that adult sensory systems retain a remarkable capacity for change, however, has raised the exciting possibility that research into the mechanisms underlying this plasticity may provide neuroscientists with tools to enhance the limited behavioral and perceptual recovery that can occur following damage to central representations or their afferent inputs.

In studies of adult reorganizational plasticity, the somatosensory system remains the model sensory system because of the great degree of specificity that can be achieved by removing afferent input to the thalamus or cortex from a discrete region of the body surface via manipulation of peripheral nerves or dorsal roots. Not only is it possible to look at the effects of peripheral nerve manipulations such as nerve cuts or nerve crushes on somatotopic maps, but there is the added advantage of being able to observe the effects of peripheral nerve regeneration on central maps.

Within the somatosensory system, the precise mechanisms through which adult reorganizational plasticity occurs are not fully understood. Although some changes have been observed acutely following experimental manipulation and indicate an unmasking of silent synapses (Merzenich et al., 1983a, 1983b), more extensive reorganizational changes appear to occur chronically and may require the growth or sprouting of new connections (Pons et al., 1991). Despite the fact that some cases of reorganization cannot be explained in terms of the normal connectivity of the system (Ergenzinger et al., 1996; Florence et al., 1998); direct anatomical evidence for such growth generally has been lacking. Recent investigations in our laboratory and others have begun to examine indirect measures of structural plasticity such as levels of growth-associated protein (GAP-43) in an attempt to determine whether growth of new connections in the adult somatosensory system is associated with reorganizational change (Dunn-Meynell et al., 1992; Glasier et al., 1997; Levin & Dunn-Meynell, 1993). Future studies in this area may even focus on the possibility that neurotrophic factors may be involved in adult somatosensory plasticity, as some researchers have proposed (Conti et al., 1996; Kaas, 1995) and initial studies suggest (Rocamora et al., 1996). In addition, nonneuronal cells such as astrocytes may provide a permissive environment for growth of new connections or may actively promote growth through the release of neurotrophic factors (Conti et al., 1996).

Plasticity in the Somatosensory System

Reorganizational changes in somatosensory cortex have been demonstrated following peripheral nerve damage (Merzenich et al., 1983a, 1983b; Wall & Cusick, 1984, 1986; Pons et al., 1991; Cusick et al., 1990; Garraghty & Kaas, 1991; Garraghty et al., 1991); central Dykes, 1990; Dykes et al., 1984), and peripheral (Calford & Tweedale, 1991a) chemical effects; select cortical ablations Pons et al., 1988; Webster et al., 1991); specific behavioral training (Jenkens et al., 1990; Recanzone et al., 1992a, 1992b); and amputations (Calford & Tweedale, 1988, 1991b; Kelahan & Doetsch, 1984; Merzenich et al., 1984; Rasmusson, 1982; Turnbull & Rasmusson, 1991). Due to the variety of experimental manipulations utilized it is not surprising that both the type and the extent of reorganizational changes observed have also varied. Differences in experimental manipulation may give rise to alternative mechanisms of reorganizational change, making direct comparison of results across studies problematic.

Initial studies of plasticity following peripheral nerve section (Merzenich et al., 1983a, 1983b) indicated that the amount of cortex that could be reactivated was on the order of 1–2 mm^2 and that this distance was the upper limit of reorganization after manipulation of peripheral nerves. However, reorganization over 5 mm or more of cortex has been observed in SII following ablations of the hand representation in SI cortex (Pons et al., 1988). In addition, Pons et al. (1991) showed that at least 1.5 cm^2 of cortical area had reorganized following a manipulation that deprived the entire upper limb representation in SI of its normal input. This was a reorganization across one-third of SI, which effectively increased the original upper limit of cortical reorganization by an order of magnitude. However, the source of the differential effects observed between these studies was obscured by the fact that several variables were not held constant, namely, (*1*) the size or extent of the denervation (a portion of the hand vs. the entire hand vs. the entire upper limb); (*2*) the site of the manipulation (peripheral vs. central); (*3*) the site where reorganizational changes were assessed (SI vs. SII); and (*4*) the time course of the reorganizational change (weeks to months in the former studies vs. years in the latter study). Such variables need to be addressed before a full understanding of the capacity of somatosensory cortical changes can be achieved.

Reorganization at the subcortical level has been more difficult to characterize since these areas are smaller than cortical representations and because changes in maps are thus harder to determine. There have been reports of limited reorganization in the dorsal spinal cord after peripheral nerve injury, but these changes are such that new receptive fields were very close in size to the original receptive fields (Snow & Wilson, 1991). At the level of the dorsal column nuclei, somatotopic reorganization has been reported after cutting of the dorsal roots before they enter the spinal cord (Dostrovsky et al., 1976). More recently, rapid reorganization (within minutes to hours) has been demonstrated in the cuneate nucleus (CN) after section of the median and ulnar nerves in primates (Xu & Wall, 1997). This procedure deprives CN of input from the glabrous portion of the hand, which normally comprises the majority of the hand representation in CN. Surprisingly, following median and ulnar nerve section, a majority of the hand representation in CN becomes responsive to stimulation of the hairy hand (72%–86%), with the rest of what would be the normal hand representation remaining unresponsive (Xu & Wall, 1997).

Thalamic plasticity has been observed in rats (Wall & Egger, 1971) and monkeys (Pollin & Albe-Fessard, 1979), in which expansions of the forelimb representation occurred following ablation of the gracile nucleus. However, these changes were too small and sparse to be widely accepted at the time they were reported (Kaas, 1995). Recent evidence from monkeys in which the median and ulnar nerves had been severed, essentially removing input from all parts of the glabrous hand, indicates that the representation of the hand in the thalamus becomes completely activated by hairy hand stimulation (Garraghty and Kaas, 1991). In addition, the large-scale expansion of the face representation into the deprived upper limb representation in cortex reported by Pons et al. (1991) has also been observed at the level of the thalamus (Jones & Pons, 1998). These findings indicate that substantial reorganizational change can occur at the level of the thalamus.

Mechanisms Mediating Reorganization

Two mechanisms have been suggested to explain the reorganizational changes described above: (*1*) the unmasking of previously existing connections and (*2*) the growth of new connections via collateral sprouting (Kaas, 1991, 1995). Because of the rapid reorganization that has been observed for a small amount of cortex in SI following peripheral nerve section, and because single thalamocortical axon arbors can cover the 1 to 2 mm of cortical area that is reorganized in some cases (Garraghty et al., 1989), the unmasking of previously existing inputs has been used to explain some of the reorganizations. In addition, since median nerve section reduces gamma-aminobutyric acid (GABA) levels in deprived cortex of monkeys

(Garraghty, et al., 1991), this indicates that some afferents that are normally laterally inhibited may become disinhibited following nerve section.

On the other hand, the massive reorganization observed by Pons et al. (1991) cannot be explained by the unmasking of previously existing thalamocortical afferent inputs (Ergenzinger et al., 1996; Florence et al., 1998). Such large scale changes seem to occur via reorganization at earlier processing stations since the large-scale expansion of the face representation into the deprived upper limb representation also occurs in the thalamus (Jones & Pons, 1998). Such large-scale reorganizations may point to the possibility of growth or sprouting of new connections as a part of a slow phase of reorganizational plasticity. A relatively small degree of axonal sprouting at the level of the thalamus would translate into a much larger reorganization at the level of the cortex (Kaas, 1995). Most likely for the large-scale reorganizations that have been observed, a combination of initial unmasking and growth of new connections may underlie these plastic changes.

Evidence of Growth of New Connections in Reorganization of Somatosensory Maps

Few studies have shown direct anatomical evidence of the growth of new connections following manipulations that are known to produce reorganizational changes in adult animals. Most studies that have provided such evidence have focused exclusively on the terminations of peripheral nerves in the spinal cord. In rats, section of peripheral nerves or dorsal roots produces an expansion of adjacent peripheral nerve terminals into the territory formerly occupied by the sectioned nerves (Molander et al., 1988; Woolf et al., 1992). In monkeys, nerve crush has also been shown to produce growth in the spinal cord such that the regenerating fibers overlap more extensively in the dorsal horn (Florence et al., 1993). Recent evidence by Florence et al. 1998) indicates that, following long-standing hand or upper limb amputations in monkeys, there is an expansion of corticocortical projections from the adjacent face representation into the deprived representation in area 3b. Examination of thalamocortical connectivity failed to indicate growth beyond the normal extent of thalamocortical axon arbors in these animals compared to normal monkeys (Taub & Florence, 1997; see also Ergenzinger et al., 1996).

Indirect evidence for the growth of new connections with regard to adult somatosensory reorganization has come from studies of the levels of GAP-43, which serves as an indirect marker of structural plasticity (Levin & Dunn-Meynell, 1993). Following vibrissae removal in rats, GAP-43 immunoreactivity has been shown to increase in the contralateral barrel cortex within 1 week (Dunn-Meynell et al., 1992). The regulation of GAP-43 messenger RNA (mRNA) has also been associated with reorganization following vibrissectomy, with an increase in mRNA in the ipsilateral trigeminal complex and contralateral barrel cortex within 1 week following surgery (Levin & Dunn-Meynell, 1993). Curiously, no changes in GAP-43 levels have been observed in the ventroposterior thalamus (Levin & Dunn-Meynell, 1993). It is unclear why presumptive structural changes associated with plasticity following vibrissectomy would occur in the brainstem and cortex but not in the thalamus of these animals.

A Role for Neurotrophic Factors in
Adult Somatosensory Plasticity?

A recent study by Rocamora and colleagues (1996) has shown upregulation of brain-derived neurotrophic factor (BDNF) mRNA in the barrel cortex of rats following whisker stimulation. Although upregulation occurred in layers II through VI of the contralateral cortex, upregulation in layer IV was confined to the barrels corresponding to the stimulated follicles. This is the first evidence of involvement of neurotrophic factors in activity-dependent plasticity of the adult somatosensory system. The possibility that neurotrophic factors might play a role in types of reorganization that would involve the growth and establishment of new connections has been proposed by other researchers (Kaas, 1995).

Neurotrophic factors are polypeptides that are important for the modification, enhancement, and stabilization of active synapses in the developing nervous system, as well as for maintaining connections in the mature nervous system (Bothwell, 1995; Théonen, 1995). Neurotrophic factors have also been implicated recently in the processes underlying learning, memory, and synaptic plasticity since their expression is regulated by neuronal activity and since they have potent effects on the signaling properties of target neurons (Lo, 1995). The most extensively studied of these factors are members of the neurotrophin family, including nerve growth factor (NGF), BDNF, neurotrophin 3 (NT-3), neurotrophin 4/5 (NT-4/5), and neurotrophin 6 (NT-6) (Eide et al., 1993; Götz et al., 1992; Lindsay et al., 1994). The receptors for the neurotrophins are members of the *trk* family of tyrosine kinases, with TrkA the high-affinity receptor for NGF, TrkB primarily the receptor for BDNF and NT-4/5, and TrkC the receptor for NT-3 (Lo, 1995).

In the peripheral nervous system, neurotrophins (especially NGF) are produced by nonneuronal cells such as fibroblasts and Schwann cells in a manner that seems to be independent of neuronal input (Rohrer et al., 1988; reviewed by Lindholm et al., 1994). However, in the central nervous system, in situ hybridization studies have indicated that NGF, BDNF, and NT-3 are produced primarily by neuronal cells under physiologically normal conditions (Ayer-Lelièvre et al., 1988; Bandtlow et al., 1990; Ernfors et al., 1990; Friedman et al., 1992; Gall & Isackson, 1989; Hofer et al., 1990; Whittemore et al., 1988). Although in situ hybridization experiments indicate that astrocytes do not express neurotrophin mRNA in vivo under normal physiological conditions, cultured astrocytes do express NGF (Furukawa et al., 1986; Lindholm et al., 1990, 1992; Lindsay, 1979; Yoshida & Gage, 1991), BDNF (Zafra et al., 1992), and NT-3 (Leingartner & Lindholm, 1994). In addition, mechanical brain injury has been shown to increase levels of NGF mRNA produced by astrocytes in the area surrounding the lesion (Lindholm et al., 1992).

Since the highest levels of NGF, BDNF, and NT-3 in the adult central nervous system are in the hippocampus, most of the research on their regulation and expression in adult animals has concentrated on this region (reviewed by Isackson, 1995; Lo, 1995). The levels of mRNA for BDNF and NGF are rapidly but transiently increased in the hippocampus following limbic seizures (Dugich-Djordjevic et al., 1992; Ernfors et al., 1991; Gall & Isackson, 1989; Isackson et al., 1991), depolarization via a high concentration of potassium (Zafra et al., 1991), or activation of kainate glutamate receptors (Bessho et al., 1993; Lindholm et al., 1993). Conditions that induce long-term potentiation (LTP) in the hippocampus also increase levels of mRNA for BDNF in vivo (Castrèn et al., 1993).

While neuronal expression of neurotrophins has been shown to be regulated in an activity-dependent manner in the adult hippocampus, the role of neurotrophins in the organization of sensory systems has been limited to developmental plasticity. In the developing visual system, the synthesis of BDNF is downregulated in an activity-dependent manner in the visual cortex of dark-reared rats, while exposure to light restores the levels of BDNF mRNA to normal (Castrèn et al., 1992). The effects of BDNF mRNA have been shown to be due specifically to a decrease in activity since intraocular injection of tetrodotoxin in rats has also decreased levels of BDNF mRNA (Castrèn et al., 1992).

The activity-dependent regulation of BDNF during development in the rat visual system indicated a possible role for this and other neurotrophins in the formation of normal patterns of connections and prompted research on their role in developmental visual system plasticity. Intraventricular injection of NGF during the critical period has been shown to prevent the ocular dominance shift produced by monocular deprivation in rats (Maffei et al., 1992). In addition, blockade of endogenous NGF via implantation of hybridoma cells secreting blocking antibodies to NGF in the lateral ventricle of rats after the critical period extends the time period during which monocular deprivation could affect the ocular dominance shift (Berardi et al., 1994; Domenici et al., 1994; reviewed by Theonen, 1995). In addition, the normal development of ocular dominance columns appears to involve the actions of certain neurotrophins, since infusion of BDNF or NT-4/5, but not NT-3 or NGF, into cat primary visual cortex prevents the formation of ocular dominance columns in the immediate vicinity of the infusion site (Cabelli et al., 1995). This suggests that these factors need to be present in limited amounts to allow for their actions on TrkB receptors to influence the segregation of geniculocortical axons into ocular dominance columns in layer 4 of primary visual cortex (Cabelli et al., 1995).

The fact that neurotrophins seem to be involved in aspects of sensory plasticity early in development, coupled with the knowledge that they are regulated in an activity-dependent manner in some areas of the adult brain, points to a potential involvement of these factors in the growth of new connections associated with some forms of adult somatosensory reorganization. The evidence that BDNF mRNA is upregulated in the barrel cortex of rats following somatosensory stimulation (Rocamora et al., 1996) also seems to support this idea. Reduced activity in a given area affected by long-term deafferentation may induce a growth state involving the release of neurotrophins to produce sprouting of adjacent axons into the deprived area (Conti et al., 1996). Such a mechanism would be related to a continuous process of neuronal growth and retraction that underlies the maintenance and restructuring of sensory maps throughout adulthood (Kaas, 1995). Further experiments are needed to determine whether the regulation of neurotrophins and other neurotrophic factors is associated with activity-dependent plasticity in the adult somatosensory system.

Astrocytic Involvement in Adult Somatosensory Plasticity

Glia comprise the majority of the overall volume of the brain, although historically they have been viewed as primarily providing structural support for neurons. Although a role for glia in neuronal migration during development and in the maintenance of ionic homeostasis has been established, a more dynamic and active role for glial cells in brain functions has been found in recent years, even indicating that they may contribute to the processes underlying activity-dependent plasticity (Müller & Best, 1993; Müller, 1992; Imamura et al., 1993; Müller et al., 1993). This is a remarkable shift in thinking regarding cells that were initially described simply as "nerve glue" by Virchow (Müller, 1992).

Part of this shift in attitude concerning the function of glia is the demonstration that they are capable of monitoring local neuronal activity and that they possess mechanisms through which they can signal those neurons (Müller, 1992). Astrocytes have been shown to depolarize in response to changes in local potassium concentrations that occur with postsynaptic neuronal activity (Kuffler, 1967; Wuttke, 1990). In addition, retrograde signals such those produced by arachidonic acid (Axelrod et al., 1988) and nitric oxide (Garthwaite, 1991) may also allow glial cells to react to levels of postsynaptic neuronal activity. Astrocytes are also capable of detecting levels of presynaptic neuronal activity since they possess receptors for many neurotransmitters including glutamate (Backus et al., 1989; Kettenman & Schachner, 1985; Pearce, 1992; Somogyi et al., 1990) and GABA (Backus et al., 1988; Hösli et al., 1990; Kettenman & Schachner, 1985). With respect to glial-neuronal signals, astrocytes have been shown to release neurotransmitters such as glutamate (Drejer et al., 1982; Parpura et al., 1994; Szatkowski et al., 1990), and they may influence neuronal activity through alterations in transmitter uptake (Barbour et al., 1989). Astrocytes have also been shown to release neurotrophic factors (Eckenstein, 1994; Hatten et al., 1988; Korsching, 1993; Lindholm et al., 1994; Martin, 1992; Yoshida & Gage, 1991) that may be important in synaptogenesis.

Collectively, these findings indicate that glia, specifically astrocytes, are capable of participating in the processes underlying the enhancement of synaptic transmission. This has led some investigators to examine this possibility within the developing visual system, where it has been shown that the end of the critical period for ocular dominance column formation coincides with the maturation of astrocytes (Engel & Müller, 1989) and that extension of the critical period induced by dark rearing also retards astrocytic maturation within the affected cortex (Müller, 1990). Müller (1992) has suggested that immature astrocytes may release growth-promoting factors during development and may even be involved in phagocytic actions necessary for cortical plasticity involving synapse elimination (Shatz &

Stryker, 1978) and formation (Swindale et al., 1981). In fact, it has been shown that transplantation of immature astrocytes from newborn kittens into the visual cortex of adult cats reinduces ocular dominance column plasticity (Müller & Best, 1993).

Glia have also recently been implicated in adult plasticity within the somatosensory system, in which section of the three sensory nerves subserving the hand in adult monkeys caused a proliferation of glutamate immunoreactive glia in the portion of SII corresponding to the hand representation but not in SI (Conti et al., 1996). These findings were interesting since, under normal conditions, cortical glial cells do not stain positive for glutamate; (Conti et al., 1987, 1989; Conti & Minelli, 1994; Dori et al., 1989; Otterson & Storm-Mathisen, 1984). In parallel electrophysiological studies of SI and SII in monkeys that had undergone the same experimental procedure, it was shown that at 6 weeks, neurons in the SII hand representation were still unresponsive, while neurons in the SI hand representation had already gained some responsiveness (Ommaya & Pons, 1991). This points to the possibility that the changes in glutamate immunoreactivity and proliferation observed in these glial cells may be related to the initial process of reorganization.

Although the precise mechanism through which glial cells may contribute to the reorganizational changes in somatosensory cortex is unknown, the glial cells appear to be astrocytes based on their size and staining characteristics (Conti et al., 1996), and the proliferation and increase in nuclear diameter observed in these cells are consistent with responses observed during reactive astrogliosis (Eng & Shiurba, 1988). Reactive astrogliosis is one of the earliest and most dominant responses of the central nervous system to tissue injury and can occur at sites distant from the injury (Norenberg, 1996). The biochemical events that trigger reactive astrogliosis are unknown, although this response has been correlated with increased expression of glial fibrillary acidic protein (GFAP) (Amaducci et al., 1981; Bignami & Dahl, 1976; Eng & Shiurba, 1988), and antisense oligonucleotides in the coding region of GFAP have been shown to inhibit GFAP synthesis in injured mouse astrocytes in vitro Ghirnikar et al., 1994; Yu et al., 1993).

It is possible that during the adult reorganizational process, the role of glia may involve the release of growth-promoting factors or phagocytic actions during development, as described above. For example, although mature astrocytes reduce the release or expression of growth or growth-permissive factors, an increase in the expression of these factors has been observed following damage and can be paralleled by glial proliferation (Müller, 1992). One such factor that is predominantly localized to astroglial cells is the S-100β protein (Müller et al., 1993), which has been shown not only to stimulate astrocyte proliferation (Selinfreund et al., 1991), but also to support neuronal survival (Bhattacharyya et al., 1992; Winningham-Major et al., 1989), stimulate neurite extension (Kligman & Marshak, 1985; van Eldick et al., 1988, 1991), and influence intracellular calcium concentration in neurons and glia (Barger & van Eldik, 1992). The Conti et al. (1996) study also suggests the possibility that a reduction of glutamate release from neurons following deafferentation may cause upregulation of glutamate-synthesizing enzymes in neighboring glial cells (resulting in glutamate immunoreactivity in these cells) that is mediated by glial glutamate receptors (Backus et al., 1989; Kettenman & Schachner, 1985; Pearce, 1992; Somogyi et al., 1990). Glutamate synthesized by glial cells would be released (Parpura et al., 1994) and would act on glutamate receptors of postsynaptic neurons, inducing increased intracellular calcium levels that could help trigger the functional and structural changes underlying reorganization (Conti et al., 1996).

Conclusions

Although many researchers concede that some reorganizational changes in the adult somatosensory system probably involve the growth of new connections, direct anatomical evidence of such growth is scarce. Some indirect evidence has emerged from GAP-43 immunostaining, and future studies in this area should address the role of neurotrophins in this process. In addition, while studies of plastic change focus on the response characteristics of neurons throughout the system, attention should also be paid to the contributions of glia in this process. A complete understanding of a mechanism for reorganizational plasticity that involves the sprouting of new connections and concomitant structural changes could provide tools with which greater functional and perceptual recovery can be achieved following stroke or injury. For this reason, further studies are needed in this area of research.

References

Amaducci, L., Forno, K.I., and Eng, L.F. (1981) Glial fibrillary acidic protein in cryogenic lesions of the rat brain. *Neuroscience Letters,* 21:27–32.

Axelrod, J., Burch, R.M., and Jelsema, C.L. (1988) Receptor-mediated activation of phospholipase A2 via GTP-binding proteins: Arachidonic acid and its metabolites as second messengers. TINS 11:117–123.

Ayer-Lelièvre, C., Olson, L., Ebendal, T., Hallböök, F., and Persson, H. (1988) Nerve growth factor mRNA and protein in the testis and epididymis of mouse and rat. *Proceedings of the National Academy of Sciences of the USA,* 85:2628–2632.

Backus, K.H., Kettenman, H., and Schachner, M. (1988) Effect of benzodiazepines and pentobarbital on the GABA-induced depolarization in cultured astrocytes. *Glia,* 1:132–140.

Backus, K.H., Kettenman, H., and Schachner, M. (1989) Pharmacological characterization of the glutamate receptor in cultured astrocytes. *Journal of Neuroscience Research,* 22:274–282.

Bandtlow, C.E., Meyer, M., Lindholm, D., Spranger, M., Heumann, R., and Theonen, H. (1990) Regional and cellular codistribution of interleukin lb and nerve growth factor mRNA in the adult rat brain: Possible relationship to the regulation of nerve growth factor synthesis. *Journal of Cell Biology,* 111:1701–1711.

Barbour, B., Szatkowski, M., Ingledew, N., and Attwell, D. (1989) Arachidonic acid induces a prolonged inhibition of glutamate uptake into glial cells. *Nature,* 342:918–920.

Barger, S.W., and van Eldik, L.J. (1992) S100β stimulates calcium fluxes in glial and neuronal cells. *Journal of Biological Chemistry,* 267:9689–9694.

Berardi, N., Cellerino, A., Domenici, L., Fagiolini, M., Pizzorusso, T., Cattaneo, A., and Maffei, L. (1994) Monoclonal antibodies to nerve growth factor affect the postnatal development of the visual system. *Proceedings of the National Academy of Sciences of the USA,* 91:684–688.

Bessho, Y., Nawa, H., and Nakanishi, S. (1993) Glutamate and quisqualate regulate expression of metabotropic glutamate receptor mRNA in cultured cerebellar granule cells. *Journal of Neurochemistry,* 60:253–259.

Bhattacharyya, A., Oppenheim, R.W., Prevette, D., Moore, B.W., Brackenbury, R., and Ratner, N. (1992) S100 is present in developing chicken neurons and Schwann cells and promotes motor neuron survival in vivo. *Journal of Neurobiology,* 23:451–466.

Bignami, A., and Dahl, D. (1976) The astroglial response to stabbing. Immunofluorescence studies with antibodies to astrocyte-specific protein (GFA) in mammalian and submammalian vertebrates. *Neuropathology and Applied Neurobiology,* 2:99–111.

Bothwell, M. (1995) Functional interactions of neurotrophins and neurotrophin receptors. *Annual Review of Neuroscience,* 18:223–253.

Cabelli, R.J., Hohn, A., and Shatz, C.J. (1995) Inhibition of ocular dominance column formation by infusion of NT-4/5 or BDNF. *Science,* 267:1662–1666.

Calford, M.B., and Tweedale, R. (1988) Immediate and chronic changes in responses of somatosensory cortex in adult flying-fox after digit amputation. *Nature,* 332:446–448.

Calford, M.B., and Tweedale, R. (1991a) C-fibres provide a source of masking inhibition to primary somatosensory cortex. *Proceedings of the Royal Society of London [B],* 243: 269–275.

Calford, M.B., and Tweedale, R. (1991b) Immediate expansion of receptive fields of neurons in area 3b of macaque monkeys after digit denervation. *Somatosensory Motor Research,* 8:249–260.

Castrèn, E., da Penha Berzaghi, M., Lindholm, D., and Theonen, H. (1993) Differential effects of MK-801 on brain-derived neurotrophic factor mRNA levels in different regions of the rat brain. *Experimental Neurology,* 122:244–252.

Castrèn, E., Zafra, F., Theonen H., and Lindholm, D. (1992) Light regulates the expression of BDNF mRNA in the rat visual cortex. *Proceedings of the National Academy of Sciences of the USA,* 89:9444–9448.

Conti, F., DeFelipe, J., Farinas, L., and Manzoni, T. (1989) Glutamate-positive neurons and axon terminals in cat sensory cortex: A correlative light and electron microscopic study. *Journal of Comparative Neurology,* 290:141–153.

Conti, F., and Minelli, A. (1994) Glutamate immunoreactivity in rat cerebral cortex is reversibly abolished by 6-diazo-5-oxo-L-norleucine (DON), an inhibitor of phosphate-activated glutaminase. *Journal of Histochemistry and Cytochemistry,* 42:717–726.

Conti, F., Minelli, A., and Pons, T.P. (1996) Lesion-induced changes in glutamate-immunoreactivity in the somatic sensory cortex of adult monkeys. *Journal of Comparative Neurology,* 368:503–515.

Conti, F., Rustioni, A., Petrusz, P., and Towle, A.C. (1987) Glutamate-positive neurons in the somatic sensory cortex of rats and monkeys. *Journal of Neuroscience,* 7:1887–1901.

Cusick, C.G., Wall, J.T., Whiting, J.J., and Wiley, R.G. (1990) Temporal progression of cortical reorganization following nerve injury. *Brain Research,* 537:355–358.

Domenici, L., Cellerino, A., Berardi, N., Cattaneo, A., and Maffei, L. (1994) Antibodies to nerve growth factor (NGF) prolong the sensitive period for monocular deprivation in the rat. *NeuroReport,* 5:2041–2044.

Dori, I., Petrou, M., and Parnavelas, J.G. (1989) Excitatory transmitter amino acid containing neurons in the rat visual cortex: A light and electron microscopic immunocytochemical study. *Journal of Comparative Neurology,* 290:169–184.

Dostrovsky, J.O., Millar, J., and Wall, P.D. (1976) The immediate shift of afferent drive of dorsal column nucleus cells following deafferentation: A comparison of acute and chronic deafferentation in gracile nucleus and spinal cord. *Experimental Neurology,* 52:480–495.

Drejer, J., Larsson, O.M., and Schousboe, A. (1982) Characterization of L-glutamate uptake into and release from astrocytes and neurons cultured from different brain regions. *Experimental Brain Research,* 47:259–269.

Dugich-Djordjevic, M.M., Tocco, G., Lapchak, P.A., Pasinetti, G.M., Najm, I., Baudry, M., and Hefti, F. (1992) Regionally specific and rapid increases in brain-derived neurotrophic factor messenger RNA in the adult rat brain following seizures induced by systemic administration of kainic acid. *Neuroscience,* 47:303–315.

Dunn-Meynell, A.A., Benowitz, L.I., and Levin, B.E. (1992) Vibrissectomy induced changes in GAP-43 immunoreactivity in the adult rat barrel cortex. *Journal of Comparative Neurology,* 315:160–170.

Dykes, R.W. (1990) Acetylcholine and neuronal plasticity in somatosensory cortex. In M. Steriade and D. Biesold (eds.), *Brain Cholinergic Systems.* New York: Oxford University Press, pp. 294–313.

Dykes, R.W., Landry, P., Metherate, R., and Hicks, T.P. (1984) Functional role of GABA in cat primary somatosensory cortex: Shaping receptive fields of cortical neurons. *Journal of Neurophysiology,* 52:1066–1093.

Eckenstein, F.P. (1994) Fibroblast growth factors in the nervous system. *Journal of Neurobiology,* 25:1467–1480.

Eide, F.F., Lowenstein, D.H., and Reichardt, L.F. (1993) Neurotrophins and their receptors—current concepts and implications for neurologic disease. *Experimental Neurology,* 121:200–214.

Eng, L.F., and Shiurba, R.A. (1988) Glial fibrillary acidic protein: A review of structure, function, and clinical application. In P.J. Marangos, I.C. Campbell, and R.M. Cohen (eds.), *Neuronal and Glial Proteins: Structure, Function, and Clinical Application.* San Diego, CA: Academic Press, pp. 339–359.

Engel, A.K., and Müller, C.M. (1989) Postnatal development of vimentin-immunoreactive radial glial cells in the primary visual cortex of the cat. *Journal of Neurocytology,* 18:437–450.

Ernfors, P., Bengzon, J., Kokaia, Z., Persson, H., and Lindvall, O. (1991) Increased levels of messenger RNAs for neurotrophic factors in the brain during kindling epileptogenesis. *Neuron,* 7:165–176.

Ernfors, P.J., Wetmore, C., Olson, L., and Persson, H. (1990) Identification of cells in rat brain and peripheral tissues expressing mRNA for members of the nerve growth factor family. *Neuron,* 5:511–526.

Ergenzinger, E.R., Findlay, K.A., Glasier, M.M., O'Boyle V.J., Jr., and Pons, T.P. (1996) Segregated thalamic labeling after tracer injections into somatosensory cortex of macaques. *Society for Neuroscience Abstracts,* 22:1056.

Florence, S.L., Garraghty, P.E., Carlson, M., and Kaas, J.H. (1993) Sprouting of peripheral nerve axons in the spinal cord of monkeys. *Brain Research,* 601:343–348.

Florence, S.L., Taub H.B., and Kaas J.H. (1998) Large-scale sprouting of cortical connections after peripheral injury in adult macaque monkeys. *Science,* 282:1117–1121.

Friedman, W.J., Olson, L., and Persson, H. (1992) Cells that express brain-derived neurotrophic factor mRNA in the developing postnatal rat brain. *European Journal of Neuroscience,* 3:688–697.

Furukawa, S., Furukawa, Y., Satayoshi, E., and Hayashi, K. (1986) Synthesis and secretion of nerve growth factor by mouse astroglial cells in culture. *Biochemical and Biophysical Research Communications,* 136:57–63.

Gall, C.M., and Isackson, P.J. (1989) Limbic seizures increase neuronal production of messenger RNA for nerve growth factor. *Science,* 245:758–761.

Garraghty, P.E., and Kaas, J.H. (1991) Functional reorganization in adult monkey thalamus after peripheral nerve injury. *NeuroReport,* 2:747–750.

Garraghty, P.E., Lachica, E.A., and Kaas, J.H. (1991) Injury-induced reorganization of somatosensory cortex is accompanied by reductions in GABA staining. *Somatosensory Motor Research,* 8:347–354.

Garraghty, P.E., Pons, T.P., Sur, M., and Kaas, J.H. (1989) The arbors of axons terminating in the middle cortical layers of somatosensory area 3b in owl monkeys. *Somatosensory and Motor Research,* 6:401–411.

Garthwaite, J. (1991) Glutamate, nitric oxide and cell-cell signalling in the nervous system. TINS 14:60–67.

Ghirnikar, R.S., Yu, A.C., and Eng, L.F. (1994) Astrogliosis in culture: III. Effect of recombinant retrovirus expressing antisense glial fibrillary acidic protein RNA. *Journal of Neuroscience Research,* 38:376–385.

Glasier, M.M., Ergenzinger, E.R., and Pons, T.P. (1997) Distribution of growth-associated phosphoprotein 43 in the somatosensory cortex and thalamus of macaques *Society for Neuroscience Abstracts,* 23:1989.

Götz, R., Koster, R., Winkler, C., Raulf, F., Lottspeich, F., Schartl, M., and Theonen, H. (1992) Neurotrophin-6 is a member of the nerve growth factor family. *Nature,* 372:266–269.

Hatten, M.E., Lynch, M., Rydel, R.E., Sanchez, J., Joseph-Silverstein, J., Moscatelli, D., and Rifkin, D.B. (1988) in vitro neurite extension by granule neurons is dependent upon astroglial-derived fibroblast growth factor. *Developmental Biology,* 125:280–289.

Hofer, M., Pagliusi, S.R., Hohn, A., Leibrock, J., and Barde, Y.-A. (1990) Regional distribution of brain-derived neurotrophic factor mRNA in the adult mouse brain, *EMBO. Journal,* 9:2459–2464.

Hösli, L., Hösli, E., Redle, S., Rojas, J., and Schramek, H. (1990) Action of baclofen, GABA and antagonists on the membrane potential of cultured astrocytes of rat spinal cord. *Neuroscience Letters,* 117:307–312.

Hubel, D.H., and Wiesel, T.N. (1970) The period of susceptibility to the physiological effects of unilateral eye closure in kittens. *Journal of Physiology* 206:419–436.

Imamura, K., Mataga, N., and Watanabe, Y. (1993) Gliotoxin-induced suppression of ocular dominance plasticity in kitten visual cortex. *Neuroscience Research,* 16:117–124.

Isackson, P.J. (1995) Trophic factor response to neuronal stimuli or injury. *Current Opinions in Neuroscience,* 5:350–357.

Isackson, P.J., Huntsman, M.M., Murray, K.D., and Gall, C.M. (1991) BDNF mRNA expression is increased in adult rat forebrain after limbic seizures: Temporal pattern of induction distinct from NGF. *Neuron,* 6:937–948.

Jenkins, W.M., Merzenich, M.M., Ochs, M.T., Allard, T., and Guic Robles, E. (1990) Functional reorganization of primary somatosensory cortex in adult owl monkeys after behaviorally controlled tactile stimulation. *Journal of Neurophysiology,* 63:82–104.

Jones, E.G., and Pons T.P. (1998). Thalamic and brainstem contributions to large-scale plasticity of primate somatosensory cortex. *Science,* 282:1121–1125.

Kaas, J.H. (1991) Plasticity of sensory and motor maps in adult mammals. *Annual Review of Neuroscience,* 14:137–167.

Kaas, J.H. (1995) The reorganization of sensory and motor maps in adult mammals. In M.S. Gazzaniga (ed.), *The Cognitive Neurosciences,* Cambridge, MA: MIT Press, pp. 51–710

Kelahan, A.M., and Doetsch, G.S. (1984) Time dependent changes in the functional organization of somatosensory cerebral cortex following digit amputation in adult raccoons. *Somatosensory Research,* 2:49–81.

Kettenman, H., and Schachner, M. (1985) Pharmacological properties of gamma amino butyric acid-, glutamate-, and aspartate-induced depolarizations in cultured astrocytes. *Journal of Neuroscience,* 5:3295–3301.

Kligman, D., and Marshak, D.R. (1985) Purification and characterization of a neurite extension factor from bovine brain. *Proceedings of the National Academy of Sciences of the USA,* 82:7136–7139.

Korsching, S. (1993) The neurotrophic factor concept: A reexamination. *Journal of Neuroscience,* 13:2739–2748.

Kuffler, S.W. (1967) Neuroglial cells: Physiological properties and a potassium mediated effect of neuronal activity on the glial membrane potential. *Proceedings of the Royal Society of London—Series* B: *Biological Science,* 168:1–21.

Leingärtner, A., and Lindholm, D. (1994) Two promoters direct transcription of the mouse NT-3 gene. *European Journal of Neuroscience,* 6:1149–1159.

Levin, B.E., and Dunn-Meynell, A. (1993) Regulation of growth-associated protein 43 (GAP-43) messenger RNA associated with plastic change in the adult rat barrel receptor complex. *Molecular Brain Research,* 18:59–70.

Lindholm, D., Castren, E., Berzaghi, M., Blochl, A., and Thoenen, H. (1994) Activity-dependent and hormonal regulation of neurotrophin mRNA levels in the brain-implications for neuronal plasticity. *Journal of Neurobiology* 25:1362–1372.

Lindholm, D., Castren, E., Kiefer, R., Zafra, F., and Thoenen, H. (1992) Transforming growth factor-beta 1 in the rat brain: Increase after injury and inhibition of astrocyte proliferation. *Journal of Cell Biology,* 117:395–400.

Lindholm, D., Dechant, G., Heisenberg, C.P., and Thoenen, H. (1993) Brain-derived neurotrophic factor is a survival factor for cultured rat cerebellar granule neurons and protects them against glutamate-induced neurotoxicity. *European Journal of Neuroscience,* 5:1455–1464.

Lindholm, D., Hengerer, B., Zafra, F., and Thoenen, H. (1990) Transforming growth factor-beta 1 stimulates expression of nerve growth factor in the rat CNS. *NeuroReport,* 1:9–12.

Lindsay, R.M. (1979) Adult rat brain astrocytes support survival of both NGF-dependent and NGF-insensitive neurones. *Nature,* 282:80–82.

Lindsay, R.M., Wiegand, S.J., Altar, C.A., and DiStefano, P.S. (1994) Neurotrophic factors: From molecule to man. TINS, 17:182–190.

Lo, D.C. (1995) Neurotrophic factors and synaptic plasticity. *Neuron,* 15:979–981.

Maffei, L., Berardi, N., Domenici, L., Parisi, V., and Pizzorusso, T. (1992) Nerve growth factor (NGF) prevents the shift in ocular dominance distribution of visual cortical neurons in monocularly deprived rats. *Journal of Neuroscience,* 12:4651–4662.

Martin, D.L. (1992) Synthesis and release of neuroactive substances by glial cells. *Glia,* 5:81–94.

Merzenich, M.M., Kaas, J.H., Wall, J.T., Nelson, R.J., Sur, M., and Felleman, D.J. (1983a) Topographic reorganization of somatosensory cortical areas 3b and 1 in adult monkeys following restricted deafferentation. *Neuroscience,* 8:33–55.

Merzenich, M.M., Kaas, J.H., Wall, J.T., Nelson, R.J., Sur, M., and Feldman, D.J. (1983b) Progression of change following median nerve section in the cortical representation of the hand in areas 3b and 1 in adult owl and squirrel monkeys. *Neuroscience,* 10:639–665.

Merzenich, M.M., Nelson, R.J., Stryker, M.P., Cynader, M.S., Schoppmann, A., and Zook, J.M. (1984) Somatosensory cortical map changes following digit amputation in adult monkeys. *Journal of Comparative Neurology,* 224:591–605.

Molander, C., Kinnman, E., and Aldskogius, H. (1988) Expansion of spinal cord primary sensory afferent projection following combined sciatic nerve resection and ruphenous nerve crush: A horseradish peroxidase study in the adult rat. *Journal of Comparative Neurology,* 276:436–11.

Müller, C.M. (1990) Dark-rearing retards the maturation of astrocytes in restricted layers of cat visual cortex. *Glia,* 3:487–494.

Müller, C.M. (1992) A role for glial cells in activity-dependent central nervous plasticity? Review and hypothesis. *International Review of Neurobiology,* 34:215–281.

Müller, C.M., Akhavan, A.C., and Bette, M. (1993) Possible role of S-100 in glia-neuronal signalling involved in activity-dependent plasticity in the developing mammalian cortex. *Journal of Chemical Neuroanatomy,* 6:215–227.

Müller, C.M., and Best, J. (1993) Ocular dominance plasticity in adult cat visual cortex after transplantation of cultured astrocytes. *Nature,* 342:427–430.

Norenberg, M.D. (1996) Reactive astrocytosis. In M.A. Ashner and H.K. Kimelberg (eds.), *The Role of Glia in Neurotoxicity.* Boca Raton, FL CRC Press, pp. 93–107.

Ommaya, A.K., and Pons, T.P. (1991) Reorganization in primary and secondary somatosensory cortex (SII) after complete deafferentation of the hand in rhesus monkeys. *Society for Neuroscience Abstracts,* 17:842.

Ottersen, O.P., and Storm-Mathisen, J. (1984) Glutamate and GABA-containing neurons in the mouse and rat brain, as demonstrated with a new immunocytochemical technique. *Journal of Comparative Neurology,* 229:374–392.

Parpura, V., Basarsky, T.A., Liu, F., Jeftinija, K., Jeftinija, S., and Haydon, P.G. (1994) Glutamate-mediated astrocyte-neuron signalling. *Nature,* 369;744–747.

Pearce, B. (1992) Amino acid receptors. In S. Murphy (ed.), *Astrocytes: Pharmacology and Function.* San Diego, CA: Academic Press, pp. 47–66.

Pollin, B., and Albe-Fessard, P. (1979) Organization of somatic thalamus in monkeys with and without section of dorsal spinal track. *Brain Research,* 173:431–449.

Pons, T.P., Garraghty, P.E., and Mishkin, M. (1988) Lesion induced plasticity in the second somatosensory cortex of adult macaques. *Proceedings of the National Academy of Sciences of the USA,* 85:5279–5281.

Pons, T.P., Garraghty, P.E., Ommaya, A.K., Kaas, J.H., Taub, E., and Mishkin, M.M. (1991) Massive cortical reorganization after sensory deafferentation in adult macaques. *Science,* 252:1857–1860.

Rasmusson, D.D. (1982) Reorganization of raccoon somatosensory cortex following removal of the fifth digit. *Journal of Comparative Neurology,* 205:313–326.

Recanzone, G.H., Jenkins, W.M., Hradek, G.T., and Merzenich, M.M. (1992a) Progressive improvement in discriminative abilities in adult owl monkeys performing a tactile frequency discrimination task. *Journal of Neurophysiology,* 67:1015–1030.

Recanzone, G.H., Merzenich, M.M., Jenkins, W.M., Grajski, K.A., and Dinse, H. (1992b) Topographic reorganization of the hand representation in cortical area 3b of owl monkeys trained in a frequency-discrimination task. *Journal of Neurophysiology,* 67:1031–1056.

Rocamora, N., Welker, E., Pascual, M., and Soriano, E. (1996) Upregulation of BDNF mRNA expression in the barrel cortex of adult mice after sensory stimulation. *Journal of Neuroscience,* 16:4411–4419.

Rohrer, H., Hofer, M., Hellweg, R., Korsching, S., Stehle, A.D., Saadat, S., and Theonen, M. (1988) Antibodies against mouse nerve growth factor interfere in vivo with the development of avian sensory and sympathetic neurones. *Development,* 103:545–552.

Selinfreund, R.H., Barger, S.W., Pledger, W.J., and van Eldik, L.J. (1991) Neurotrophic protein S-100β stimulates glial cell proliferation. *Proceedings of the National Academy of Sciences of the USA,* 88:3554–3558.

Shatz, C.J., and Stryker, M.P. (1978) Ocular dominance in layer IV of the cat's visual cortex and the effects of monocular deprivation. *Journal of Physiology,* 281:267–283.

Snow, P.J., and Wilson, P. (1991) Plasticity in the somatosensory system of developing and mature mammals. *Progress in Sensory Physiology,* Vol. II. New York: Springer-Verlag.

Somogyi, P., Eshhar, N., Teichberg, V.I., and Roberts, J.D. (1990) Subcellular localization of a putative kainate receptor in Bergmann glial cells using a monoclonal antibody in the chick and fish cerebellar cortex. *Neuroscience,* 35:9–30.

Swindale, N.V., Vital-Durand F., and Blakemore, C. (1981) Recovery from monocular deprivation in the monkey. III. Reversal of anatomical effects in the visual cortex. *Proceedings of the Royal Society of London, Series B.* 213:435–450.

Szatkowski, M., Barbour, B., and Attwell, D. (1990) Non-vesicular release of glutamate from glial cells by reversed electrogenic glutamate uptake. *Nature,* 348:443–446.

Theonen, H. (1995) Neurotrophins and neuronal plasticity. *Science,* 270:593–598.

Turnbull, B.G., and Rasmusson, D.D. (1991) Chronic effects of total or partial digit denervation on raccoon somatosensory cortex. *Somatosensory and Motor Research,* 8:201–213.

Van Eldik, L.J., Christie-Pope, B., Bolin, L.M., Shooter, E.M., and Whetsell, W.O., Jr. (1991) Neurotrophic activity of S-100 beta in cultures of dorsal root ganglia from embryonic chick and fetal rat. *Brain Research,* 542:280–285.

Van Eldik, L.J., Staecker, J.L., and Winningham-Major, F. (1988) Synthesis and expression of a gene coding for the calcium-modulated protein S100 beta and designed for cassette-based, site-directed mutagenesis. *Journal of Biological Chemistry,* 263:7830–7837.

Wall, J.T., and Cusick, C.G. (1984) Cutaneous responsiveness in primary somatosensory (S-I) hindpaw cortex before and after partial hindpaw deafferentation in adult rats. *Journal of Neuroscience,* 4:1499–1515.

Wall, J.T., and Cusick, C.G. (1986) The representation of peripheral nerve inputs in the S-1 hindpaw cortex of rats raised with incompletely innervated hindpaws. *Journal of Neuroscience,* 6:1129–1147.

Wall, P.P., and Egger, M.D. (1971) Formulation of new connections in adult rat brains after partial deafferentation. *Nature,* 232:542–545.

Webster, H.H., Hanisch, U.K., Dykes, R.W., and Biesold, D. (1991) Basal forebrain lesions with or without reserpine injection inhibit cortical reorganization in rat hindpaw primary somatosensory cortex following sciatic nerve section. *Somatosensory and Motor Research,* 8:327–346.

Whittemore, S.R., Friedmann, P.L., Larhammer, D., Persson, H., Gonzales-Carvajal, M., and Holets, V.R. (1988) Rat beta-nerve growth factor sequence and site of synthesis in the adult hippocampus. *Journal of Neuroscience Research,* 20:403–410.

Winningham-Major, F., Staecker, J.L., Barger, S.W., Coats, S., and Van Eldik, L.J. (1989) Neurite extension and neuronal survival activities of recombinant S100 beta proteins that differ in the content and position of cysteine residues. *Journal of Cell Biology,* 109:3063–3071.

Woolf, C.J., Shortland, P., and Coggeshall, R.E. (1992) Peripheral nerve injury triggers central sprouting of myelinated afferents. *Nature,* 355:75–78.

Wuttke, W.A. (1990) Mechanism of potassium uptake in neuropile glial cells in the central nervous system of the leech. *Journal of Neurophysiology,* 63:1089–1097.

Yoshida, K., and Gage, F.H. (1991) Fibroblast growth factors stimulate nerve growth factor synthesis and secretion by astrocytes. *Brain Research,* 538:118–126.

Yu, A.C., Lee, Y.L., and Eng, L.F. (1993) Astrogliosis in culture: I. The model and the effect of antisense oligonucleotides on glial fibrillary acidic protein synthesis. *Journal of Neuroscience Research,* 34:295–303.

Zafra, F., Castren, E., Thoenen, H., and Lindholm, D. (1991) Interplay between glutamate and gamma-aminobutyric acid transmitter systems in the physiological regulation of brain-derived neurotrophic factor and nerve growth factor synthesis in hippocampal neurons. *Proceedings of the National Academy of Sciences of the USA,* 88:10037–10041.

Zafra, F., Lindholm, D., Castren, E., Hartikka, J., and Thoenen, H. (1992) Regulation of brain-derived neurotrophic factor and nerve growth factor mRNA in primary cultures of hippocampal neurons and astrocytes. *Journal of Neuroscience,* 12:4793–4799.

5

Neuroanatomic Basis for Reorganization of Function After Prefrontal Damage in Primates

HELEN BARBAS

Neural connections in primates constitute an extensive communication network underlying all neural processes, ranging from simple reflexes to complex executive functions. Consequently, damage to a specific neural structure and functional compensation, when it occurs, are not isolated events but rather change the network of which the structure is a part.

Understanding the numerous circuits of the cortex is a daunting task. However, evidence has emerged from nonhuman primate studies that neural connections can be described by a set of rules, suggesting that connectional relationships can be inferred in humans when invasive procedures are precluded. This chapter explores the basic patterns of neural connections in nonhuman primates and the implications of these connections for normal neural function and for human disease. The central premise is that an understanding of the organization of the limbic cortices is key to understanding the circuits of the cortex. The major inputs and outputs of prefrontal areas may underlie their capacity to undergo the modifications necessary for learning and memory, and their potential for plasticity and functional compensation after brain injury or disease.

Significance of the Concept of the Limbic System

Appreciation of the fact that the prefrontal cortex has a limbic component marked a turning point in, understanding its organization and function. The prefrontal region, which makes up a large proportion of the cortical mantle in primates, was previously thought to be the seat of high-order cognitive processes. The demonstration by Broca (1878), Papez (1937), and, more recently, Yakovlev (1948) and

Nauta (1979) that the posterior medial and orbitofrontal cortices belong to the cortical limbic system has several important implications. From a functional point of view, it implies that the prefrontal cortex has a role in emotional and mnemonic processes, which previously were thought to be the exclusive domain of the cingulate cortex and a set of temporal limbic structures, including the amygdala and the hippocampus. Prefrontal limbic cortices have widespread connections with neighboring areas and with distant sensory, premotor, and other association cortices. The strong connections between limbic and association neocortices suggest that networks underlying cognitive, mnemonic, and emotional processes are intricately linked in the cortex. In contrast to medial and orbitofrontal limbic cortices, the lateral prefrontal areas have a different set of connections and functional characteristics.

Evidence is presented demonstrating that connections and their pattern distinguish prefrontal limbic from lateral eulaminate cortices. The differences in connections have widespread implications for the regional specialization of prefrontal cortices and their preferential involvement in dynamic processes including learning, memory, and emotion. The connectional and neurochemical characteristics established in development may determine the extent to which a given prefrontal area is able to support complex cognitive processes and to adapt after injury.

Prefrontal Limbic and Eulaminate Cortices are Structurally Distinct

There are fundamental structural differences between limbic and eulaminate cortices in primates. The most prominent difference is in the number of layers in these cortices, which can be readily observed in Nissl-stained brain sections. In eulaminate areas, it is possible to identify readily more layers than in limbic cortices. According to modern methods used for numbering layers, eulaminate areas are those that have six layers and limbic cortices are those that have fewer than six layers. Cajal described more than six layers for those areas that are now considered eulaminate, having numbered individually the subdivisions of each layer. Nevertheless, regional differences in the number of layers were noted by Cajal (Arendt et al., 1997; see also DeFelipe & Jones, 1988). However, it was not until much later that Sanides observed that the architectonic differences in cortices are systematic (Sanides, 1969, 1970). Thus, gradual changes in cortical lamination are observed in a radial direction from agranular cortices, which have three layers, to eulaminate cortices, which have six layers. Systematic differences in cortical structure have been observed in all cortical systems (for review see Pandya et al., 1988). Here the focus is on the prefrontal cortices.

Prefrontal limbic cortices have either three distinguishable layers, and thus belong to the agranular type of cortex, or four layers, including a poorly developed granular layer 4, and thus belong to the dysgranular cortical type (Barbas & Pandya, 1989). Collectively called *limbic,* agranular and dysgranular cortices are found in two parts of the prefrontal cortex: one is situated around the anterior part of the

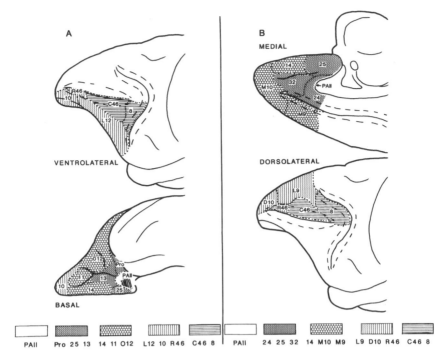

Figure 5-1. Map of the (A) basoventral and (B) mediodorsal prefrontal sectors, where areas are subdivided into five structural types. In both sectors the number of layers and laminar definition increase in cortices listed in rectangles from left to right: far left (PAll) shows agranular cortices, which have three layers (white areas); adjacent dysgranular areas have four layers (cuboidal pattern). The central to far right rectangles show eulaminate cortices, which have six layers but differ in the degree of their laminar definition, ranging from low (third from left, honeycomb pattern) to intermediate (wavy pattern) to high (horizontal stripes). Agranular and dysgranular cortices are collectively called *limbic*. Abbreviations: PAll, periallocortex; Pro, proisocortex. Letter abbreviations appearing before architectonic areas: C, caudal; D, dorsal; L, lateral; M, medial; O, orbital; R, rostral. Reprinted with permission from Barbas and Pandya (1989) by Wiley-Liss, a division of John Wiley and Sons, Inc.

corpus callosum on the medial surface, and the other is found on the posterior orbitofrontal surface (Fig. 5-1). All other prefrontal cortices have six layers and thus can be considered eulaminate. However, eulaminate areas show regional differences in the distinction of their layers as well. Figure 5-1 illustrates the parceling of prefrontal cortices into five structural types based on the number and definition of the cortical layers in each area.

The above structural analysis is used to classify areas into cortical types on the basis of their general laminar features. Cytoarchitectonic parceling, by contrast, is a more detailed process through which cortices belonging to each type are further subdivided into distinct architectonic areas on the basis of the unique cellular features of each area. For example, the dysgranular cortical type includes areas that have four layers. Dysgranular areas, in turn, can be subdivided into specific cyto-architectonic areas. Thus, prefrontal areas 25, 32, and 13 are dysgranular by their laminar structure, yet they can be subdivided into distinct cytoarchitectonic areas on the basis of specific cellular features unique to each area.

The concept of cortical type is useful in summarizing the connectional organization of the prefrontal cortices and in distinguishing between the topography and pattern of connections of prefrontal limbic and eulaminate cortices, as described below. In turn, major differences in connections underlie the distinct functions of these cortices determined in physiologic and behavioral studies. Finally, the patterns of connections of prefrontal limbic and eulaminate cortices have implications for the extent to which these cortices exhibit plasticity after injury, as well as for their relative vulnerability in neurologic and psychiatric disease.

Connections with Subcortical and Cortical Areas Distinguish Limbic from Eulaminate Prefrontal Cortices

Thalamic Connections

The thalamus is a major relay and processing center and is connected with all parts of the cortex (for review see Jones, 1985). In the sensory systems, the thalamus conveys signals from the sensory periphery to the respective sensory cortices. The prefrontal cortices, however, are not primarily sensory in nature, and their thalamic input is likely to be associated with the cognitive, mnemonic, and emotional functions of prefrontal cortices. This section summarizes the differences in the thalamic connections of prefrontal limbic and eulaminate cortices, and a subsequent section discusses their functional implications.

Classic studies associated prefrontal cortices with the mediodorsal (MD) nucleus of the thalamus (for reviews see Le Gros Clark, 1932; Nauta, 1971; Reep, 1984) and have provided more detailed topographic information by associating the magnocellular sector (MDmc) with the orbitofrontal cortices, the parvicellular sector (MDpc) with the lateral prefrontal cortices, and the multiform sector (MDmf) with the frontal eye fields. Subsequent studies, however, ascertained that thalamic nuclei other than MD project to prefrontal cortices as well (Asanuma et al., 1985; Baleydier & Mauguiere, 1985; Barbas & Mesulam, 1981; Bos & Benevento, 1975; Carmel, 1970; Ilinsky et al., 1985; Ilinsky & Kultas-Ilinsky, 1987; Jones & Leavitt, 1974; Kievit & Kuypers, 1977; Trojanowski & Jacobson, 1974).

Studies using quantitative neural tracing procedures demonstrated substantial differences in the relative proportion of projection neurons from MD that project to lateral eulaminate cortices, such as areas 8 and 46, than to limbic areas, such as the posterior orbitofrontal areas (Barbas et al., 1991; Dermon & Barbas, 1994). Thus, whereas MD includes the majority (over 80%) of thalamic neurons directed to lateral eulaminate areas, it contributes about half or fewer of the projection neurons directed to prefrontal limbic cortices. In addition, while projection neurons in midline, intralaminar, medial pulvinar, and ventral anterior nuclei project to all prefrontal cortices, they target the limbic cortices most heavily. Moreover, the specific topography of thalamic projection neurons directed to limbic and eulaminate prefrontal cortices differs. The posterior parts of MD project to orbital and medial limbic cortices, while its anterior parts project to eulaminate areas.

Another connectional feature that distinguishes prefrontal limbic from eulaminate areas is in the degree of their connections with the contralateral thalamus. Although thalamocortical axons generally innervate the ipsilateral cortex, a few neurons from the contralateral thalamus project to the cortex as well (Andersen et al., 1985; Preuss & Goldman-Rakic, 1987; Tigges et al., 1982) and target preferentially the prefrontal limbic cortices (Dermon & Barbas, 1994). Moreover, thalamic nuclei that project to limbic as well as to eulaminate areas issue bilateral projections to limbic areas but issue only ipsilateral projections to eulaminate areas. This evidence suggests that bilateral thalamic projections depend on the interaction of thalamic nuclei with specific cortices and are not peculiar to specific thalamic nuclei. In sum, eulaminate areas receive topographically restricted projections from the thalamus that are strictly ipsilateral. This pattern is in sharp contrast to the prefrontal limbic cortices, which receive widespread ipsilateral as well as contralateral thalamic projections.

Projections from the Hippocampus and the Amygdala

Among prefrontal cortices, the medial limbic and orbitofrontal cortices are the preferential targets of the hippocampus and the amygdala, two limbic structures found in the depths of the temporal lobe. The hippocampal formation in the rhesus monkey projects most robustly to medial areas, followed by orbitofrontal areas (Barbas & Blatt, 1995). Neurons from the entire rostrocaudal extent of the hippocampal formation project to prefrontal cortices, although most projection neurons are found rostrally. The subiculum has been implicated in cortical projections in both cats and monkeys (Cavada et al., 1983; Irle & Markowitsch, 1982; Rosene & Van Hoesen, 1977; Schwerdtfeger, 1979). Recent evidence, however, indicates that whereas the subiculum and prosubiculum project to medial and orbitofrontal cortices, the CA1 ammonic field includes a significant proportion of the projection neurons directed to these cortices as well (Barbas & Blatt, 1995).

In contrast to the limbic areas, lateral prefrontal areas receive only sparse projections from the hippocampal formation, and these are limited to the subiculum (Barbas & Blatt, 1995). However, lateral prefrontal cortices receive substantial projections from the presubiculum and from area 29a–c (Barbas & Blatt, 1995; Goldman-Rakic et al., 1984). On a regional basis, projection neurons from the presubiculum and area 29a–c are directed preferentially to lateral prefrontal cortices, particularly those around the banks of the principal sulcus, followed by orbital cortices and then by medial cortices. With respect to density of projection neurons, the order is the reverse of that seen for projections from the hippocampal formation.

The amygdala targets preferentially prefrontal limbic cortices as well. The orbitofrontal cortices, in particular, receive the most robust projections from the amygdala (Amaral & Price, 1984; Barbas & De Olmos, 1990; Morecraft et al., 1992).

This input originates from a diverse set of amygdaloid nuclei, including the baso-lateral, basomedial (also known as *accessory basal*), lateral, and cortical nuclei. Medial prefrontal cortices receive projections from the amygdala, although from a smaller population of projection neurons than the orbitofrontal cortices. In con-trast to both orbitofrontal and medial prefrontal cortices, lateral eulaminate areas receive few and topographically restricted projections from the amygdala (Barbas & De Olmos, 1990).

Corticocortical Connections

A prominent feature distinguishing between prefrontal limbic and eulaminate cor-tices is the extent of their intrinsic and extrinsic cortical connections. Prefrontal cortices, in general, have distributed connections (for review see Goldman-Rakic, 1988). However, by comparison with the eulaminate areas, the connections of limbic cortices are more widespread (for review see Barbas, 1995a). For example, whereas all prefrontal cortices are connected with their immediate neighbors, the intrinsic connections of limbic cortices extend to more distant prefrontal cortices as well (Barbas & Pandya, 1989). In addition, prefrontal limbic cortices have the most robust connections with other limbic cortices (Barbas, 1988, 1993). In contrast, eulaminate cortices, such as areas 46 and 8, have comparatively restricted connec-tions with limbic cortices (Barbas, 1988; Barbas & Mesulam, 1981, 1985; Barbas & Pandya, 1989). Furthermore, prefrontal limbic areas can be distinguished from culaminate areas by the diversity of the input they receive in terms of both topog-raphy and modality. Thus, prefrontal limbic cortices receive projections from di-verse occipital, temporal, and parietal cortices that process input from several sen-sory modalities. Orbitofrontal areas, in particular, receive projections from primary olfactory areas (Barbas, 1993; Carmichael et al., 1994; Potter & Nauta, 1979) with which they have been classically associated (for review see Takagi, 1986), but they also receive highly distributed input from gustatory, visual, auditory, and somato-sensory association areas (Barbas, 1993). Moreover, orbitofrontal limbic cortices have a variety of autonomic functions (Kaada et al., 1949), suggesting a strong interoceptive input as well.

Medial limbic areas receive input from cortices associated with several sensory modalities as well, but not to the same extent as the orbitofrontal areas. Rather, there appears to be a bias toward projections from auditory cortices to medial limbic ar-eas (Barbas, 1988, 1992; Barbas et al, 1999). Both orbitofrontal and medial limbic cortices receive robust projections from other limbic cortices (for review see Bar-bas, 1995a).

In contrast to the prefrontal limbic areas, projections to lateral eulaminate areas are comparatively restricted with respect to the number of modalities repre-sented (for review see Barbas, 1992). For example, even though projections to area 8 are topographically widespread, there is a preponderance of projections from visual areas to posterior area 8 and from auditory cortices to anterior area 8 (Barbas, 1988; Barbas & Mesulam, 1981). In addition, robust projections from auditory cortices reach area 10 on the frontal pole (for review see Barbas, 1992).

Finally, in contrast to prefrontal limbic cortices, lateral eulaminate cortices receive only sparse projections from limbic cortices.

Pattern of Corticocortical Connections. As described above, there are major differences in the topography of the subcortical and cortical connections of prefrontal limbic, and eulaminate cortices in primates. In addition, there are differences in the pattern of corticocortical connections. *Pattern* in this context refers to the laminar origin and termination of connections. The significance of identifying the pattern of corticocortical connections is based on physiologic findings indicating that there are differences in the response properties of neurons in different layers (e.g. Hubel & Wiesel, 1968). Consequently, one might expect different layers to transmit signals of a different nature within the cortex.

Corticocortical connections in primates have been divided into two large classes: those that originate predominantly in the upper layers (2 and 3) and those that originate mostly in the deep layers (5 and 6). In the sensory cortices, projection neurons directed away from the primary cortices originate largely in the upper layers. In functional terms, they originate in cortices concerned with elementary sensory processing and can be considered ascending, or feedforward projections. In contrast, neurons projecting in the opposite direction, from sensory association toward the primary cortices, originate mostly in the deep layers. The latter have been described as feedback or descending because of their relationship to the direction of flow of sensory information (Friedman et al., 1986; Rockland & Pandya, 1979).

How do cortices that are not unimodal sensory communicate within the cortex? One of the first clues to the pattern of communication of association cortices, such as the prefrontal cortices, emerged with the observation that limbic and eulaminate cortices issue projections from different layers when they communicate with each other (Barbas, 1986). Thus, limbic cortices issue projections to eulaminate cortices mostly from neurons in the deep layers, and their axons terminate in the upper layers of eulaminate cortices (Barbas & Rempel-Clower, 1997). In contrast, when eulaminate cortices project to limbic cortices, the projection neurons are found mostly in the upper layers (2 and 3), and the fibers terminate in the deep layers of limbic cortices (Fig. 5-2).

The classification of connections into feedforward and feedback categories, however, appears to be an oversimplification. In the past, connections that did not fit strictly into the above pattern were considered "intermediate" (for review see Felleman & Van Essen, 1991). However, even the addition of a third category does not capture the complexity of the pattern of corticocortical connections, whose relative distribution in layers varies from area to area (Barbas & Mesulam, 1981).

An intriguing question is whether specific rules apply to the patterns of corticocortical connections. The fundamental difference between limbic and eulaminate cortices, which issue projections from different layers when they are interconnected, is in their cortical structure. This observation suggests that cortical structure may be key to understanding the pattern of corticocortical connections. Moreover, the structure of prefrontal cortices varies systematically, ranging from areas that have only three identifiable layers, to those that have six layers. This feature made it

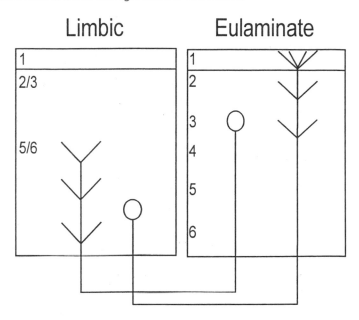

Figure 5-2. The predominant pattern of origin and termination linking limbic and eulaminate cortices. Projection neurons from limbic cortices originate mostly in the deep layers, and their axons terminate in the upper layers (1–3) of eulaminate cortices. In contrast, most projection neurons from eulaminate cortices originate in the upper layers, and their axons terminate in the deep layers (5 and 6) of limbic cortices.

possible to test the hypothesis that cortical structure underlies the pattern of corticocortical connections (Barbas & Rempel-Clower, 1997). The prefrontal cortex was used as a model system, and each area was assigned a numerical rating based on the number and definition of its cortical layers (level 1, lowest; level 5, highest). Connections were described in terms of the difference between the level of origin and termination of each pair of connected areas, a relationship expressed as delta, Δ (Δ = level of origin − level of termination).

The above analysis indicates that when an area with fewer layers or lower laminar definition communicates with an area with more layers or higher laminar definition, the projection neurons originate mostly in the deep layers and their axons terminate mostly in the upper layers (Fig. 5-3). The opposite pattern applies to the reciprocal connections. In addition, the proportion of projection neurons or efferent terminals in the upper to the deep layers varies with the number of levels between the interconnected cortices. The structural relationship of two cortices thus appears to be the best indicator of the pattern of connection of any pair of prefrontal cortices (Fig. 5-3). The power of this structural model lies in its potential to predict patterns of connections in the human cortex, where invasive procedures are precluded (Barbas & Rempel-Clower, 1997).

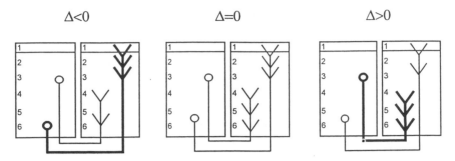

Figure 5-3. The pattern of origin and termination of neurons linking two cortices can be predicted by Δ (Δ = level of the cortex of origin minus level of the cortex of termination; the level of each architectonic area is shown in Figure 5-1 for each sector: far left = 1, far right = 5). The laminar distribution of connections predicted for connections originating in a cortex with a lower (Δ < 0), equal (Δ = 0) and higher (Δ > 0) laminar definition than the cortex of termination. The predominant pattern is indicated by thick lines.

Functional Implications of Connections

Specific Memory-Related Domains in the Prefrontal Cortex

The connectional differences between prefrontal limbic and eulaminate cortices suggest that they have distinct roles in mnemonic processes. Prefrontal limbic cortices receive robust projections from three structures known to be important for long-term memory, including specific thalamic nuclei, the hippocampal formation, and perirhinal cortices (Fig. 5-4). The first major connection of prefrontal limbic cortices with memory-related structures involves thalamic midline nuclei, MDmc, and the caudal part of MDpc (Barbas et al., 1991; Dermon & Barbas, 1994; Goldman-Rakic & Porrino, 1985; Morecraft et al., 1992; Ray & Price, 1993). All of these thalamic nuclei have been implicated in memory, and their damage leads to the classic amnesic syndrome (Aggleton & Mishkin, 1983; Isseroff et al., 1982; for review see Markowitsch, 1982).

The second important connection of prefrontal limbic cortices is with the hippocampal formation, which has classically been associated with mnemonic processes (Mahut, 1971, 1972; Mahut et al., 1982; Murray and Mishkin, 1986; Parkinson et al., 1988; Zola-Morgan et al., 1989a, 1989b; for reviews see Amaral et al., 1990; Squire, 1992; Squire and Zola-Morgan, 1988; Zola-Morgan and Squire, 1993). In humans, damage to the hippocampus results in severe anterograde amnesia, which is characterized by selective inability to remember information acquired after the lesion (Cummings et al., 1984; DeJong et al., 1968; Muramoto & Kuru, 1979; Scoville & Milner, 1957). In their classic study, Scoville and Milner (1957) suggested that the amnesic syndrome could be attributed to the hippocampal lesion. This hypothesis has been substantiated by recent findings of anterograde mnemonic deficits after restricted lesions in the hippocampus in both humans and

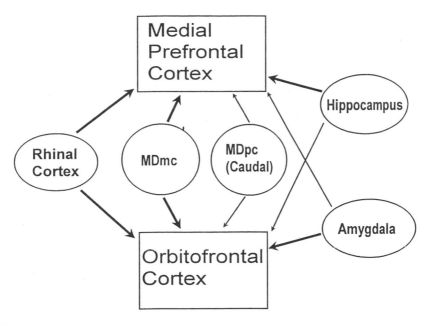

Figure 5-4. Circuits associated with long-term memory. Connections of prefrontal limbic cortices with the principal memory-related structures of the thalamus, the hippocampus, and the rhinal cortices, as well as with the amygdala, which has a role in emotional memory. The strength of the projection is indicated by the thickness of the arrows. The diagram is simplified and shows only unidirectional projections to prefrontal cortices, even though most connections are reciprocal.

monkeys (Alvarez et al., 1995; Beason-Held, 1994; Rempel-Clower, 1994; Zola-Morgan et al., 1986). Moreover, recent evidence indicates that selective bilateral damage to CA1 in humans is sufficient to produce marked anterograde amnesia (Rempel-Clower, 1994; Rempel-Clower et al., 1996; Zola-Morgan et al., 1986). Recent findings indicate that CA1 includes more projection neurons innervating prefrontal limbic areas than any other hippocampal field (Barbas & Blatt, 1995).

The third memory-related structure innervating prefrontal limbic cortices is the cortex around the rhinal sulcus. Animals with damage to the perirhinal area are unable to remember information acquired after the lesion much like those with hippocampal damage (George et al., 1989; Horel et al., 1984; Meunier et al., 1993; Zola-Morgan et al., 1989c, 1993). The perirhinal cortices issue strong projections to both orbitofrontal and medial limbic cortices in the rhesus monkey (Barbas, 1988, 1993; Morecraft et al., 1992) but not to lateral prefrontal cortices.

The above pathways from the thalamus, the hippocampal formation, and the perirhinal areas to prefrontal limbic cortices implicate these networks in remembering events on a long-term basis. The idea that prefrontal limbic cortices, and particularly the medial cortices, share mnemonic functions with the hippocampus is supported by behavioral studies as well. For example, lesions of the ventromedial prefrontal cortices in monkeys result in visual recognition deficits (Bachevalier & Mishkin, 1986; Voytko, 1985). In humans, vascular lesions affecting the anterior communicating artery, which supplies the ventromedial prefrontal areas (Crowell & Morawetz, 1977), result in severe anterograde amnesia comparable to the classic amnesic syndrome seen after hippocampal lesions (Alexander & Freedman, 1984; Talland et al., 1967). The areas affected in such vascular accidents include Brodmann's area 25 and the parts of areas 32 and 24 situated adjacent to the genu and the rostrum of the corpus callosum. The mnemonic deficits observed in both monkeys and humans (Alexander & Freedman, 1984; Bachevalier & Mishkin, 1986; Chapter 2, this volume; Talland et al., 1967; Voytko, 1985) may be due to interruption of a pathway linking the hippocampus with ventromedial prefrontal cortices. Ventromedial prefrontal areas in the rhesus monkey receive the most robust projections from the hippocampal formation (Barbas & Blatt, 1995).

In marked contrast to medial and orbitofrontal cortices, lateral eulaminate cortices do not receive significant input from structures associated with long-term memory. The lateral prefrontal cortices receive projections from a distinct set of thalamic nuclei, and they receive only a sparse input from the amygdala, the hippocampal formation, and the cortical limbic areas. The thalamic projections to lateral prefrontal cortices originate most prominently from the multiform (mf) part of MD and the anterior part of MDpc (Barbas et al., 1991; Dermon & Barbas, 1994; Fig. 5-5). Unlike the prefrontal limbic areas, lateral eulaminate cortices receive only sparse projections from the hippocampal formation that are restricted to the subiculum.

Lateral eulaminate cortices at the caudal part of the principal sulcus and in the arcuate concavity are distinguished by the robust projections they receive from cortical and subcortical structures associated with attentional processes and eye movements. For example, the intraparietal visuomotor cortex targets area 8 and caudal area 46 heavily (Andersen et al., 1985; Barbas & Mesulam, 1981, 1985; Cavada & Goldman-Rakic, 1989; Huerta et al., 1987; Petrides and Pandya, 1984). Several thalamic nuclei that project to prefrontal area 8, including MDmf, the suprageniculate, and the limitans, receive projections from the superior colliculus and the lateral part of the substantia nigra, both of which have been implicated in eye movement (Benevento & Fallon, 1975; Hikosaka & Wurtz, 1983a–1983d; Ilinsky & Kultas-Ilinsky, 1987; Ilinsky et al., 1985; Wurtz & Albano, 1980). Other thalamic nuclei which have visual and visuomotor properties, including the upper parts of the central lateral and paracentral nuclei (Schlag and Schlag-Rey, 1984; Schlag-Rey and Schlag, 1984) project to area 8 as well.

Finally, lateral prefrontal cortices receive input from a substantial population of projection neurons from the presubiculum and area 29a–c (Goldman-Rakic et al., 1984), which equals or surpasses a similar projection to prefrontal limbic cortices (Barbas & Blatt, 1995). Like the parietal cortices, cingulate areas have a prominent role in attentional processes (Mesulam, 1981, 1990).

The above connectional pattern of lateral prefrontal cortices is consistent with their involvement in cognitive tasks where attention is critical in keeping stimuli

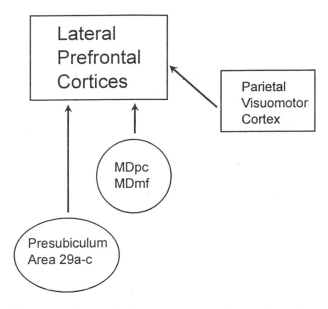

Figure 5-5. Circuits associated with short-term memory. Connections of lateral prefrontal cortices with principal cortical and subcortical structures associated with visuomotor and attentional processes, which may underlie their role in working memory.

and responses in temporary memory in order to perform a sequential task (for reviews see Fuster, 1993; Goldman-Rakic, 1988; Petrides, 1989). Lesions of lateral prefrontal cortices do not render nonhuman or human primates amnesic (Janowsky et al., 1989; Milner & Petrides, 1984; Petrides, 1989). However, damage to lateral prefrontal cortices around the principal sulcus impairs the performance of nonhuman primates when they must remember information after a short delay. The lateral prefrontal cortices thus have a role in working memory during cognitive tasks (Bauer & Fuster, 1976; Funahashi et al., 1989; Fuster, 1973; Jacobsen, 1936; Kojima & Goldman-Rakic, 1982; Kubota & Niki, 1990; Kubota et al., 1980; Sawaguchi & Goldman-Rakic, 1991; Sawaguchi et al., 1988; for reviews see Fuster, 1989; Goldman-Rakic, 1988;). It is possible that this type of mnemonic processing is supported by a pathway linking lateral prefrontal areas with the intraparietal, MDpc, and MDmf thalamic nuclei, as well as with the presubiculum and area 29a–c (Fig. 5-5).

Emotional Processing in the Prefrontal Cortex

Prefrontal limbic cortices receive strong projections from the amygdala. There is evidence from classic and recent studies that the amygdala has a predominant role in emotional processes and emotional memory (for reviews see Damasio, 1994; Davis, 1992; LeDoux, 1994). The orbitofrontal cortices, in particular, followed by the medial limbic cortices, receive robust projections from the amygdala (Fig. 5-4). In addition, the orbitofrontal cortices receive input from sensory cortices where the emphasis in processing appears to be on the features of stimuli and their memory (for reviews see Barbas, 1992, 1995a). The coupling of sensory and amygdaloid signals in orbitofrontal cortices may be related to remembering emotionally significant events. Behavioral studies suggest a functional interrelationship between the orbitofrontal cortices and the amygdala. Monkeys with damage to the orbitofrontal cortex or the amygdala do not exhibit appropriate emotional responses and are unable to engage in normal social interactions (for review see Kling & Steklis, 1976).

Finally, both the orbitofrontal cortex and the amygdala in primates are robustly interconnected with the thalamic MDmc nucleus (Aggleton & Mishkin, 1984; Aggleton et al., 1980; Nauta, 1961; Russchen et al., 1987). Recent evidence implicates the MDmc in emotional memory as well (Oyoshi et al., 1996), a function which may be mediated by the strong interconnections of the MDmc and the amygdala.

The Role of Feedback Systems in Neural Function

The pattern of projections from limbic to eulaminate cortices, originating in the deep layers and terminating in the upper layers, matches the pattern of feedback connections in sensory cortices (Rockland & Pandya, 1979). In the sensory systems, feedback projections from the deep layers are directed from sensory association areas back to the primary cortices or from the cortex to subcortical structures (for references see Barbas, 1986). By the above criteria, the cortical limbic system can be considered the ultimate feedback system to the rest of the neocortex.

There is evidence that feedback projections are critical in all systems and have a role in tasks ranging from sensory perception to learning and memory (Sakai & Miyashita, 1994; Ullman, 1995). What is the role of the massive feedback projections issued from prefrontal limbic cortices to the neuraxis? As indicated above, prefrontal limbic cortices receive rich projections from distributed pathways associated with sensory perception and with associative mnemonic and emotional processes. Limbic areas may have an essential role in integrating this information and in comparing external sensory signals with internal perceptual representations. In addition, because limbic cortices have a fundamental role in monitoring the internal emotional environment, they may provide the appropriate context for interpreting events in a behavioral setting. Disruption of feedback projections from limbic cortices may account for the cognitive and emotional deficits observed in several neurologic and psychiatric diseases that affect limbic cortices prominently (Gloor et al., 1982; Hooper & Vogel, 1976; Reynolds, 1989; Weinberger, 1988). The prefrontal cortices, in particular, have been implicated in schizophrenia (Weinberger, 1988), a disease affecting limbic areas preferentially (Reynolds, 1989; Roberts et al., 1983). The pathology in schizophrenia may be a consequence of a breakdown of a massive feedback system issued from limbic areas that have a role in the integration of distributed pathways associated with sensory perception, associative mnemonic, and emotional processes.

The Pattern of Connections and Neurochemical
Features May Underlie the Extent of Plasticity
in Distinct Prefrontal Cortices

The above findings suggest that cortical areas communicate with each other according to a pattern that appears to depend on the types of cortices participating in connections. Moreover, this pattern of communication appears to be general in all cortical systems (for review see Barbas, 1995a).

How is the adult pattern of connections established? The organized pattern of connections observed in adult animals emerges from a more chaotic state in development when exuberant connections are observed in several neural systems (e.g., Chalupa & Killackey, 1989; Innocenti, 1981; Innocenti et al., 1977, 1986; Ivy et al., 1979; Laemle & Sharma, 1986; Minciacchi & Granato, 1989; O'Leary et al., 1981; Rodman & Consuelos, 1994; Scheibel & Scheibel, 1967; Takada et al., 1987; Wise & Jones, 1976), albeit to a different extent (see Schwartz & Goldman-Rakic, 1991). Connections eventually appear to settle into the organized pattern seen in the adult. An intriguing question concerns the factors that contribute to the establishment of consistent connectional patterns. One hypothesis is that distinct prefrontal cortices develop and establish connections at different times in the genesis of the cortex. Differences in temporal developmental factors (for reviews see Allendoerfer & Shatz, 1994; O'Leary et al., 1994; Sur & Cowey, 1995) may explain the structural differences in these cortices, since the time of onset or duration of neurogenesis has profound effects on neural density (e.g. Caviness et al., 1995). Even small differences in the onset or duration of ontogeny would affect the pattern of connections as a consequence of the developmental constraints imposed during different ontogenetic periods. In this context it is interesting that exuberant connections, observed transiently during development in all areas, are seen preferentially in limbic cortices in adulthood, both from the thalamus and from a small population of neurons that project via divergent axons (Barbas, 1995b; Dermon & Barbas, 1994). In addition, in adult primates, even though the connections of prefrontal cortices in general are distributed, they are more widespread and diverse for prefrontal limbic than for eulaminate cortices.

It is also intriguing that the developmentally associated proteins growth-associated protein 43 (GAP-43) and nitric oxide synthase (NOS) are found at considerably higher levels in limbic and associative areas that have a role in learning and memory than in other cortices in adult animals (Benowitz & Routtenberg, 1987; Dombrowski & Barbas, 1996; Lovinger et al., 1985; Skene & Willard, 1981a, 1981b; for reviews see Benowitz & Routtenberg, 1987; Benowitz et al., 1989; Dani et al., 1991; De la Monte et al., 1989; Kruger et al., 1992; Nelson et al., 1987; Routtenberg, 1985; Snipes et al., 1987;). These observations raise the possibility that some connectional and neurochemical features seen in development may be retained in limbic and associative cortices to a greater extent than in other cortices.

The above connectional and neurochemical characteristics suggest that the extent of plasticity may differ for limbic and eulaminate cortices. The parallels in the connectional and neurochemical characteristics noted in limbic areas and in all areas during development may help explain the great plasticity of limbic areas, their involvement in learning and memory, and their selective ability to regenerate after neonatal damage, at least in rats (Chapter 6, this volume). In turn, the properties that render prefrontal limbic cortices plastic may also contribute to their preferential vulnerability in several neurologic disorders including epilepsy and Alzheimer's disease (Braak & Braak, 1991; Gloor et al., 1982; Hooper & Vogel, 1976; Hyman et al., 1984; Kromer Vogt et al., 1990; Penfield & Jasper, 1954; Reynolds, 1989; Roberts et al., 1983; Vogt et al., 1990; Weinberger, 1988). In fact, GAP-43 and the precursor of the Alzheimer amyloid β protein show a similar distribution in the human cortex (Neve et al., 1988).

In the rhesus monkey, connections of prefrontal cortices are established prenatally (Schwartz et al., 1991). If the highly ordered corticocortical connections are guided by developmental factors, abnormalities that disturb their sequence are likely to have a profound effect on their establishment and function in the mature organism. Several human disorders, including dyslexia, learning disabilities, schizophrenia, and certain forms of epilepsy, appear to have their origin in development (Akbarian et al., 1993; for review see Mischel et al., 1995). Cortical structure and connections are likely to be altered in these disorders (e.g., Galaburda & Kemper, 1979). Disruption of organized pathways may also account for the complex cognitive and mnemonic deficits observed in Alzheimer's disease, which appears to affect preferentially neurons participating in corticocortical connections (Arnold et al., 1991; Hyman et al., 1984; Lewis et al., 1987; Morrison et al., 1990; Pearson et al., 1985; Van Hoesen et al., 1991). The structural and neurochemical differences between limbic and eulaminate areas may provide clues to an understanding of why limbic areas are so vulnerable in neurologic and psychiatric diseases. This is prerequisite for developing rational approaches to facilitate recovery of function.

When the nervous system is damaged by injury or affected by disease, it may revert to a more chaotic pattern of synaptic contacts perhaps comparable to that seen in development. Both GAP-43 and NOS, which are expressed at a high rate during development, are also expressed preferentially in the adult brain after neural injury (for review see Benowitz & Routtenberg, 1987; Vizzard et al., 1995). Like the sequence of events in development, the nervous system may eventually settle into a more orderly pattern of local circuits, which may account for the recovery seen after brain injury. The challenge in future research is to determine the specific factors that facilitate the establishment of appropriate connections, which may, in turn, result in functional compensation after neural damage.

Studies comparing the pattern of connections of fetal, neonatal, and adult animals have focused on eulaminate sensory or association cortices (Andersen et al., 1985; Chalupa & Killackey, 1989; Innocenti, 1981; Innocenti et al., 1977; Ivy et al., 1979; Schwartz & Goldman-Rakic, 1984). Further studies are necessary to determine whether limbic cortices in mammals retain features observed in development to a greater extent than in the eulaminate areas, which may increase their capacity for compensation after injury.

Conclusion

The prefrontal region in primates is composed of limbic and eulaminate cortices that differ in their structure and connections. Prefrontal limbic cortices have widespread connections with thalamic and temporal structures associated with long-term memory and emotional memory. In contrast, lateral eulaminate cortices are the targets of input from a distinct set of thalamic nuclei and are connected with parietal visuomotor cortices and posterior cingulate areas associated with attentional processes and working memory. The connections of prefrontal cortices show a consistent pattern whereby the laminar origin and terminations of connections seem to depend on the structure of the connected cortices. Damage to the nervous system in development or in adults is likely to upset these consistent connectional patterns. Prefrontal limbic cortices have several connectional and neurochemical features that are seen in all areas during development. These connectional and neurochemical features may account for the plasticity of limbic cortices and their involvement in learning and memory, their preferential vulnerability in neurologic and psychiatric diseases, and their potential for recovery after brain injury or disease.

ACKNOWLEDGMENTS
I thank my collaborators whose work is cited in this review and Mr. Troy Ghashghaei for help with the graphics. This work was supported by NIH Grants NS24760 (NINDS) and NS57414 (NIMH).

References

Aggleton, J.P., Burton, M.J., and Passingham, R.E. (1980) Cortical and subcortical afferents to the amygdala of the rhesus monkey (*Macaca mulatta*). *Brain Reserch,* 190:347–368.

Aggleton, J.P., and Mishkin, M. (1983) Visual recognition impairment following medial thalamic lesions in monkeys. *Neuropsychologia,* 21:189–197.

Aggleton, J.P., and Mishkin, M. (1984) Projections of the amygdala to the thalamus in the cynomolgus monkey. *Journal of Comparative Neurology,* 222:56–68.

Akbarian, S., Bunney, W.E., Potkin, S.G., Wigal, S.B., Hagman, J.O., Sandmen, C.A. and Jones, E.G. (1993) Altered distribution of nicotinamide-adenine-dinucleotide phosphate-diaphorase cells in frontal lobes of schizophrenics implies disturbances of cortical development. *Archives of General Psychiatry,* 50:169–177.

Alexander, M.P., and Freedman, M. (1984) Amnesia after anterior communicating artery aneurysm rupture. *Neurology,* 34:752–757.

Allendoerfer, K.L., and Shatz, C.J. (1994) The subplate, a transient neocortical structure: Its role in the development of connections between thalamus and cortex. *Annual Review of Neuroscience,* 17:185–218.

Alvarez, P., Zola-Morgan, S., and Squire, L.R. (1995) Damage limited to the hippocampal region produces long-lasting memory impairment in monkeys. *Journal of Neuroscience,* 15:3796–3807.

Amaral, D.G., Insausti, R., Zola-Morgan, S., Squire, L.R., and Suzuki, W.A. (1990) The perirhinal and parahippocampal cortices and medial temporal lobe memory function. In

Vision, Memory, and the Temporal Lobe. New York: Elsevier, Iwai, E. & Mishkin, M. (eds) pp. 149–161.

Amaral, D.G., and Price, J.L. (1984) Amygdalo-cortical projections in the monkey *(Macaca fascicularis). Journal of Comparative Neurology,* 230:465–496.

Andersen, R.A., Asanuma, C., and Cowan, W.M. (1985) Callosal and prefrontal associational projecting cell populations in area 7a of the macaque monkey: A study using retrogradely transported fluorescent dyes. *Journal of Comparative Neurology,* 232:443–455.

Arendt, T., Schindler, C., Bruckner, M.K., Eschrich, K., Bigl, V., Zedlick, O, Mercova, L. (1997) Plastic neuronal remodeling is impaired in patients with Alzheimer's disease carrying apolipoprotein E4 Allele. *Journal of Neuroscience,* 17(2):516–529.

Arnold, S.E., Hyman, B.T., Flory, J., Damasio, A.R., and Van Hoesen, G.W. (1991) The topographical and neuroanatomical distribution of neurofibrillary tangles and neuritic plaques in the cerebral cortex of patients with Alzheimer's disease. *Cerebral Cortex,* 1:103–116.

Asanuma, C., Andersen, R.A., and Cowan, W.M. (1985) The thalamic relations of the caudal inferior parietal lobule and the lateral prefrontal cortex in monkeys: Divergent cortical projections from cell clusters in the medial pulvinar nucleus. *Journal of Comparative Neurology,* 241:357–381.

Bachevalier, J., and Mishkin, M. (1986) Visual recognition impairment follows ventromedial but not dorsolateral prefrontal lesions in monkeys. *Behavioral Brain Research,* 20: 249–261.

Baleydier, C., and Mauguiere, F. (1985) Anatomical evidence for medial pulvinar connections with the posterior cingulate cortex, the retrosplenial area, and the posterior parahippocampal gyrus in monkeys. *Journal of Comparative Neurology,* 232:219–228.

Barbas, H. (1986) Pattern in the laminar origin of corticocortical connections. *Journal of Comparative Neurology,* 252:415–422.

Barbas, H. (1988) Anatomic organization of basoventral and mediodorsal visual recipient prefrontal regions in the rhesus monkey. *Journal of Comparative Neurology,* 276:313–342.

Barbas, H. (1992) Architecture and cortical connections of the prefrontal cortex in the rhesus monkey. In P. Chauvel, A.V. Delgado-Escueta, E. Halgren, and J. Bancaud (eds.), *Advances in Neurology, Vol. 57* New York: Raven Press, pp. 91–115.

Barbas, H. (1993) Organization of cortical afferent input to orbitofrontal areas in the rhesus monkey. *Neuroscience,* 56:841–864.

Barbas, H. (1995a) Anatomic basis of cognitive-emotional interactions in the primate prefrontal cortex. *Neuroscience and Biobehavioral Reviews,* 19:499–510.

Barbas, H. (1995b) Pattern in the cortical distribution of prefrontally directed neurons with divergent axons in the rhesus monkey. *Cerebral Cortex,* 5:158–165.

Barbas, H., and Blatt, G.J. (1995) Topographically specific hippocampal projections target functionally distinct prefrontal areas in the rhesus monkey. *Hippocampus,* 5:511–533.

Barbas, H., and De Olmos, J. (1990) Projections from the amygdala to basoventral and mediodorsal prefrontal regions in the rhesus monkey. *Journal of Comparative Neurology,* 301:1–23.

Barbas, H., Ghashghaei, H., Dombrowski, S.M. and Rempel-Clower, N.L. Medial prefrontal cortices are unified by common connections with superior temporal cortices and distinguished by input from memory-related areas in the rhesus monkey. J. *Comp. Neurol.* 410:343–367, 1999.

Barbas, H., Henion, T.H., and Dermon, C.R. (1991) Diverse thalamic projections to the prefrontal cortex in the rhesus monkey. *Journal of Comparative Neurology,* 313:65–94.

Barbas, H., and Mesulam, M.-M. (1981) Organization of afferent input to subdivisions of area 8 in the rhesus monkey. *Journal of Comparative Neurology,* 200:407–431.

Barbas, H., and Mesulam, M.-M. (1985) Cortical afferent input to the principalis region of the rhesus monkey. *Neuroscience,* 15:619–637.

Barbas, H., and Pandya, D.N. (1989) Architecture and intrinsic connections of the prefrontal cortex in the rhesus monkey. *Journal of Comparative Neurology,* 286:353–375.

Barbas, H., and Rempel-Clower, N. (1997) Cortical structure predicts the pattern of cortico-cortical connections. *Cerebral Cortex,* 7:635–646.

Bauer, R.H., and Fuster, J.M. (1976) Delayed-matching and delayed-response deficit from cooling dorsolateral prefrontal cortex in monkeys. *Journal of Comparative and Physiological Psychology,* 90:299–302.

Beason-Held, L.L. (1994) Contributions of the hippocampus and related ventromedial temporal cortices to memory in the rhesus monkey. Ph.D. thesis, Boston University.

Benevento, L.A., and Fallon, J.H. (1975) The ascending projections of the superior colliculus in the rhesus monkey *(Macaca mulatta). Journal of Comparative Neurology,* 160: 339–362.

Benowitz, L.I., Perrone-Bizzozero, N.I., Finklestein, S.P., and Bird, E.D. (1989) Localization of the growth-associated phosphoprotein GAP-43 (B-50, F1) in the human cerebral cortex. *Journal of Neuroscience,* 9:990–995.

Benowitz, L.I., and Routtenberg, A. (1987) A membrane phosphoprotein associated with neural development, axonal regeneration, phospholipid metabolism, and synaptic plasticity. *Trends in Neuroscience,* 10:527–532.

Bos, J., and Benevento, L.A. (1975) Projections of the medial pulvinar to orbital cortex and frontal eye fields in the rhesus monkey *(Macaca mulatta). Experimental Neurology,* 49: 487–496.

Braak, H., and Braak, E. (1991) Alzheimer's disease affects limbic nuclei of the thalamus. *Acta Neuropathologica,* 81:261–268.

Broca, P. (1878) Anatomie compareée des enconvolutions cérébrales: Le grand lobe limbique et la scissure limbique dans la serie des mammifères. *Revue Anthropologie,* 1:385–498.

Carmel, P.W. (1970) Efferent projections of the ventral anterior nucleus of the thalamus in the monkey. *American Journal of Anatomy,* 128:159–184.

Carmichael, S.T., Clugnet, M.-C. and Price, J.L. (1994) Central olfactory connections in the macaque monkey. *Journal of Comparative Neurology,* 346:403–434.

Cavada, C., and Goldman-Rakic, P.S. (1989) Posterior parietal cortex in rhesus monkey: II. Evidence for segregated corticocortical networks linking sensory and limbic areas with the frontal lobe. *Journal of Comparative Neurology,* 287:422–445.

Cavada, C., Llamas, A., and Reinoso-Suarez, F. (1983) Allocortical afferent connections of the prefrontal cortex in the cat. *Brain Research,* 260:117–120.

Caviness, V.S., Jr., Takahashi, T., and Nowakowski, R.S. (1995) Numbers, time and neocortical neuronogenesis: A general developmental and evolutionary model. *Trends in Neuroscience,* 18:379–383.

Chalupa, L.M., and Killackey, H.P. (1989) Process elimination underlies ontogenetic change in the distribution of callosal projection neurons in the postcentral gyrus of the fetal rhesus monkey. *Proceedings of the National Academy of Sciences of the USA,* 86:1076–1079.

Crowell, R.M., and Morawetz, R.B. (1977) The anterior communicating artery has significant branches. *Stroke,* 8:272–273.

Cummings, J.L., Tomiyasu, U., Read, S., and Benson, D.F. (1984) Amnesia with hippocampal lesions after cardiopulmonary arrest. *Neurology,* 34:679–681.

Damasio, A.R. (1994) *Descarte's Error: Emotion, Reason, and the Human Brain.* New York: G.P. Putnam's Sons.

Dani, J.W., Armstrong, D.M., and Benowitz, L.I. (1991) Mapping the development of the rat brain by GAP-43 immunocytochemistry. *Neuroscience,* 40:277–287.

Davis, M. (1992) The role of the amygdala in fear and anxiety. *Annual Review of Neuroscience,* 15:353–375.

DeFelipe, J., and Jones, E.G. (1988) *Cajal on the Cerebral Cortex. An Annotated Translation of the Complete Writings.* New York and Oxford: Oxford University Press.

DeJong, R.N., Itabashi, H.H., and Olson, J.R. (1968) "Pure" memory loss with hippocampal lesions: A case report. *Transactions of the American Neurological Association,* 93:31–34.

De la Monte, S., Federoff, H.J., Ng, S.-C., Grabczyk, E., and Fishman, M.C. (1989) GAP-43 gene expression during development: Persistence in a distinctive set of neurons in the mature central nervous system. *Developmental Brain Research,* 46:161–168.

Dermon, C.R., and Barbas, H. (1994) Contralateral thalamic projections predominantly reach transitional cortices in the rhesus monkey. *Journal of Comparative Neurology,* 344:508–531.

Dombrowski, S.M., and Barbas, H. (1996) Differential expression of NADPH diaphorase in functionally distinct prefrontal cortices in the rhesus monkey. *Neuroscience,* 72: 49–62.

Felleman, D.J., and Van Essen, D.C. (1991) Distributed hierarchical processing in the primate cerebral cortex. *Cerebral Cortex,* 1:1–47.

Friedman, D.P., Murray, E.A., O'Neill, J.B., and Mishkin, M. (1986) Cortical connections of the somatosensory fields of the lateral sulcus of macaques: Evidence for a cortico-limbic pathway for touch. *Journal of Comparative Neurology,* 252:323–347.

Funahashi, S., Bruce, C.J., and Goldman-Rakic, P.S. (1989) Mnemonic coding of visual space in the monkey's dorsolateral prefrontal cortex. *Journal of Neurophysiology,* 61:331–349.

Fuster, J.M. (1973) Unit activity in prefrontal cortex during delayed-response performance: Neuronal correlates of transient memory. *Journal of Neurophysiology,* 36:61–78.

Fuster, J.M. (1989) *The Prefrontal Cortex,* 2nd ed. New York: Raven Press.

Fuster, J.M. (1993) Frontal lobes. *Current Opinion in Neurobiology,* 3:160–165.

Galaburda, A.M., and Kemper, T.L. (1979) Cytoarchitectonic abnormalities in developmental dyslexia: A case study. *Annals of Neurology,* 6:94–100.

George, P.J., Horel, J.A., and Cirillo, R.A. (1989) Reversible cold lesions of the parahippocampal gyrus in monkeys result in deficits on the delayed match-to-sample and other visual tasks. *Behavioral Brain Research,* 34:163–178.

Gloor, P., Olivier, A., Quesney, L.F., Andermann, F., and Horowitz, S. (1982) The role of the limbic system in experiential phenomena of temporal lobe epilepsy. *Annals of Neurology,* 12:129–144.

Goldman-Rakic, P.S. (1988) Topography of cognition: Parallel distributed networks in primate association cortex. *Annual Review of Neuroscience,* 11:137–156.

Goldman-Rakic, P.S., and Porrino, L.J. (1985) The primate mediodorsal (MD) nucleus and its projection to the frontal lobe. *Journal of Comparative Neurology,* 242:535–560.

Goldman-Rakic, P.S., Selemon, L.D., and Schwartz, M.L. (1984) Dual pathways connecting the dorsolateral prefrontal cortex with the hippocampal formation and parahippocampal cortex in the rhesus monkey. *Neuroscience,* 12:719–743.

Hikosaka, O., and Wurtz, R.H. (1983a) Visual and oculomotor functions of monkey substantia nigra pars reticulata, I. Relation of visual and auditory responses to saccades. *Journal of Neurophysiology,* 49:1230–1253.

Hikosaka, O., and Wurtz, R.H. (1983b) Visual and oculomotor functions of monkey sub-stantia nigra pars reticulata. II. Visual responses related to fixation of gaze. *Journal of Neurophysiology*, 49:1254–1267.

Hikosaka, O., and Wurtz, R.H. (1983c) Visual and oculomotor functions of monkey sub-stantia nigra pars reticulata. III. Memory-contingent visual and saccade responses. *Journal of Neurophysiology*, 49:1268–1284.

Hikosaka, O., and Wurtz, R.H. (1983d) Visual and oculomotor functions of monkey sub-stantia nigra pars reticulata. IV. Relation of substantia nigra to superior colliculus. *Journal of Neurophysiology*, 49:1285–1301.

Hooper, M.W., and Vogel, F.S. (1976) The limbic system in Alzheimer's disease. *American Journal of Pathology*, 85:1–20.

Horel, J.A., Voytko, M.L., and Salsbury, K.G. (1984) Visual learning suppressed by cool-ing the temporal pole. *Behavioral Neuroscience*, 98:310–324.

Hubel, D.H., and Wiesel, T.N. (1968) Receptive fields and functional architecture of mon-key striate cortex. *Journal of Physiology (London)*, 195:215–243.

Huerta, M.F., Krubitzer, L.A., and Kaas, J.H. (1987) Frontal eye field as defined by intra-cortical microstimulation in squirrel monkeys, owl monkeys, and macaque monkeys II. Cortical connections. *Journal of Comparative Neurology*, 265:332–361.

Hyman, B.T., Van Hoesen, G.W., Damasio, A.R., and Barnes, C.L. (1984) Alzheimer's dis-ease: Cell-specific pathology isolates the hippocampal formation. *Science*, 225:1168–1170.

Ilinsky, I.A., Jouandet, M.L., and Goldman-Rakic, P.S. (1985) Organization of the nigro-thalamocortical system in the rhesus monkey. *Journal of Comparative Neurology*, 236:315–330.

Ilinsky, I.A., and Kultas-Ilinsky, K. (1987) Sagittal cytoarchitectonic maps of the *Macaca mulatta* thalamus with a revised nomenclature of the motor-related nuclei validated by observations on their connectivity. *Journal of Comparative Neurology*, 262:331–364.

Innocenti, G.M. (1981) Growth and reshaping of axons in the establishment of visual cal-losal connections. *Science*, 212:824–827.

Innocenti, G.M., Clarke, S., and Kraftsik, R. (1986) Interchange of callosal and association projections in the developing cortex. *Journal of Neuroscience*, 6:1384–1409.

Innocenti, G.M., Fiore, L., and Caminiti, R. (1977) Exuberant projection into the corpus callosum from the visual cortex of newborn cats. *Neuroscience Letters*, 4:237–242.

Irle, E., and Markowitsch, H.J. (1982) Widespread cortical projections of the hippocampal formation in the cat. *Neuroscience*, 7:2637–2647.

Isseroff, A., Rosvold., H.E., Galkin, T.W., and Goldman-Rakic, P.S. (1982) Spatial memory impairments following damage to the mediodorsal nucleus of the thalamus in rhesus monkeys. *Brain Research*, 232:97–113.

Ivy, G.O., Akers, R.M., and Killackey, H.P. (1979) Differential distribution of callosal pro-jection neurons in the neonatal and adult rat. *Brain Research*, 173:532–537.

Jacobsen, C.F. (1936) Studies of cerebral function in primates: I. The functions of the frontal association area in monkeys. *Comparative Psychology Monographs*, 13:3–60.

Janowsky, J.S., Shimamura, A.P., Kritchevsky, M., and Squire, L.R. (1989) Cognitive im-pairment following frontal lobe damage and its relevance to human amnesia. *Behavioral Neuroscience*, 103:548–560.

Jones, E.G. (1985) *The Thalamus*. New York: Plenum Press.

Jones, E.G., and Leavitt, R.Y. (1974) Retrograde axonal transport and the demonstration of non-specific projections to the cerebral cortex and striatum from thalamic intralaminar nuclei in the rat, cat, and monkey. *Journal of Comparative Neurology*, 154:349–378.

Kaada, B.R., Pribram, K.H., and Epstein, J.A. (1949) Respiratory and vascular responses in monkeys from temporal pole, insula, orbital surface and cingulate gyrus. *Journal of Neurophysiology,* 12:347–356.

Kievit, J., and Kuypers, H.G.J.M. (1977) Organization of the thalamo-cortical connexions to the frontal lobe in the rhesus monkey. *Experimental Brain Research,* 29:299–322.

Kling, A., and Steklis, H.D. (1976) A neural substrate for affiliative behavior in nonhuman primates. *Brain Behavior and Evolution,* 13:216–238.

Kojima, S., and Goldman-Rakic, P.S. (1982) Delay-related activity of prefrontal neurons in rhesus monkeys performing delayed response. *Brain Research,* 248:43–49.

Kromer Vogt, L.J., Van Hoesen, G.W., Hyman, B.T., and Damasio, A.R. (1990) Pathological alterations in the amygdala in Alzheimer's disease. *Neuroscience,* 37:377–385.

Kruger, L., Bendotti, C., Rivolta, R., and Samanin, R. (1992) GAP-43 mRNA localization in the rat hippocampus CA3 field. *Molecular Brain Research,* 13:267–272.

Kubota, K., and Niki, H. (1990) Prefrontal cortical unit activity and delayed alternation performance in monkeys. *Journal of Neurophysiology,* 34:337–347.

Kubota, K., Tonoike, M., and Mikami, A. (1980) Neuronal activity in the monkey dorsolateral prefrontal cortex during a discrimination task with delay. *Brain Research,* 183:29–42.

Laemle, L.K., and Sharma, S.C. (1986) Bilateral projections of neurons in the lateral geniculate nucleus and nucleus lateralis posterior to the visual cortex in the neonatal rat. *Neuroscience Letters,* 63:207–214.

LeDoux, J.E. (1994) Emotion, memory and the brain. *Scientific American,* 270:50–57.

Le Gros Clark, W.E. (1932) The structure and connections of the thalamus. *Brain,* 35:406–470.

Lewis, D.A., Campbell, M.J., Terry, R.D., and Morrison, J.H. (1987) Laminar and regional distributions of neurofibrillary tangles and neuritic plaques in Alzheimer's disease: A quantitative study of visual and auditory cortices. *Journal of Neuroscience,* 7:1799–1808.

Lovinger, D.M., Akers, R.F., Nelson, R.B., Barnes, C.A., McNaughton, B.L., and Routtenberg, A. (1985) A selective increase in phosporylation of protein F1, a protein kinase C substrate, directly related to three day growth of long term synaptic enhancement. *Brain Research,* 343:137–143.

Mahut, H. (1971) Spatial and object reversal learning in monkeys with partial temporal lobe ablations. *Neuropsychologia,* 9:409–424.

Mahut, H. (1972) A selective spatial deficit in monkeys after transection of the fornix. *Neuropsychologia,* 10:65–74.

Mahut, H., Zola-Morgan, S., and Moss, M. (1982) Hippocampal resections impair associative learning and recognition memory in the monkey. *Journal of Neuroscience,* 2:1214–1229.

Markowitsch, H.J. (1982) Thalamic mediodorsal nucleus and memory: A critical evaluation of studies in animals and man. *Neuroscience and Biobehavioral Reviews,* 6:351–380.

Mesulam, M.-M. (1981) A cortical network for directed attention and unilateral neglect. *Annals of Neurology,* 10:309–325.

Mesulam, M.-M. (1990) Large-scale neurocognitive networks and distributed processing for attention, language, and memory. *Annals of Neurology,* 28:597–613.

Meunier, M., Bachevalier, J., Mishkin, M., and Murray, E.A. (1993) Effects on visual recognition of combined and separate ablations of the entorhinal and perirhinal cortex in rhesus monkeys. *Journal of Neuroscience,* 13:5418–5432.

Milner, B., and Petrides, M. (1984) Behavioural effects of frontal-lobe lesions in man. *Trends in Neuroscience,* 7:403–407.

Minciacchi, D., and Granato, A. (1989) Development of the thalamocortical system: Transient-crossed projections to the frontal cortex in neonatal rats. *Journal of Comparative Neurology,* 281:1–12.

Mischel, P.S., Nguyen, L.P., and Vinters, H.V. (1995) Cerebral cortical dysplasia associated with pediatric epilepsy: review of neuropathologic features and proposal for a grading system. *Journal of Neuropathology and Experimental Neurology,* 54:137–153.

Morecraft, R.J., Geula, C., and Mesulam, M.-M. (1992) Cytoarchitecture and neural afferents of orbitofrontal cortex in the brain of the monkey. *Journal of Comparative Neurology,* 323:341–358.

Morrison, J.H., Hof, P.R., Campbell, M.J., De Lima, A.D., Voigt, T., Bouras, C., Cox, K., Young, W.G. (1990) Cellular pathology in Alzheimers disease: Implications for corticocortical disconnection and differential vulnerability. In (S.R.) Rapoport, H. Petit, D. Leys, and Y. Christen (eds.), *Imaging, Cerebral Topography and Alzheimer's Disease.* Berlin and Heidelberg: Springer-Verlag, pp. 19–40.

Muramoto, O., and Kuru, Y. (1979) Pure memory loss with hippocampal lesions. *Archives of Neurology,* 36:54–56.

Murray, E.A., and Mishkin, M. (1986) Visual recognition in monkeys following rhinal cortical ablations combined with either amygdalectomy or hippocampectomy. *Journal of Neuroscience,* 6:1991–2003.

Nauta, W.J.H. (1961) Fibre degeneration following lesions of the amygdaloid complex in the monkey. *Journal of Anatomy,* 95:515–531.

Nauta, W.J.H. (1971) The problem of the frontal lobe: A reinterpretation. *Journal of Psychiatric Research,* 8:167–187.

Nauta, W.J.H. (1979) Expanding borders of the limbic system concept. In T. Rasmussen and R. Marino (eds.), *Functional Neurosurgery.* New York: Raven Press, pp. 7–23.

Nelson, R.B., Friedman, D.P., O'Neill, J.B., Mishkin, M., and Routtenberg, A. (1987) Gradients of protein kinase C substrate phosphorylation in primate visual system peak in visual memory storage areas. *Brain Research,* 416:387–392.

Neve, R.L., Finch, E.A., Bird, E.D., and Benowitz, L.I. (1988) Growth-associated protein GAP-43 is expressed selectively in associative regions of the adult human brain. *Proceedings of the National Academy of Sciences of the USA,* 85:3638–3642.

O'Leary, D.D., Schlaggar, B.L., and Tuttle, R. (1994) Specification of neocortical areas and thalamocortical connections. *Annual Review of Neuroscience,* 17:419–439.

O'Leary, D.D.M., Stanfield, B.B., and Cowan, W.M. (1981) Evidence that the early postnatal restriction of the cells of origin of the callosal projection is due to the elimination of axonal collaterals rather than to the death of neurons. *Developmental Brain Research,* 1:607–617.

Oyoshi, T., Nishijo, H., Asakura, T., Takamura, Y., and Ono, T. (1996) Emotional and behavioral correlates of mediodorsal thalamic neurons during associative learning in rats. *Journal of Neuroscience,* 16:5812–5829.

Pandya, D.N., Seltzer, B., and Barbas, H. (1988) Input-output organization of the primate cerebral cortex. In H.D. Steklis, and J. Erwin (eds.), *Comparative Primate Biology, Vol. IV: Neurosciences.* New York: Alan R. Liss, pp. 39–80.

Papez, J.W. (1937) A proposed mechanism of emotion. *American Medical Association Archives of Neurology and Psychiatry,* 38:725–743.

Parkinson, J.K., Murray, E.A., and Mishkin, M. (1988) A selective mnemonic role for the hippocampus in monkeys: Memory for the location of objects. *Journal of Neuroscience,* 8:4159–4167.

Pearson, R.C.A., Esiri, M.M., Hiorns, R.W., Wilcock, G.K., and Powell, T.P.S. Anatomical correlates of the distribution of the pathological changes in the neocortex in Alzheimer's disease. *Proceedings of the National Academy of Sciences of the USA,* 82:4531–4534.

Penfield, W., and Jasper, H. (1954) *Epilepsy and the Functional Anatomy of the Human Brain.* Boston: Little, Brown.

Petrides, M. (1989) Frontal lobes and memory. In F. Boller, and J. Grafman (eds.), *Handbook of Neuropsychology, Vol. III.* New York: Elsevier (Biomedical Division), pp. 75–90.

Petrides, M., and Pandya, D.N. (1984) Projections to the frontal cortex from the posterior parietal region in the rhesus monkey. *Journal of Comparative Neurology,* 228:105–116.

Potter, H., and Nauta, W.J.H. (1979) A note on the problem of olfactory associations of the orbitofrontal cortex in the monkey. *Neuroscience,* 4:361–367.

Preuss, T.M., and Goldman-Rakic, P.S. (1987) Crossed corticothalamic and thalamocortical connections of macaque prefrontal cortex. *Journal of Comparative Neurology,* 257: 269–281.

Ray, J.P., and Price, J.L. (1993) The organization of projections from the mediodorsal nucleus of the thalamus to orbital and medial prefrontal cortex in macaque monkeys. *Journal of Comparative Neurology,* 337:1–31.

Reep, R. (1984) Relationship between prefrontal and limbic cortex: A comparative and anatomical review. *Brain Behavior and Evolution,* 25:1–80.

Rempel-Clower, N. (1994) *Human amnesia and the hippocampal region: neuropsychological and neuropathological findings from two new patients. Ph.D. thesis, University of California at San Diego.*

Rempel-Clower, N.L., Zola, S.M., Squire, L.R., and Amaral, D.G. (1996) Three cases of enduring memory impairment after bilateral damage limited to the hippocampal formation. *Journal of Neuroscience,* 16:5233–5255.

Reynolds, J.P. (1989) Beyond the dopamine hypothesis. The neurochemical pathology of schizophrenia. *British Journal of Psychiatry,* 155:305–316.

Roberts, G.W., Ferrier, I.N., Lee, Y., Crow, E.C.J., and Bloom, S.R. (1983) Peptides, the limbic lobe and schizophrenia. *Brain Research,* 288:199–211.

Rockland, K.S., and Pandya, D.N. (1979) Laminar origins and terminations of cortical connections of the occipital lobe in the rhesus monkey. *Brain Research,* 179:3–20.

Rodman, H.R., and Consuelos, M.J. (1994) Cortical projections to anterior inferior temporal cortex in infant macaque monkeys. *Visual Neuroscience,* 11:119–133.

Rosene, D.L., and Van Hoesen, G.W. (1977) Hippocampal efferents reach widespread areas of cerebral cortex and amygdala in the rhesus monkey. *Science,* 198:315–317.

Routtenberg, A. (1985) Protein kinase C and substrate protein F1 (47 kD, 4.5 pI): Relation to synaptic plasticity and growth. *Advances in Behavioral Biology,* 28:107–117.

Russchen, F.T., Amaral, D.G., and Price, J.L. (1987) The afferent input to the magnocellular division of the mediodorsal thalamic nucleus in the monkey, *Macaca fascicularis. Journal of Comparative Neurology,* 256:175–210.

Sakai, K., and Miyashita, Y. (1994) Visual imagery: An interaction between memory retrieval and focal attention. *Trends in Neuroscience,* 17:287–289.

Sanides, F. (1969) Comparative architectonics of the neocortex of mammals and their evolutionary interpretation. *Annals of the New York Academy of Science,* 167:404–423.

Sanides, F. (1970) Functional architecture of motor and sensory cortices in primates in the light of a new concept of neocortex evolution. In C.R. Noback and W. Montagna (eds.), *The Primate Brain: Advances in Primatology,* Vol. 1 Appleton-Century-Crofts, N.Y. pp. 137–208.

Sawaguchi, T., and Goldman-Rakic, P.S. (1991) D1 dopamine receptors in prefrontal cortex: Involvement in working memory. *Science,* 251:947–950.

Sawaguchi, T., Matsumura, M., and Kubota, K. (1988) Dopamine enhances the neuronal activity of spatial short-term memory task in the primate prefrontal cortex. *Neuroscience Research,* 5:465–473.

Scheibel, M.E., and Scheibel, A.B. (1967) Structural organization of nonspecific thalamic nuclei and their projection toward cortex. *Brain Research,* 6:60–94.

Schlag, J., and Schlag-Rey, M. (1984) Visuomotor functions of central thalamus in monkey. II. Unit activity related to visual events, targeting, and fixation. *Journal of Neurophysiology,* 51:1175–1195.

Schlag-Rey, M., and Schlag, J. (1984) Visuomotor functions of central thalamus in monkey. I. Unit activity related to spontaneous eye movements. *Journal of Neurophysiology,* 51:1149–1174.

Schwartz, M.L., and Goldman-Rakic, P.S. (1984) Callosal and intrahemispheric connectivity of the prefrontal association cortex in rhesus monkey: Relation between intraparietal and principal sulcal cortex. *Journal of Comparative Neurology,* 226:403–420.

Schwartz, M.L., and Goldman-Rakic, P.S. (1991) Prenatal specification of callosal connections in rhesus monkey. *Journal of Comparative Neurology,* 307:144–162.

Schwartz, M.L., Rakic, P., and Goldman-Rakic, P.S. (1991) Early phenotype expression of cortical neurons—evidence that a subclass of migrating neurons have callosal axons. *Proceedings of the National Academy of Sciences of the USA,* 88:1354–1358.

Schwerdtfeger, W.K. (1979) Direct efferent and afferent connections of the hippocampus with the neocortex in the marmoset monkey. *American Journal of Anatomy,* 156:77–82.

Scoville, W.B., and Milner, B. (1957) Loss of recent memory after bilateral hippocampal lesions. *Journal of Neurology, Neurosurgery, and Psychiatry,* 20:11–21.

Skene, J.H., and Willard, M. (1981a) Changes in axonally transported proteins during axon regeneration in toad retinal ganglion cells. *Journal of Cell Biology,* 89:86–95.

Skene, J.H., and Willard, M. (1981b) Axonally transported proteins associated with axon growth in rabbit central and peripheral nervous systems. *Journal of Cell Biology,* 89:96–103.

Snipes, G.J., Chan, S.Y., McGuire, C.B., Costello, B.R., Norden, J.J., Freeman, J.A., Routtenberg, A. (1987) Evidence for the coidentification of GAP-43, a growth-associated protein, and F1, a plasticity-associated protein. *Journal of Neuroscience,* 7:4066–4075.

Squire, L.R. (1992) Memory and the hippocampus: A synthesis from findings with rats, monkeys, and humans. *Psychological Review,* 99:195–231.

Squire, L.R., and Zola-Morgan, S. (1988) Memory: Brain systems and behavior. *Trends in Neuroscience,* 11:170–175.

Sur, M., and Cowey, A. (1995) Cerebral cortex: Function and development. *Neuron,* 15:497–505.

Takada, M., Fishell, G., Li, Z.K., Van Der Kooy, D., and Hattori, T. (1987) The development of laterality in the forebrain projections of midline thalamic cell groups in the rat. *Developmental Brain Research,* 35:275–282.

Takagi, S.F. (1986) Studies on the olfactory nervous system of the old world monkey. *Progress in Neurobiology,* 27:195–250.

Talland, G.A., Sweet, W.H., and Ballantine, T. (1967) Amnesic syndrome with anterior communicating artery aneurysm. *Journal of Nervous and Mental Disease,* 145:179–192.

Tigges, J., Tigges, M., Cross, N.A., McBride, R.L., Letbetter, W.D., and Anschel, S. (1982) Subcortical structures projecting to visual cortical areas in squirrel monkey. *Journal of Comparative Neurology,* 209:29–40.

Trojanowski, J.Q., and Jacobson, S. (1974) Medial pulvinar afferents to frontal eye fields in rhesus monkey demonstrated by horseradish peroxidase. *Brain Research,* 80:395–411.

Ullman, S. (1995) Sequence seeking and counter streams: A computational model for bidirectional information in the visual cortex. *Cerebral Cortex,* 5:1–11.

Van Hoesen, G.W., Hyman, B.T., and Damasio, A.R. (1991) Entorhinal cortex pathology in Alzheimer's disease. *Hippocampus,* 1:1–8.

Vizzard, M.A., Erdman, S.L., and de Groat, W.C. (1995) Increased expression of neuronal nitric oxide synthase (NOS) in visceral neurons after nerve injury. *Journal of Neuroscience,* 15(5):4033–4045.

Vogt, B.A., Van Hoesen, G.W., and Vogt, L.J. (1990) Laminar distribution of neuron degeneration in posterior cingulate cortex in Alzheimer's disease. *Acta Neuropathologica,* 80:581–589.

Voytko, M.L. (1985) Cooling orbital frontal cortex disrupts matching-to-sample and visual discrimination learning in monkeys. *Physiological Psychology,* 13:219–229.

Weinberger, D.R. (1988) Schizophrenia and the frontal lobe. *Trends in Neuroscience,* 11: 367–370.

Wise, S.P., and Jones, E.G. (1976) The organization and postnatal development of the commissural projection of the rat somatic sensory cortex. *Journal of Comparative Neurology,* 168:313–344.

Wurtz, R.H., and Albano, J.E. (1980) Visual-motor function of the primate superior colliculus, *Annual Review of Neuroscience,* 3:189–226.

Yakovlev, P.I. (1948) Motility, behavior and the brain: Stereodynamic organization and neurocoordinates of behavior. *Journal of Nervous and Mental Disease,* 107:313–335.

Zola-Morgan, S., and Squire, L.R. (1993) Neuroanatomy of memory. *Annual Review of Neuroscience,* 16:547–563.

Zola-Morgan, S., Squire, L.R., and Amaral, D.G. (1986) Human amnesia and the medial temporal region: Enduring memory impairment following a bilateral lesion limited to field CA1 of the hippocampus. *Journal of Neuroscience,* 6:2950–2967.

Zola-Morgan, S., Squire, L.R., and Amaral, D.G. (1989a) Lesions of the amygdala that spare adjacent cortical regions do not impair memory or exacerbate the impairment following lesions of the hippocampal formation. *Journal of Neuroscience,* 9:1922–1936.

Zola-Morgan, S., Squire, L.R., and Amaral, D.G. (1989b) Lesions of the hipppocampal formation but not lesions of the fornix or the mammillary nuclei produce long-lasting memory impairment in monkeys. *Journal of Neuroscience,* 9:898–913.

Zola-Morgan, S., Squire, L.R., Amaral, D.G., and Suzuki, W.A. (1989c) Lesions of perirhinal and parahippocampal cortex that spare the amygdala and hippocampal formation produce severe memory impairment. *Journal of Neuroscience,* 9:4355–4370.

Zola-Morgan, S., Squire, L.R., Clower, R.P., and Rempel, N.L. (1993) Damage to the perirhinal cortex exacerbates memory impairment following lesions to the hippocampal formation. *Journal of Neuroscience,* 13:251–265.

6

Reorganization of Function After Cortical Lesions in Rodents

BRYAN KOLB AND IAN Q. WHISHAW

One of the major accomplishments of neuropsychology in the twentieth century has been to establish that functions are relatively localized in the cerebral cortex. There can be little doubt anymore that damage to the primary motor cortex will produce a specific loss of certain motor abilities or that damage to the occipital areas will produce specific alterations in visual functions. This localization of function presents a major clinical problem, however, for it implies that there is little hope for functional restitution after cortical injury. But this is not entirely true, as it has become clear that partial restitution of function may be possible, at least under some circumstances. Indeed, it has been known since 1868 that damage to the left hemisphere of children does not necessarily lead to permanent language deficits. Even Broca was apparently aware of this possibility, as he wrote: "I am convinced that a lesion of the left third frontal convolution, apt to produce lasting aphemia (aphasia) in an adult, will not prevent a small child from learning to talk" (Finger & Almli, 1988, p. 122). Since there was little doubt that language ought to have been affected by the injuries in Broca's young patients, it was reasonable for him to presume that there had been a fundamental change in the cortical organization of these children. Although such extensive reorganization is not seen in adults after cerebral injury, there is growing evidence that at least some recovery is possible in certain types of cerebral injury and that it may be possible to influence recovery processes by intervention.

Routes to Recovery

In principle, there are three ways in which the brain could show plastic changes that might support recovery. First, there could be reorganization of remaining circuits. Since it seems unlikely that a localized structure like the cerebral cortex could undergo a wholesale reorganization of cortical connectivity in the adult, we assume that recovery from cortical damage will most likely result from a change in the intrinsic organization of local cortical circuits in regions directly or indirectly disrupted by the injury. We recognize, however, that it might be possible to produce significant reorganization of cortical connectivity in the developing brain. Indeed, Broca's young patients seem to provide evidence in support of this possibility. We also assume that the best place to look for evidence of cortical reorganization is the output cells (i.e., pyramidal cells). This does not preclude changes in the intrinsic cortical neurons, but our focus has been on the pyramidal neurons, largely layers III and V. These cells are easily visualized using Golgi-type stains, and both their dendritic morphology and their distribution of spines, which are the presumptive site of a majority of their excitatory synapses, are clearly visible with the light microscope.

A second route to cerebral reorganization could be stimulated by the exogenous application of different treatments. This could take the form of behavioral therapy or it might involve pharmacological treatment that would influence reparative processes in the remaining brain. Once again, it seems most likely that the induced changes would occur in the intrinsic organization of the cortex, although the changes might be more widespread than in endogenous change, in part because the treatment could act on the whole brain. Thus, a pharmacological agent introduced into either the cerebral ventricles or the bloodstream could influence the entire brain. Similarly, a behavioral therapy would focus on neural regions involved in the behaviors produced by the therapy.

Finally, it should be possible, at least in principle, to replace lost neurons and at least some functions. This logic has led to considerable work on neural transplantation, although the utility of this approach is far from proven. There is, in addition, another and even less developed possibility: to stimulate the injured brain to replace its own neurons. The adult mammalian brain maintains a quiescent population of stem cells in the subventricular zone, and it may be possible to induce these cells to divide after a cerebral injury. This route to recovery is far more speculative, but we shall see that recent findings are encouraging.

We shall consider each of these routes to functional reorganization and restitution in turn. In addition, we shall separate our discussion of the changes in the adult and developing brain since there are important differences between the reparative processes in the adult and infant brain.

Endogenous Change after Cortical Injury

It is a general principle that when neurons lose synapses, there is a retraction of dendritic arborization; conversely, when neurons gain synapses, there is an extension of dendritic arborization (Figure 6-1). This principle can be seen clearly in the extensive studies by Oswald Steward and his colleagues on the effects of entorhinal lesions on spatial learning and the structure of hippocampal neurons. These studies show that animals with unilateral entorhinal cortex lesions exhibit an initial deficit

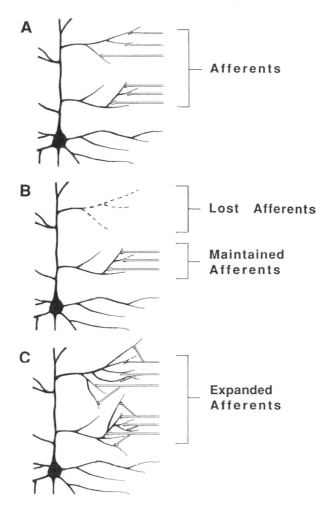

Figure 6-1. Putative changes to neurons with loss or increase of afferents. (A) Standard neuron. (B) Retraction of dendrites with loss of afferents. (C) Extension of dendrites with addition of afferents.

in spatial learning that disappears over time. This recovery is correlated with changes in hippocampal connectivity and the dendritic morphology of hippocampal neurons (e.g., Steward, 1991). The Steward studies show clearly that there are endogenous changes in cerebral connectivity after cortical lesions and that these changes have a behavioral correlate. Rather than looking at the effects of damage to hippocampal formation, we have focused on the effect of unilateral or bilateral lesions of the neocortex. We began by developing an extensive neuropsychological test battery for the rat (Whishaw et al., 1983). We then characterized the chronic behavioral effects of lesions throughout the neocortical mantle (for a review, see Kolb & Whishaw, 1989).

Our first studies on the anatomical correlates of recovery of function looked at the effects of bilateral frontal lesions on the performance of spatial navigation tasks in rats. Rats with large midline frontal lesions show severe deficits in various tests of spatial navigation followed by slow improvement (for a review, see Kolb, 1995). When we analyzed the dendritic morphology in these studies, our general finding was that there is initial atrophy in dendritic fields of cortical pyramidal cells in adjacent sensorimotor cortex, followed by regrowth of dendritic material such that there is a net gain in dendritic space (Kolb, 1995; Kolb & Gibb, 1991). These dendritic changes are temporally correlated with recovery of performance on cognitive tasks, such as the Morris water task (Kolb, 1995). That is, in the early postinjury period there is dendritic atrophy in areas adjacent to the injury, and the animals perform the spatial tasks very poorly. Later, as the neurons expand their dendritic fields, there is marked improvement in spatial learning. This temporal correlation between anatomical and behavioral changes after cortical injury was encouraging and led us to pursue this line of inquiry.

One difficulty with studies using maze tasks is that training is usually extensive and it is difficult to make a rapid assessment of functional recovery. Thus, more recently, our studies have focused on the effect of motor cortex lesions. Rats can be trained preoperatively to use their forepaws to retrieve small pieces of food and, once trained, they remain efficient indefinitely (e.g., (Whishaw & Pellis 1992); Whishaw et al., 1986. Thus, animals can then be given various lesions and tested quickly, and routinely, for functional recovery. Our studies of rats with motor cortex lesions have led us to several conclusions.

First, animals with lesions restricted to the forelimb region of the motor cortex show substantial improvement in reaching efficiency (Fig. 6-2). However, recovery is far from complete. Thus, when we have studied the kinematics of the movements of animals with similar lesions, we have found that the animals make markedly different movements than they did preoperatively (Whishaw et al., 1991). Thus, the apparent recovery in achieving accuracy reflects not only some behavioral recovery but also behavioral compensation.

Second, the extent of functional recovery varies directly with the size of the lesion. Animals with restricted lesions, such as those summarized in Figure 6-2, show substantial recovery, whereas animals with larger lesions, which remove most of the motor cortex, show far less improvement. Indeed, animals with lesions that include most of the sensorimotor cortex show virtually no improvement in using the limb contralateral to the lesion, even when they are given extensive training.

One experimental advantage of the observed variance in the extent of recovery with lesions of different sizes is that it allows us to make predictions about the relationship between dendritic reorganization and recovery. Hence, if dendritic growth is related in some way to postinjury improvement, then animals with significant improvement should show dendritic growth, whereas animals without recovery should probably show dendritic atrophy. This is the case. In our studies of reaching in rats with restricted motor cortex injuries, we found initial atrophy of dendritic fields of pyramidal neurons in the remaining motor cortex, followed by expansion of the dendritic fields of the pyramidal neurons in the remaining motor cortex

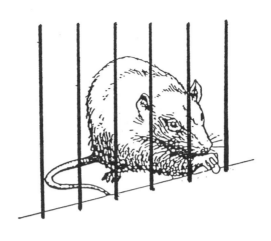

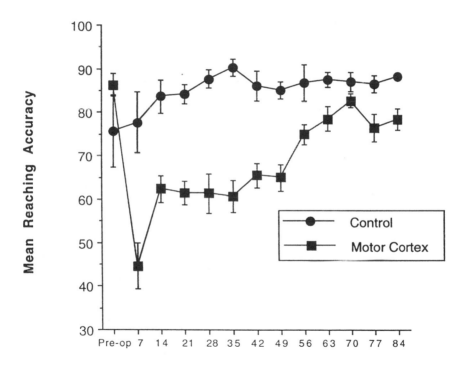

Figure 6-2. Top: the Whishaw reaching task. Bottom: recovery of forelimb reaching accuracy after small motor cortex lesions.

(Kolb et al., 2000a; Rowntree & Kolb, 1997). We can speculate that this increased dendritic space reflects an increase in the number of synapses on the dendrites, although we have not yet measured this directly. In contrast, when we analyzed the changes in rats with large sensorimotor cortex lesions, we found only atrophy in the remaining pyramidal neurons in the residual motor cortex (e.g, Kolb et al., 1997). Furthermore, when we studied animals with transections of the pyramidal tract, which cuts the spinal cord–projecting axons of pyramidal cells in motor cortex, we found no functional restitution and no change in cortical pyramidal neurons in motor cortex (Whishaw et al., 1993).

In sum, it appears that recovery of spatial learning after medial frontal lesions and forelimb use after restricted motor cortex lesions is correlated with an expansion of dendritic fields in regions adjacent to the lesion. Furthermore, this dendritic expansion is seen only in animals with an improved behavioral outcome. It is reasonable to predict, therefore, that treatments that act to potentiate dendritic growth might be correlated with an enhanced functional outcome (see below).

Endogenous Change After Cortical Injury in the Developing Brain

The first systematic studies of the effects of early cortical injury on behavior in adulthood were done by Margaret Kennard in the late 1930s. She created unilateral motor cortex lesions in infant and adult monkeys and studied their subsequent ability to use their forelimbs to locomote, climb, and retrieve objects. Her most important observation was that the impairments in the infant monkeys appeared to be milder than those in the adults. This led Kennard to hypothesize that there had been a change in cortical organization in the infants and that this reorganization supported the behavioral recovery. In particular, she hypothesized that if some synapses were removed as a consequence of brain injury, "others would be formed in less usual combinations" and that "it is possible that factors which facilitate cortical organization in the normal young are the same by which reorganization is accomplished in the imperfect cortex after injury" (Kennard, 1942, p. 239). Although Kennard had much to say about the limitations of functional recovery after early brain injury (see the review by Finger & Almli, 1988), it was her demonstration that the consequences of motor cortex lesions in infancy were less severe than those of similar injuries, in adulthood that is usually associated with her name and is commonly referred to as the *Kennard principle.*

Kennard was aware that early brain damage might actually produce more severe deficits than expected, but it was Hebb (1949) who focused on this issue. "It appears . . . that an early injury may prevent the development of some intellectual capacities that an equally extensive injury, at maturity, would not have destroyed . . . Physiologically, the matter may be put as follows: some types of behaviour that require a large amount of brain tissue for their first establishment can then persist when the amount of available tissue has been decreased. This of course is consistent with the theory of cell-assemblies . . . . It has been postulated that, with the enlargement of synaptic knobs, the number of fibers necessary for transmission at the synapse decreases. In the first establishment of an assembly, then, more fibers are necessary than for its later functioning" (Hebb, 1949, pp. 292–293).

The difference between the views of Kennard and Hebb is important in the current context, for it provides an important starting point for studies looking for a relationship between synaptic change and behavior. Whereas Kennard hypothesized that recovery from early brain damage was associated with a reorganization into novel neural networks, Hebb postulated that the failure to recover was correlated with a failure of initial organization of basic neural networks. Hebb also made an important point about recovery from cerebral injury in adulthood. He expected that recovery would be possible since he believed that less neural tissue would be needed to support at least certain types of behavior, once learned, than for the initial learning. Hebb recognized, however, that the functioning of partially damaged cell assemblies might be less reliable and more easily subject to disruption.

We are left with several behavioral and anatomical predictions that follow from both Kennard's and Hebb's hypotheses. First, from Kennard, we should be able to demonstrate functional recovery of some types of behavior after injury during development. Second, from Hebb, we should be able to show a worsened effect of brain injury at other times during development. Finally, it follows from both Kennard and Hebb that we ought to be able to identify a synaptic correlate of these two functional outcomes. In addition, as a corollary, if we are able to manipulate the synaptic correlate, function should also be affected. In sum, studies of the functional and anatomical consequences of cerebral injury at different ages ought to provide a window on the general mechanism by which synaptic plasticity is related to behavioral and cognitive flexibility.

The resolution of the Kennard-Hebb predictions is related to the precise developmental status of the brain at the time of injury. This developmental status varies considerably relative to the time of birth for different mammalian species. The neurological status of different species is easily inferred from the behavioral capacity at birth. Precocial species such as cows and horses are born able to walk and to investigate the world, whereas other species such as cats and dogs are born blind and with limited motor capacities. Rats are born even less developed than kittens and thus provide an excellent subject for developmental studies because much of their neurological development is ex utero and thus can be manipulated fairly easily. We note that humans and monkeys fall somewhere between rats and the more precocial species. Thus, in order to compare the effects of lesions to the cortex of rats and primates, we must match the developmental status at the time of injury (Fig 6-3).

Over the past 20 years, we have removed virtually every region of the cortical mantle of rats at varying ages ranging from birth to adolescence. Our general finding is that cortical injury during the first few days of life is functionally devastating, whereas similar damage at 7–12 days of age allows remarkable sparing and/or recovery of function (for reviews, see Kolb, 1995; Kolb & Whishaw, 1989; Kolb et al., 1996b). For example, rats with medial frontal lesions on the first days of life are severely impaired in adulthood at a wide range of cognitive and motor tasks, including tasks for which adults with similar lesions would not be impaired. Similarly, rats with motor cortex lesions on the day of birth show very poor development of motor skills with their forelimbs, and they too are impaired in performing cognitive tasks that would present no difficulty for adult rats (Fig 6-4). Thus, rats

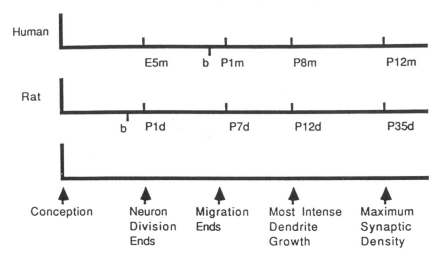

Figure 6-3. Schematic illustration of the comparable developmental ages of rat and human brain. Note that the day of birth in the rat is much earlier in embryonic development than the day of birth in the human. Rhesus monkeys are born even more developed than humans. Abbreviations: E, embryonic day; P, postnatal day; b, day of birth.

with cortical injuries in the first days of life show a functional outcome that is reminiscent of retardation in human infants with injuries in the third trimester of gestation. In contrast, rats with medial frontal or motor cortex injuries at 7–10 days of age show behavioral capacities in adulthood that exceed those of animals with similar lesions at any other time. In fact, on some behavioral tests, these animals show recovery that is virtually complete. Importantly, this recovery is far more extensive on cognitive tasks, such as the learning of various spatial navigation problems, than it is on tests of species-typical behaviors (Kolb & Whishaw, 1981). This difference is important and probably reflects the relative ease of reorganized cortical circuitry in supporting different types of behavior. We must note here that the extent of functional recovery is not equivalent in animals with lesions in different cortical regions. The most extensive recovery is associated with lesions of the frontal regions, and the least extensive recovery is associated with damage to the primary sensory areas. For example, rats with occipital lesions on day 10 show no recovery of visually guided behaviors. In contrast, they show an enhanced somatosensory capacity that is not observed after similar lesions on day 4, which is consistent the general idea that there is something special about the sequelae of injuries around 10 days of age (Kolb et al., 1996a).

We have analyzed the morphological changes associated with early lesions in two ways. First, we have examined the dendritic fields of cortical pyramidal cells after lesions at different ages. We predicted that if dendritic changes were supporting recovery of function, then animals with lesions on day 10 should show dendritic hypertrophy, whereas animals with lesions on days 1–5 should show dendritic atrophy. This prediction was confirmed. Rats with lesions in either frontal,

Whishaw Reaching Task

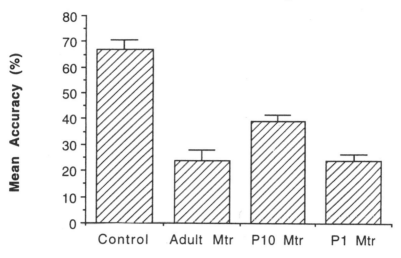

Morris Water Task

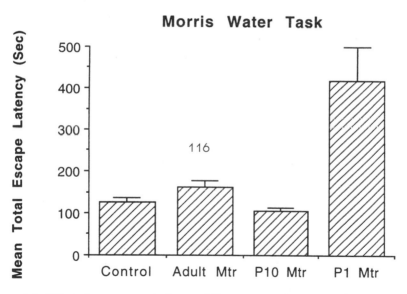

Figure 6-4. Effect of motor cortex lesions at different postnatal ages on performance of the Whishaw reaching task and the Morris water task. Rats with lesions on postnatal day 10 show significant recovery of function relative to rats with similar lesions in adulthood. Rats with lesions on postnatal day 1 show both motor impairments and impairments on the Morris water task.

Day 1   Day 10

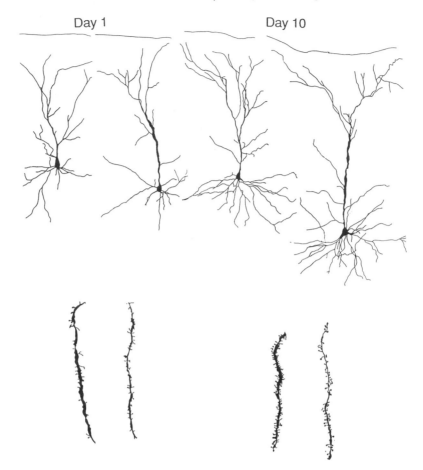

Figure 6-5. Representative examples of layer III pyramidal neurons (top) and representative terminal dendritic segments (bottom) from the brains of rats with medial frontal lesions on either postnatal day 1 or 10. The cell from the day 1 rat illustrates both atrophy of dendrites and decreased spine density, whereas the cell from the day 10 rat illustrates hypertrophy of dendrites and increased spine density.

parietal, or occipital cortex at 10 days of age all showed increased dendritic arborization and increased spine density, whereas those with similar lesions prior to 5 days of age showed decreased dendritic arborization and decreased spine density (Fig. 6-5). These findings parallel directly our findings from studies in adults. Furthermore, these findings provide an anatomical explanation for the Kennard and Hebb effects: Increased synaptic formation is correlated with a good functional outcome, whereas decreased synaptic formation is correlated with a very poor functional outcome.

Our second morphological analysis has examined the possibility that early lesions allow significant reorganization of cortical connectivity with subcortical

Control   P10 Bilateral   P1 Bilateral

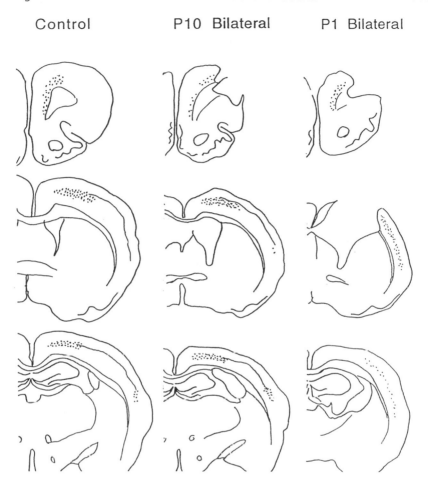

Figure 6-6. Summary of representative examples of the pattern of retrograde labeling of corticospinal neurons in rats with bilateral motor cortex lesions or postnatal day 10 (P10) or day 1 (P1). The labeling pattern is far more extensive in the P1 animals. This was correlated with a disruption of performance on tasks not normally affected by motor cortex lesions.

structures. In one series of studies, we focused on the corticospinal projections following motor cortex injury on day 1, day 10, or in adulthood (Kolb & et al., 2000b; Whishaw & Kolb, 1988). Rats were given unilateral or bilateral, motor cortex injuries, tested 90 days later in a series of behavioral tests, and then injected with a fluorescent retrograde tracer into the lower cervical spinal cord. This allowed us to determine the source of the corticospinal projections arising from the motor cortex. The principal findings of these studies were that (*1*) there was an expansion of the ipsilateral corticospinal projection of rats with both day 1 and day 10 lesions and (*2*) there was an additional expansion of corticospinal projections from the injured hemisphere of rats with day 1 but not day 10 lesions (Fig. 6-6). This latter enhancement was from an extensive region of cortex that included virtually all of the somatosensory cortex and in some animals extended anteriorly into the prefrontal regions. The enhanced projection from the normal hemisphere is thus correlated with enhanced recovery in the day 10–injured rats, whereas the additional enhanced projection from the injured hemisphere is correlated with poor recovery in the day 1–injured rats. Furthermore, since the day 1 rats were also impaired at a spatial navigation task, we can speculate that the expanded projection from the somatosensory and prefrontal cortices may have interfered with the normal functioning of the remaining hemisphere. Parallel studies of corticocortical and corticosubcortical projections in rats with medial frontal injuries at 1 or 10 days of age showed parallel findings. The earliest lesions produced widespread abnormalities in cortical connectivity, which correlated with a very poor behavioral outcome (Kolb et al., 1994).

In sum, we have found that functional recovery is correlated with enhanced dendritic growth as well as will specific expansions of corticospinal pathways after cortical lesions at 10 days of age. In contrast, we have found that a very poor functional outcome is correlated with dendritic atrophy and an apparently pathological expansion of cortical connectivity. This latter observation was somewhat surprising, but it is consistent with the general hypothesis that recovery of function is probably associated with reorganization of intrinsic neural circuitry rather than extensive reorganization of cortical afferents and efferents.

Stimulation of Neuronal Change after Cortical Injury

We have seen that if a cerebral injury is followed by an increase in dendritic space, then there is a good functional outcome, whereas if an injury leads to atrophy of dendritic space, then there is a poor functional outcome. It follows that if we can potentiate dendritic growth in animals showing poor recovery of function, we should enhance functional recovery. The treatments for potentiated growth could take several forms, including behavioral therapy or a chemical treatment that would influence reparative processes in the remaining brain. Chemical treatments could include growth factors (e.g., nerve growth factor), hormones (e.g., sex steroids), or chemicals that influence transmitters, especially the neuromodulators such as acetylcholine and noradrenaline. We will focus here on behavioral therapy and growth factors and consider other factors only briefly.

Behavioral Therapy and Recovery of Function

There is now considerable evidence that environmental treatments can lead to enhanced dendritic growth that is correlated with enhanced behavioral abilities (e.g., Greenough & Chang, 1989). It follows that environmental manipulation might influence both morphological change and the functional outcome after cortical injury. Although there have been many studies of the effects of experience on functional outcome after cerebral injury in adulthood, the findings have been inconsistent at best (for reviews see Shulkin, 1989, and Will & Kelche, 1992). We have therefore focused on the effects of environmental therapies on recovery from cortical lesions in the first week of life. We reasoned that animals with the worst functional outcomes would probably have the most potential to benefit from environmental treatments. We also recognized that the age at which treatment is initiated might be important, so we began treatments in infancy, adolescence, and adulthood.

It has been shown that tactile stimulation of premature human babies with a brush leads to faster growth and earlier hospital discharge (e.g., Field et al., 1986; Schanberg & Field, 1987; Solkoff & Matuszak, 1975). In addition, studies in infant rats have shown that similar treatment alters the structure of olfactory bulb neurons and affects later behavior (e.g., Leon, 1992). We therefore stroked infant rats with a camel hair paintbrush three times daily from day 7 to day 21 of life. The rats were subsequently raised in standard laboratory cages and were sacrificed in adulthood. Golgi analysis revealed that the early experience had no effect on dendritic length in adulthood but did produce a significant *drop* in spine density (Kolb & Gibb, 2000). Curiously, this anatomical change was correlated with significant improvement in both the reaching task and the Morris water task.

Having shown that early experience could alter both the brain and behavior, we repeated our experiments with animals with frontal or posterior parietal injuries at 4 days of age, followed by tactile stimulation until weaning. The rats with the tactile stimulation showed an unexpectedly large reduction in behavioral deficits, and this was correlated with a reversal of the atrophy of cortical neurons normally associated with these lesions. Furthermore, in contrast to the decrease in spine density observed in the normal rats, the treated brain-injured rats showed an increase in spine density relative to the untreated injured animals. Thus, not only did the early experience alter the brain and ameliorate the effects of the early brain injury, the experience actually had different effects on the brains of normal and brain-injured animals.

In another series of experiments, we placed animals with lesions on postnatal days 1, 5, or 7 in enriched environments for 3 months, beginning at the time of weaning. We anticipated that the animals with the earliest injuries would show the greatest functional benefit because the experience would reverse the neuronal atrophy. In contrast, we expected that the animals with the best recovery would show the least benefit because their neurons had already expanded their dendritic fields after the injury. This was indeed the case. Animals with day 1 or day 5 lesions showed a dramatic reversal of functional impairments that was correlated with a reversal of dendritic atrophy (e.g., Kolb & Elliott, 1987; Kolb, et al., 2000c). Animals with day 7 lesions showed only a small enhancement of recovery and neural structure. The dramatic improvement in the animals with the earliest injuries carries an important message: It suggests that even the young animal with substantial neural atrophy and behavioral dysfunction is capable of considerable neuroplasticity and functional recovery in response to behavioral therapy. The important remaining therapeutic questions relate to the nature of the most beneficial therapy and the optimal timing for initiating therapy.

Growth Factors

Basic neurobiological research over the past decade has shown that several proteins have the ability to stimulate neuromitosis as well as synaptogenesis during development and childhood. These compounds have generated considerable interest because of their potential for treatment of dementing diseases (e.g., Hefti et al., 1991) as well as recovery from injuries (e.g., Hagg, et al., 1993). We will illustrate this potential with a study of the effects of nerve growth factor (NGF) on recovery from motor cortex injury.

We noted earlier that rats with large lesions of the motor cortex show limited recovery of function and a correlated atrophy of the remaining cortical neurons. We therefore injected NGF into the ventricles of rats with large devascularizing lesions of the motor cortex (Kolb et al., 1997a). The principal findings were that the NGF treatment (*1*) reduced the behavioral deficits and (*2*) stimulated a reversal of the dendritic atrophy and a marked increase in spine density. Thus, once again, we found that behavioral outcome and dendritic morphology are tightly linked. It therefore appears that the reparative capacity of the brain can be stimulated by providing appropriate growth factors. Indeed, more recently, we have shown that basic fibroblast growth factor (bFGF), which increases the endogenous production of NGF by astrocytes, can also influence both functional recovery and cell morphology (Rowntree & Kolb, 1997). In this experiment, we took advantage of the good recovery of rats with restricted motor cortex lesions. Some animals were allowed to recover without interference, whereas others had neutralizing antibodies to bFGF placed in the lesion cavity. Rats treated with the antibodies showed only limited recovery accompanied by atrophy of cortical neurons. The results of this experiment imply that endogenous factors such NGF or bFGF may play a role in the recovery, albeit limited, that occurs in the absence of treatment.

One of the difficulties in treating brain-injured people with trophic factors is that these substances do not pass the blood-brain barrier easily. There is, therefore, considerable interest in developing compounds that might stimulate the brain to produce trophic factors. Recently, it has been shown that the production of trophic factors may be stimulated by experience. For example, we have shown that animals placed in an enriched environment have increased bFGF activity if they subsequently have cortical injury (Kolb et al., 1997b). Similarly, Hamm and colleagues (Chapter 3) have shown that another trophic factor (brain-derived neurotrophic factor, BDNF) is also increased by enriched experience. In other words, experience appears to stimulate the brain's endogenous production of trophic factors and this trophic activation may play an important role in the effects of behavioral therapies on recovery from an injury. Indeed, it may be possible to enhance the effects of behavioral therapies by coadministration of trophic factors such as NGF or BDNF.

Other Treatments

Various other treatments have been proposed to enhance endogenous recovery. These include especially sex hormones and neuromodulators. We consider each briefly.

There is now considerable evidence that sex hormones play a significant role in defining the dendritic structure of cortical neurons (e.g., Gould et al., 1990; Stewart & Kolb, 1994; Woolley et al., 1990). Furthermore, in a series of studies, we have shown that the presence or absence of testosterone during development affects recovery from early frontal cortex injury as well as the subsequent dendritic structure (Kolb & Stewart, 1995). Rats were given medial frontal lesions on postnatal day 7 and studied behaviorally and anatomically in adulthood. Hormonally-intact male rats showed recovery of function that was correlated with increased spine density in cortical pyramidal neurons. Recovery and the associated anatomical changes were abolished in animals gonadectomized at birth. Thus, it appears that endogenous sex hormones play an important role in processes related to recovery. The role of estrogens appears to be more complicated than that of androgens. The removal of ovaries in adult female rats leads to hypertrophy of dendritic fields, which was an unexpected finding (Stewart & Kolb, 1994). Future studies will need to look more closely at the role of hormone replacement in postmenopausal women.

The brain has several diffusely projecting fiber systems that appear to regulate neuronal activity by releasing "modulatory" transmitters in the forebrain. These modulatory systems include the noradrenergic and serotonergic inputs from the brain stem and the cholinergic input from the basal forebrain. Neuromodulatory systems have been implicated in the facilitation of virtually all types of learning, ranging from habituation and imprinting to complex cognitive learning (e.g., Kolb and Whishaw, 1998). The prevalent view on the role of neuromodulators is that they facilitate or inhibit the activity and formation of neural circuits. It seems likely, therefore, that these neuromodulators could influence processes related to recovery of function. Thus, when we depleted the cerebrum of noradrenaline in infant rats, we were able to block recovery of function (Kolb & Sutherland, 1992; Sutherland et al., 1982). This functional blockade was correlated with a blockage of the dendritic changes that are hypothesized to support the recovery (Kolb et al., 1997e). Recently, in a parallel set of studies, we found that if pregnant female rats are fed high-choline diets from conception until weaning of their pups, then the effects of subsequent frontal removals on postnatal day 4 can be reduced. Furthermore, this functional improvement is correlated with a partial reversal of the dendritic atrophy (B. Kolb and R. Tees, unpublished). The high-choline diets are associated not only with an increase in acetylcholinesterase activity in the cortex but also with increased mRNA for NGF. Thus, there may be a relationship between the level of neuromodulatory activity and neurotrophins.

In sum, it appears that both sex hormones and neuromodulators can also influence the extent of functional recovery and that this is correlated with changes in dendritic arborization.

Stimulation of Cortical Regeneration

The demonstration that there are quiescent stem cells in the adult mammalian brain has important implications for the study of recovery of function (Craig et al., 1994; Morshead et al., 1994; Reynolds & Weiss, 1992). Several studies have now shown that these cells can be removed from the adult human brain, placed in culture, and stimulated to divide and produce both neurons and glia (Kirschenbaum, et al., 1994). Furthermore, it now appears that at least two brain regions, the olfactory

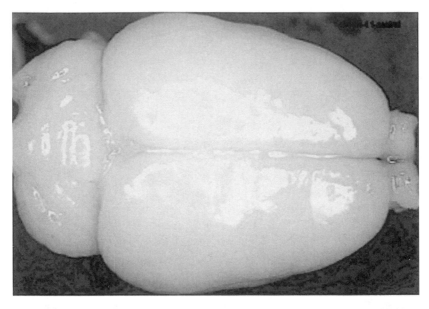

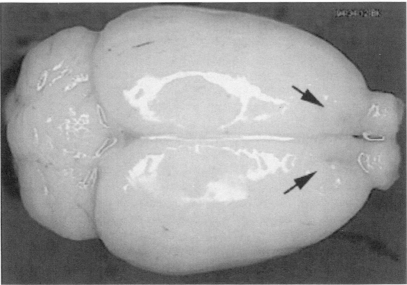

Figure 6-7. Photographs of the brains of a representative control rat (top) and a rat with a medial frontal lesion (bottom). The lesion cavity has been filled with newly generated neurons in the lesioned brain. Arrows point to the lesion scar.

bulb and the hippocampus, produce new neurons throughout the lives of mammals, including primates (e.g., Altman & Bayer, 1993; Lois & Alvarez-Buylla, 1994). Thus, the mammalian brain not only has the potential to develop new neurons in adulthood, but it actually does. In principle, therefore, it should be possible to stimulate these cells to produce new neurons after an injury. Recently, we have found that the brain may not only be capable of generating new neurons after an injury, but also that these neurons may be capable of connecting with the existing brain and supporting recovery of function.

Our first experiments evolved from our studies on the effects of restricted lesions of the midline frontal region in infancy. We noticed that in rats with restricted medial frontal lesions, no lesion cavity was visible in adulthood (Fig. 6-7). Although this cavity loss might have been due to mechanical shifting of the remaining neural tissue, we have now shown that the cavity fills with neurons that are created after the injury and that the new neurons develop appropriate connections with the rest of the brain. Furthermore, animals with this regrowth show virtually complete restitution of function, and if we block the regrowth process with a substance that interferes with stem cell activity, we block the recovery of function. This is an exciting discovery because it implies not only that it is possible to regrow lost neural regions, but also that these neural regions are functional.

The next step in these studies is to find a way to stimulate neurogenesis in the adult brain. Weiss and his colleagues (e.g., Weiss et al., 1996) have shown that the introduction of trophic factors into the ventricles of adult rats does indeed stimulate mitotic activity in the stem cells of the subventricular zone. Recently we have shown that this activity is enhanced in animals with cortical lesions and that neurons are not only generated after such treatment but also that they can migrate into a region of cortical lesion (Kolb et al., 1998, b; 1998c). These neurons do not differentiate normally, however, and thus do not sustain recovery. Our next task is to provide additional trophic support to encourage the cells to differentiate and, it is hoped, connect with the rest of the brain. We believe that long corticosubcortical connections are unlikely to be re-formed, and in view of the apparently interfering effects of abnormal connectivity after lesions in infancy, such attempted reformation may not be desirable. On the other hand, connections with the more proximal cerebral regions may be established, and these may be capable either of supporting recovery directly or of stimulating the remaining brain to reorganize its intrinsic circuitry to enhance recovery.

Conclusions

1. Functional recovery after cerebral injury is correlated with a reorganization of intrinsic cortical circuits. This reorganization can be inferred from changes in the dendritic morphology of cortical neurons.
2. Functional recovery after neocortical injury is not normally associated with significant changes in corticosubcortical connectivity. Indeed, such changes may prove disruptive.

3. The functional sequelae of cortical injury during development vary with the developmental status of the brain. Injuries during the time when the neurons are undergoing maximal dendritic growth and synaptogenesis are associated with the best functional outcomes, whereas injuries occurring earlier, during the time of neuron migration, are associated with very poor behavioral outcomes.

4. Processes that enhance dendritic growth lead to enhanced recovery, whereas processes that retard such growth lead to reduced recovery.

5. Reorganization of dendritic arborizations can be potentiated by various treatments including behavioral therapy, trophic factors, sex steroids, and other pharmacological agents.

6. Preliminary evidence suggests that it may be possible to induce neural regeneration in the injured brain and that the regenerated tissue is functional.

References

Altman, J., and Bayer, S. (1993) Are new neurons formed in the brains of adult mammals? A progress report, 1962–1992. In A.C. Cuello (ed.), *Neuronal Cell Death and Repair.* New York: Elsevier, pp. 203–225.

Craig, C.G., Morshead, C., Roach, A., and van der Kooy, D. (1994) Evidence for a relatively quiescent stem cell in the subependyma of the adult mammalian forebrain. *Journal of Cell Biochemistry Supplement 18B;* 176.

Field, T., Schanberg, S.M., Scafidi, F., Bauer, C.R., Vega-Lahr, N., Garcia, R., Nystrom, J., and Kuhn, C.M. (1986) Tactile/kinesthetic stimulation effects on preterm neonates. *Pediatrics,* 77:654–658.

Finger, S., and Almli, C.R. (1988) Margaret Kennard and her "principle" in historical perspective. In S. Finger, C.R. Almli, T.E. LeVere, and D.G. Stein, (eds.), *Brain Injury and Recovery: Controversial and Theoretical Issues.* New York: Plenum Press, pp. 117–132.

Gould, E., Woolley, C.S., Frankfurt, M., and McEwen, B.S. (1990) Gonadal steroids regulate dendritic spine density in hippocampal pyramidal cells in adulthood. *Journal of Neuroscience,* 10:1286–1291.

Greenough, W.T., and Chang, F.F. (1989) Plasticity of synapse structure and pattern in the cerebral cortex. In A. Peters, and E.G. Jones (eds.), *Cerebral Cortex,* Vol. 7. New York: Plenum Press, pp. 391–440.

Hagg, T., Louis, J.-C., and Varon, S. (1993) Neurotrophic factors and CNS regeneration. In A. Gorio (ed.), *Neuroregeneration.* New York: Raven Press, pp. 265–288.

Hebb, D.O. (1949) *The Organization of Behavior.* New York: Wiley.

Hefti, F., Brachet, P., Will, B., and Christen, Y. (eds.). (1991) *Growth Factors and Alzheimer's Disease.* Berlin: Springer-Verlag.

Kennard, M.A. (1942) Cortical reorganization of motor function: Studies on a series of monkeys of various ages from infancy to maturity. *Archives of Neurology and Psychiatry,* 48:227–240.

Kirschenbaum, B., Nedergaard, M., Preuss, A., Barami, K., Fraser, F.A.R., and Goldman, S.A. (1994) In vitro neuronal production and differentiation by precursor cells derived from the adult human forebrain. *Cerebral Cortex,* 4:576–589.

Kolb, B. (1995) *Brain Plasticity and Behavior.* Mahwah, NJ: Erlbaum.

Kolb, B., Cioe, J., and Whishaw, I.Q. (2000a) Is there an optimal age for recovery from unilateral motor cortex lesions? Restorative Neurology and Neuroscience, in press.

Kolb, B., Cioe, J., and Whishaw, I.Q. (2000b) Behavioral and anatomical sequelae of bilateral motor cortex lesions in rats on postnatal days 1, 10, and adulthood. Submitted.

Kolb, B., Cote, S., Ribeiro-da-Silva, A., and Cuello, A.C. (1997a) NGF stimulates recovery
of function and dendritic growth after unilateral motor cortex lesions in rats. Neuroscience, 76:1139–1151.

Kolb, B., and Elliott, W. (1987) Recovery from early cortical damage in rats, II. Effects of
experience on anatomy and behavior following frontal lesions at 1 or 5 days of age. Behavioural Brain Research, 26:47–56.

Kolb, B., Forgie, M., Gibb, R., Gorny, G., and Rowntree, S. (1998a) Age, experience and
the changing brain. Neuroscience and Biobehavioural Reviews, 22:143–159.

Kolb, B., and Gibb, R. (1991) Environmental enrichment and cortical injury: Behavioural
and anatomical consequences of frontal cortex lesions. Cerebral Cortex, 1:189–198.

Kolb, B., and Gibb, R. (2000) Experience dependent changes in dendritic arbor and spine
density in neocortex vary with age and sex. In submission

Kolb, B., Gibb, R., and Gorny, G. (2000c) Therapeutic effects of enriched rearing after
frontal lesions in infancy vary with age and sex. In submission.

Kolb, B., Gibb, R., Gorny, G., and Whishaw, I.Q. (1998b) Submitted. Possible brain regrowth after cortical lesions in rats. Behavioural Brain Research, 91:127–141.

Kolb, B., Gibb, R., and van der Kooy, D. (1994) Neonatal frontal cortical lesions in rats
alter cortical structure and connectivity. Brain Research, 645:85–97.

Kolb, B., Gibb, R., Biernaskie, J., Dyck, R.H. and Whishaw, I.Q. (1998c) Regeneration of
olfactory bulb or frontal cortes in adult or infant rats. Society for Neuroscience Abstracts, 24:518.4.

Kolb, B., Ladowsky, R., Gibb, R., and Gorny, G. (1996a) Does dendritic growth underlay
recovery from neonatal occipital lesions in rats? Behavioural Brain Research, 77:125–
133.

Kolb, B., Petrie, B., and Cioe, J. (1996b) Recovery from early cortical lesions in rats. VII.
Comparison of the behavioural and anatomical effects of medial prefrontal lesions at
different ages of neural maturation. Behavioural Brain Research, 79:1–13.

Kolb, B., and Stewart, J. (1995) Changes in the neonatal gonadal hormonal environment
prevent behavioral sparing and alter cortical morphogenesis after early frontal cortex lesions in male and female rats. Behavioural Neuroscience, 109:285–294.

Kolb, B., Stewart, J., and Sutherland, R.J. (1997e) Recovery of function is associated with
increased spine density in cortical pyramidal cells after frontal lesions or noradrenaline
depletion in neonatal rats. Behavioural Brain Research, 89:61–70.

Kolb, B., and Sutherland, R.J. (1992) Noradrenaline depletion blocks behavioural sparing
and alters cortical morphogenesis after neonatal frontal cortex damage in rats. Journal
of Neuroscience, 12:2221–2330.

Kolb, B., and Whishaw, I.Q. (1981) Neonatal frontal lesions in the rat: Sparing of learned
but not species-typical behavior in the presence of reduced brain weight and cortical
thickness. Journal of Comparative and Physiological Psychology, 95:863–879.

Kolb, B., and Whishaw, I.Q. (1989) Plasticity in the neocortex: Mechanisms underlying recovery from early brain damage. Progress in Neurobiology, 32:235–276.

Kolb, B., and Whishaw, I.Q. (1998) Brain plasticity and behavior. Annual Review of Psychology, 49:43–64.

Leon, M. 1992. Neuroethology of olfactory preference development. Journal of Neurobiology, 23:1557–1573.

Lois, C., and Alvarez-Buylla, A. (1994) Long-distance neuronal migration in the adult mammalian brain. *Science,* 264:1145–1148.

Morshead, C.M., Reynolds, B.A., Craig, C.G., McBurney, M.W., Staines, W.A., Morassutti, D., Weiss, S., and van der Kooy, D. (1994) Neural stem cells in the adult mammalian forebrain: A relatively quiescent subpopulation of subependymal cells. *Neuron,* 13: 1071–1082.

Purpura, D.P. (1974) Dendritic spine "dysgenesis" and mental retardation. *Science* 186: 1126–1128.

Reynolds, B., and Weiss, S. (1992) Generation of neurons and astrocytes from isolated cells of the adult mammalian central nervous system. *Science,* 255:1727–1710.

Rowntree, S., and Kolb, B. (1997) Blockade of basic fibroblast growth factor retards recovery from motor cortex injury in rats. *European Journal of Neuroscience,*

Schanberg, S.M., and Field, T.M. (1987) Sensory deprivation stress and supplemental stimulation in the rat pup and preterm human neonate. *Child Development,* 58:1431–1447.

Shulkin, J. (ed.). (1989) *Preoperative Events: Their Effects on Behavior Following Brain Damage.* Hillsdale, NJ: Erlbaum.

Solkoff, N., and Matuszak, D. (1975) Tactile stimulation and behavioural development among low-birthweight infants. *Child Psychiatry. Human Development,* 6:33–37.

Steward, O. (1991) Synapse replacement on cortical neurons following denervation. In A. Peters and E.O. Jones (eds.), *Cerebral Cortex,* Vol. 9. New York: Plenum Press, pp. 81–131.

Stewart, J., and Kolb, B. (1994) Dendritic branching in cortical pyramidal cells in response to ovariectomy in adult female rats: Suppression by neonatal exposure to testosterone. *Brain Research,* 654:149–154.

Sutherland, R.J., Kolb, B., Whishaw, I.Q., and Becker, J. (1982) Cortical noradrenaline depletion eliminates sparing of spatial learning after neonatal frontal cortex damage in the rat. *Neuroscience Letters,* 32:125–130.

Weiss, S., Reynolds, B.A., Vescovi, A.L., Morshead, C., Craig, C.G., and vand der Kooy, D. (1996) Is there a neural stem cell in the mammalian forebrain? *Trends in Neuroscience,* 19:387–393.

Whishaw, I.Q., and Kolb, B. (1988) Sparing of skilled forelimb reaching and corticospinal projections after neonatal motor cortex removal or hemidecortication in the rat: support for the Kennard doctrine. *Brain Research,* 451:97–114.

Whishaw, I.Q., Kolb, B., and Sutherland, R.J. (1983) The behavior of the laboratory rat. In T.E. Robinson (ed.), *Behavioral Contributions to Brain Research.* New York: Oxford University Press, pp. 141–211.

Whishaw, I.Q., O'Connor, W.T., and Dunnett, S.B. (1986) The contributions of motor cortex, nigrostriatal dopamine and caudate-putámen to skilled forelimb use in the rat. *Brain,* 109:805–843.

Whishaw, I.Q., and Pellis, S.M. (1992) The structure of skilled forelimb reaching in the rat: A proximally driven movement with a single distal rotatory component. *Behavioural Brain Research,* 41:49–59.

Whishaw, I.Q., Pellis, S.M., Gorny, B.P., and Pellis, V.C. (1991) The impairments in reaching and the movements of compensation in rats with motor cortex lesions: an endpoint, videorecording, and movement notation analysis. *Behavioural Brain Research,* 42: 277–91.

Whishaw, I.Q., Pellis, S.M., Gorny, B.P., Kolb, B., and Tetzlaff, W. (1993) Proximal and distal impairments in rat forelimb use in reaching following unilateral pyramidal tract lesions. *Behavioural Brain Research,* 56:59–76.

Will, B., and Kelche, C. (1992) Environmental approaches to recovery of function from brain damage: A review of animal studies (1981 to 1991). In F.D. Rose and D.A. Johnson (eds.), *Recovery from Brain Damage: Reflections and Directions.* New York: Plenum Press, pp. 79–104.

Woolley, C.S., Gould, E., Frankfurt, M., and McEwen, B.S. (1990) Naturally occurring fluctuation in dendritic spine density on adult hippocampal pyramidal neurons. *Journal of Neuroscience,* 10:4035–4039.

7

Rapid Reorganization of Subcortical and Cortical Maps in Adult Primates

J. XU AND J.T. WALL

The somatosensory system has its beginning in sensory nerves that transmit signals from the body to the spinal cord and brainstem. From these levels, information is then processed in the thalamus before reaching cortical areas. This system is organized somatotopically and, as a result, each level contains a map or representation of cutaneous inputs from the body. It was long thought that these maps were formed during development and thereafter were unable to change for the remainder of life. Thus, peripheral injuries in adults were believed to cause loss of functioning in related parts of central maps (see Chapter 1, this volume). This view has been disproven by studies of peripheral injuries which show that cortical maps in adult humans and animals can reorganize, so that parts of maps that lose inputs due to injury become activated by remaining, noninjured inputs (e.g., Birbaumer et al., 1997; Calford & Tweedale, 1991; Kaas, 1995; Kaas et al., 1983; Merzenich & Jenkins, 1993; Mogilner et al., 1993; Turnbull & Rasmusson, 1991; Wall, 1988). Following injuries to important parts of the body, like the hand, cortical reorganization can be quite extensive (see Chapter 4); in addition, initial cortical changes appear quite rapidly—within minutes or hours (Buchner et a., 1995; Calford & Tweedale, 1991; Kolarik et al., 1994; Merzenich et al., 1983; Silva et al., 1996). The rapidity of this initial reorganization dictates involvement of existing circuits; however, the central locations of these changes remain hotly debated. This chapter outlines some of our recent attempts to identify the substrates of early central reorganization after hand injuries in adult primates.

Rapid Reorganization of Cortical and Subcortical Substrates

The adult primate somatosensory system contains a multilevel "stack" of interconnected maps of the hand (Fig. 7-1). Given this organization, there are different

130

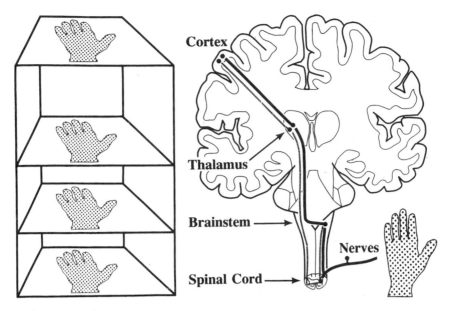

Figure 7-1. Somatosensory circuits that process inputs from the hand. Tactile and other inputs from the median, ulnar, and radial nerves project to the spinal cord and main cuneate nucleus in the brainstem. Major projections from the cuneate nucleus are to the ventroposterior lateral nucleus (VPL) in the thalamus. Projections from the spinal cord are to the cuneate nucleus via the postsynaptic dorsal column system and to the VPL. Major VPL projections are to the primary (area 3b) cortex. Inputs from the hand are organized somatotopically as they ascend this system; consequently, spinal, cuneate, VPL, and cortical area 3b levels all contain maps of the hand that together form a "stack" of maps that the brain uses to interpret inputs from the hand.

ways in which reorganization could spread across this stack after injuries of the hand. For example, if cortical substrates have greater capacities for change, initial reorganization might occur only intracortically. From this viewpoint, injury would not result in map reorganization at subcortical levels, producing a "disjunct" spread of rapid reorganization between the peripheral site of injury and intracortical locations of change. Alternatively, capacities for change may not be specific to cortical substrates. In this case, injury might result in reorganization in one or more subcortical substrates, producing a more continuous spread of rapid changes across subcortical and cortical maps. Speculations aside, there is little consensus on which of these possibilities hold.

The brainstem nucleus for processing cutaneous inputs from the hand is the main cuneate nucleus. Defining how cuneate organization is affected by injury is thus an important step in understanding subcortical central changes. Studies in nonprimates present mixed views on whether the cuneate and other brainstem sensory nuclei (i.e., gracile and trigeminal nuclei) reorganize after injuries or other manipulations of peripheral inputs. For example, acute transections of *nerves* resulted in no immediate reorganization in either the gracile (McMahon & Wall, 1983) or trigeminal (Waite, 1984) nuclei of adult rats. In contrast, transection of sensory axons in *dorsal roots* or *dorsal spinal columns* resulted in immediate changes in receptive fields of neurons in the gracile nucleus of adult cats (Dostrovsky & Millar, 1997; Dostrovsky et al., 1976; Millar et al., 1976). Studies that used temporary functional blockade of sensory inputs, rather than injury, also present mixed findings (Dostrovsky et al., 1976; Faggin et al., 1997; Northgrave & Rasmusson, 1996; Panetsos et al., 1997; Pettit & Schwark, 1993, 1996; Zhang & Rowe, 1997). Overall, these studies provide no general consensus on whether brainstem substrates have the capacity to reorganize rapidly, and leave uncertain whether cuneate changes contribute to central reorganization after hand injuries in primates.

Studies of Rapid Postinjury Reorganization in Cortical and Cuneate Maps of Primates

To evaluate the capacities of cortical and brainstem substrates to reorganize rapidly after hand injury, we performed wrist-level transections of nerves to the hands of adult monkeys. We then used neurophysiological mapping techniques to evaluate how normal functional organization in cortical area 3b and the cuneate nucleus changes during the first minutes to hours after injury (Kolarik et al., 1994; Wall et al., 1993; Xu & Wall, 1996, 1997).

Cortical Hand Maps

The area 3b cortex in adult squirrel and marmoset monkeys normally contains a map of cutaneous mechanoreceptor inputs from the hand. Inputs from glabrous digits, palmar pads, and hairy surfaces activate specific areas within the map and, with some variation, form a recognizably similar pattern of somatotopy in maps of different individuals (Fig. 7-2A,B; Wall et al., 1992, 1993). The hand is innervated by the median, ulnar, and radial nerves. Nerve recording studies have defined the peripheral mechanoreceptor innervation territory of each nerve, and cortical mapping studies have defined related band- and patch-like aggregates of neurons within the hand map that are dominantly activated by tactile inputs from each nerve (Wall et al., 1993). The radial nerve normally provides low-threshold cutaneous innervation to hairy skin on most or all of the dorsal aspect of the hand while normally activating discontinuous, patch-like cortical zones that occupy about 12% of the hand map (Fig. 7-2E,H). In contrast, the median and ulnar nerves innervate the entire glabrous hand and a small fraction of the little finger side of the hairy hand while activating the remaining large percentage of the cortical hand map area (Fig. 7-2C,D,F,G).

To assess rapid changes in the cortical hand map after injury, we acutely transected the median and ulnar nerves at the wrist, thus depriving the hand skin and cortical hand map of these inputs (i.e., Fig. 7-2C,D,F,G) but leaving radial nerve inputs intact (Fig. 7-2E,H). Several changes were seen in the area 3b hand map

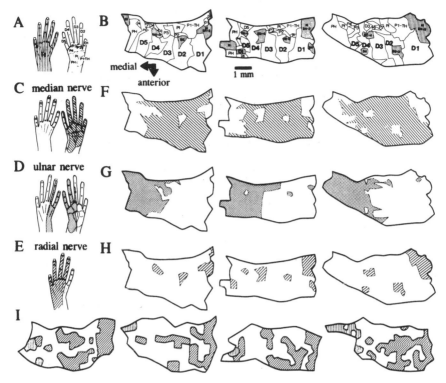

Figure 7-2. The cortical area 3b map of the hand in adult squirrel monkeys. (A) The hand has hairy (left) and glabrous (right) surfaces that can be subdivided further as indicated: H: hairy hand between knuckles and wrist; D1–D5: digits 1–5; P: palmar pads. (B) Three cortical hand maps illustrating normal somatotopic organization. Cortical areas activated by inputs from parts of hairy (hatching) and glabrous (clear) hand surfaces are indicated (abbreviations as in A). (C–E) Angled hatching or stippling on hands indicates common peripheral innervation territories of the median (C), ulnar (D), and radial (E) nerves. (F–H) Corresponding to the peripheral territories in (C–E), angled hatching or stippling indicates cortical areas in three normal hand maps (same as in B) that were activated by median (F), ulnar (G), or radial (H) nerve inputs. Clear areas in (F–H) were activated by the other hand nerves (i.e., by ulnar and radial nerves in F, by median and radial nerves in G, and by median and ulnar nerves in H). (I): Cortical hand maps in four monkeys with acute wrist-level section of the median and ulnar nerves, leaving only the radial nerve intact. After injury, (1) cortical areas activated by radial nerve inputs are larger than normal (compare angled hatching in I versus H), (2) sizable areas of the hand map are not responsive to cutaneous inputs (clear areas in I), (3) small areas are activated by forelimb inputs (vertical hatching in I), and (4) a similar pattern of the above map changes is produced in each individual. Spatial orientation and calibration in B apply to all maps. [Based on Kolarik et al., 1994, and Wall et al., 1993].

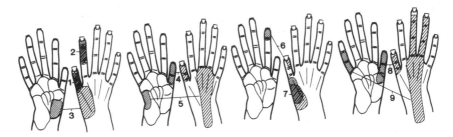

Figure 7-3. Examples of receptive field shifts associated with enlargements of radial nerve cortical areas. Each number indicates a preinjury (stippled) and postinjury (hatched) receptive field that was recorded at an identified cortical site before and after transection of the median and ulnar nerves. Changes in locations of pre- versus postinjury fields varied from little or no shift in location (e.g., 1, 2, 7), to shifts around a digit (e.g., 4, 6, 8), to shifts around the hand (e.g., 3, 5, 9). Preinjury fields were either inside (e.g., 1, 2, 7) or outside (e.g., 3–6) the radial nerve peripheral territory, whereas postinjury fields were always inside the radial nerve peripheral territory (compare to Fig. 7-2E). These shifts occurred during the first several minutes to hours after injury. Based on Kolarik et al., 1994.

after this injury (Kolarik et al., 1994). First, the large representation of the glabrous hand, which normally received inputs from the injured nerves, was missing. Second, the normally discontinuous, patch-like representations of radial nerve dorsal inputs increased in size from a normal mean area of 12% of the hand map to a mean area of 37% after injury (Fig. 7-2; compare the angled hatching in parts H and I). Third, neurons at recording sites occupying a mean area of 58% of the hand map became unresponsive to cutaneous inputs after injury (Fig. 7-2I, clear areas). This contrasts with normal conditions in which neurons at virtually all recording sites are responsive to cutaneous inputs. Fourth, a small mean area of about 5% of the hand map became activated by cutaneous inputs from the forelimb (Fig. 7-2I, vertical hatching). Fifth, the above pattern of changes (i.e., enlargements of the radial nerve, cutaneously unresponsive, and forelimb areas) was consistently produced in different individuals (Fig. 7-2I). Finally, the enlargements of radial nerve cortical areas involved rapid shifts in the locations of receptive fields from denervated skin to the peripheral territory of the radial nerve (Fig. 7-3). These shifts initially appeared within minutes after injury and remained apparent or continued to develop for several hours after injury (Kolarik et al., 1994).

Brainstem Hand Maps

Using the mapping techniques employed in cortex, attention was next shifted to the cuneate nucleus. The normal cuneate nucleus contains an organized map of inputs from the hand, forelimb, and trunk. Main features of this normal map include the following (Xu & Wall, 1996, 1997). In transverse planes through the nucleus, cutaneous inputs from the glabrous and dorsal hand activate central locations of

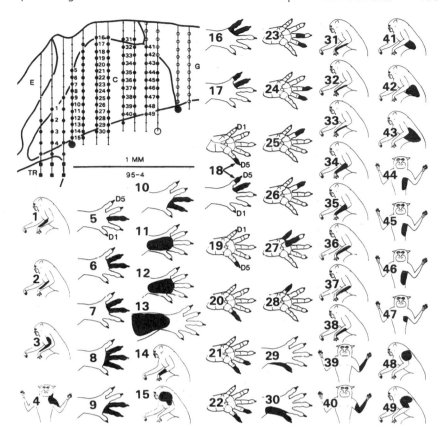

Figure 7-4. Examples of cutaneous receptive fields defined in a mapping study of the cuneate nucleus in a normal marmoset monkey. At the upper left is a camera lucida drawing of a brainstem transverse section showing a reconstruction of a mediolateral row of penetrations (vertical lines). The cuneate nucleus (C) is located between the gracile (G), trigeminal (TR), and external cuneate (E) nuclei. Numbers 1–49 illustrate examples of relationships between cuneate recording sites (black dot to the left of each number in the transverse section) and receptive field locations (black area on the body picture). The hand pictures for 18 orient the D1 (thumb) and D5 (little finger) sides of the glabrous (top) and hairy (bottom) hand surfaces. Based on Xu & Wall, 1996, 1997.

the nucleus (Figs. 7-4 and 7-5A–D). The representation of inputs from the glabrous side of the hand is continuous, whereas the representation of inputs from the dorsal hairy side of the hand is discontinuous and distributed in small patches adjacent to the glabrous representation (Fig. 7-5B–D). The hand representation, in turn, is bordered medially and laterally by representations of the forelimb and trunk (Figs. 7-4 and 7-5A–D). Finally, at rostrocaudal levels where the nucleus is largest in the transverse extent, all but about 3% of recording sites are normally responsive to cutaneous stimuli (Figs. 7-5B–D and 7-6).

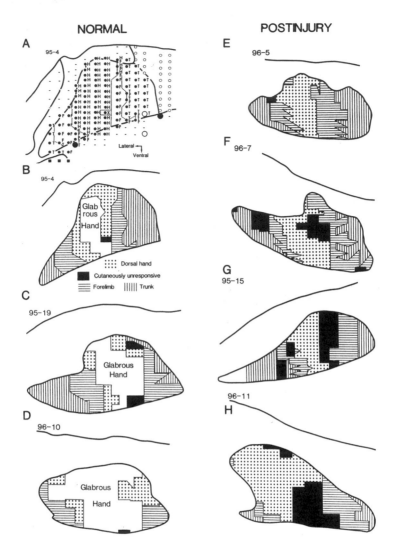

NORMAL　　　　　　　　**POSTINJURY**

Figure 7-5. Cuneate maps under normal and postinjury conditions. (A) Procedures used to define maps. Neurophysiological techniques were used to define the responsiveness and cutaneous receptive fields of neurons recorded across a grid of recording sites (e.g., Fig. 7-4). Cutaneously responsive sites were then identified by their receptive field location on the hand (H), forelimb (F), and/or trunk (T). Cutaneously unresponsive sites are indicated by X. Borders (dotted lines) between representations of different body parts were established either by halving the distance between adjacent recording sites with inputs from different body parts (e.g. H vs. F) or by placing the border at recording sites with inputs that spanned different body parts (e.g., T–F). These procedures were used to define the maps shown in (B) to (H) (A and B illustrate the case shown in Fig. 7-4). *Normal* maps from marmoset (B and C) and squirrel (D) monkeys are shown in the left column, and *postinjury* maps from marmoset (E–G) and squirrel (H) monkeys are shown in the right column. The spatial orientation in (A) and the key for shading in (B) apply to all maps. After injury, (1) the normal, centrally located representation of the glabrous hand is lost, (2) the representation of the dorsal hairy hand is more continuous and enlarged, and (3) cutaneously unresponsive areas are enlarged. Based on Xu & Wall, 1996, 1997.

Dorsal Hand

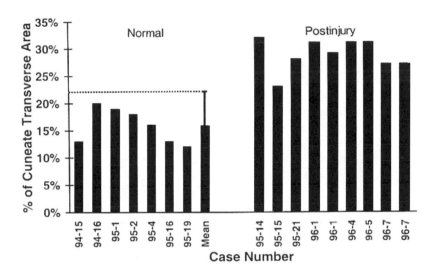

Cutaneously Unresponsive

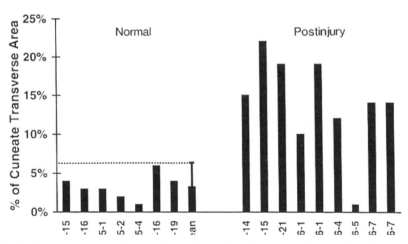

Figure 7-6. Bar graphs comparing the sizes of dorsal hand representations (top) and cutaneously unresponsive areas (bottom) in the cuneate nucleus of marmoset monkeys under normal (left) and postinjury (right) conditions. Each numbered bar is a measure from one transverse plane map. A repeated number reflects measures from transverse plane maps at different rostrocaudal levels in one nucleus. The right bars show means of each sample. The upper 95% confidence limits for the normal samples are indicated by the lines above these samples.

Immediately after wrist-level transections of the median and ulnar nerves, leaving intact only radial nerve inputs from the hairy dorsal hand, normal features of cuneate maps changed in several ways (Xu & Wall, 1997). First, the representation of the glabrous hand was missing (Fig. 7-5B–D vs. 7-5E–H). Second, the normal discontinuous, patch-like representation of radial nerve dorsal hand inputs became more continuous and increased significantly in size from a normal mean area of 16% of the cuneate transverse area to a mean area of 29% after injury (Fig. 7-6). Third, neurons at recording sites occupying a mean area of 14% of the cuneate transverse area became unresponsive to cutaneous inputs, whereas normally cutaneously unresponsive areas occupied a mean area of 3% (Fig. 7-6). Fourth, the larger, more continuous representations of dorsal hand inputs and larger, cutaneously unresponsive areas were seen consistently at different transverse planes in the same nucleus and in planes from the nuclei of different individuals (e.g., Figs. 7-5 and 7-6). Finally, these changes initially appeared, and were maintained or continued to develop, during the first minutes to hours after injury (Xu & Wall, 1997).

Significance of These Findings for Understanding Rapid Central Reorganization

Explanations of postinjury central reorganization require a knowledge of the substrates of changes; moreover, early changes are important because they reflect beginning points from which slower changes develop. Given this perspective, our results suggest, first, that nerve injury in adult primates results in reorganization of substrates at at least two levels of the neuraxis, i.e., brainstem and cortical levels. Second, initial reorganization is rapid (within minutes to hours) and occurs concurrently at both levels. Third, consistent general patterns of rapid changes are produced in different individuals at each level. Fourth, the receptive field changes seen in the cuneate are reiterated, to some degree, in cortical area 3b. Taken together, these findings suggest that injury initiates rapid, concurrent, consistent, and reiterative (to some degree) changes in brainstem and cortical maps.

The cuneate nucleus provides major lemniscal inputs to the ventroposterior lateral nucleus (VPL), which, in turn, provides major inputs to the area 3b cortical map of the hand. Given these connectivities, and the above-mentioned rapid changes in cuneate and area 3b maps, it is reasonable to predict that VPL maps also undergo some degree of rapid reorganization. Consistent with this view, a recent study of VPL in *normal* monkeys found that tactile receptive fields of some VPL neurons changed within minutes after presentation of noxious stimuli (Apkarian & Shi, 1994). Rapid (minutes to hours) response changes have also been seen in primate spinothalamic neurons following tissue damage in the hindlimb (e.g., Lin et al., 1996). Thus, thalamic and spinal substrates in adult primates also appear to have the capacity to reorganize rapidly. Together with our findings, this suggests that injury triggers rapid, concurrent changes in cortical and multiple subcortical substrates.

This view differs sharply from views of cortical theories suggesting that post-injury central changes are largely or entirely determined intracortically. In these views, cortical changes are dictated by substrates and mechanisms relating to the spatial extent of thalamocortical arbors (e.g., Garraghty & Kaas, 1992; Merzenich, 1987; Rausell & Jones, 1995), corticocortical axons (Jones, 1993), intracortical inhibition (e.g., Garraghty et al., 1991; Jones, 1993), intracortical N-methyl-D-aspartate (NMDA) receptor functions (Kano et al., 1991), and temporal correlations of signals at thalamocortical synapses (Merzenich, 1987; Merzenich et al., 1988). Although these substrates and mechanisms certainly contribute to central reorganization, our findings indicate an increased need to understand how subcortical substrates and mechanisms interact with cortical changes. This issue has received little attention in explanations of postinjury somatosensory reorganization (e.g., Garraghty & Kaas, 1992; Kaas, 1885; Merzenich & Jenkins, 1993; O'Leary et al., 1994; Weinberger, 1995; also see Darian-Smith & Gilbert, 1995, for a visual system view).

Cellular and Molecular Mechanisms of Rapid Subcortical Plasticity

The rapid onset of the cuneate changes in our studies suggests that these changes result from synaptic changes in existing brainstem substrates. Recent studies of spinal neurons in adult primates and rats provide evidence of rapid mechanisms of synaptic change that appear pertinent to the rapid cuneate changes we observe (e.g., Coderre et al., 1993; Lin et al., 1996; McMahon et al., 1993; Silvotti & Woolf, 1994; Urban et al., 1994; Woolf & Doubell, 1994). In this regard, peripheral injury has been shown to trigger activation of nociceptive C-fiber inputs that corelease neuropeptides and excitatory amino acids (EAAs). This results in coactivation of neurokinin and metabotropic glutamate receptors on postsynaptic spinal cells, which, in turn, results in intracellular cascades that produce sensitization and disinhibition of postsynaptic responses to sensory inputs. In one cascade, coactivation is proposed to be linked to G-protein activation, which, through activation of phospholipase C and production of diacylglycerol, elevates protein kinase C (PKC). Elevation of PKC, in turn, sensitizes (facilitates) the opening of NMDA receptor channels, thus increasing the response to EAAs; in addition, elevation of PKC desensitizes gamma-aminobutyric acid (GABA) and glycine receptors, thus decreasing inhibitory responses. In a second cascade, coactivation is proposed to produce sustained postsynaptic depolarization, which, by relieving Mg^{2+} blockade of NMDA receptor channels, either primes or makes these receptors more accessible; as a consequence, EAAs produce larger excitatory responses. In still another cascade, coactivation is proposed to increase intracellular Ca^{2+}, which, in turn, results in activation of PKC (and the above effects), activation of nitric oxide synthase, and expression of c-*fos* or other proto-oncogenes. Thus, in the spinal cord, injury-triggered activity of nociceptive C-fiber inputs rapidly modulates the efficacy of existing excitatory and inhibitory synapses to rapidly increase responses to sensory inputs, including A-fiber tactile inputs.

The cuneate and gracile nuclei have long been known to receive tactile inputs from A fibers; less well recognized is the fact that these nuclei also receive nociceptive inputs that project directly or indirectly up the dorsal columns and that converge functionally on neurons with tactile inputs (Al-Chaer et al., 1996; Berkley & Hubscher, 1995; Briner et al., 1988; Cliffer & Willis, 1994; Cliffer et al., 1992; Fabri & Conti, 1990; Ferrington et al., 1988; Garrett et al., 1992; Rustioni & Weinberg, 1989). Thus, the cuneate appears to contain substrates similar to those underlying rapid postinjury changes in the spinal cord. This suggests that rapid cuneate sensitization and disinhibition may occur via the above mechanisms. These subcortical changes then interact with intracortical substrates and mechanisms of change (see above).

Implications for Understanding Sensory Disorders

Injuries of the body and peripheral nervous system cause changes in perceptions of innocuous and painful stimuli, many of which become apparent soon after injury. Numerous studies have related postinjury changes in perception to postinjury functional changes at a specific central level, most often the cortex (e.g., Birbaumer et al., 1997; Flor et al., 1995; Merzenich & Jenkins, 1993; Mogilner et al., 1993; Ramachandran, 1993; Wall & Kaas, 1985) or the spinal cord (e.g., Coderre et al., 1993; Dubner & Ruda, 1992; Sivilotti & Woolf, 1994; Urban et al., 1994; Willis, 1992; Woolf, 1991). Although acknowledging changes at other levels in general ways, these studies do not address potential multilevel central contributions to sensory disorders. Our studies suggest that cuneate and cortical area 3b maps reorganize rapidly after peripheral injury; thus, the brain's perspective in the minutes to hours after injury appears to be one of simultaneous functional reorganization involving these and (as discussed above) other (e.g. spinal, thalamic) substrates. Clearly, explanations of postinjury sensory disorders, and improved therapeutic management of these disorders, must be based on a vision of these multilevel changes.

Summary

Injury in the adult peripheral nervous system causes central maps in distant parts of the brain to reorganize. There is little understanding of how reorganization proceeds across central substrates from a site of peripheral injury. Our studies suggest that central changes spread in a rapid, concurrent, multilevel fashion across brainstem and cortical substrates. This multilevel perspective of brain reorganization is important for understanding both the cellular and molecular substrates of postinjury central reorganization and the central correlates of disorders in sensory perception.

ACKNOWLEDGMENTS
We thank Dr. Richard Lane and Dr. Robert Rhoades for helpful comments on the manuscript and Jessica Nguyen and Marshonna Forgues for their contributions to this work. This research was supported by NIH Grant NS21105.

References

Al-Chaer, E.D., Lawand, N.B., Westlund, K.N., and Willis, W.D. (1996) Pelvic visceral input into the nucleus gracilis is largely mediated by the postsynaptic dorsal column pathway. *Journal of Neurophysiology,* 76:2675–2690.

Apkarian, A.V., and Shi, T. (1994) Squirrel monkey lateral thalamus. I. Somatic nociresponsive neurons and their relation to spinothalamic terminals. *Journal of Neuroscience,* 14:6779–6795.

Berkley, K.J., and Hubscher, C.H. (1995) Are there separate central nervous system pathways for touch and pain? *Nature Medicine,* 1:766–773.

Birbaumer, N., Lutzenberger, W., Montoya, P., Larbig, W., Unertil, K., Topfner, S., Grodd, W., Taub, E., and Flor, H. (1997) Effects of regional anesthesia on phantom limb pain are mirrored in changes in cortical reorganization. *Journal of Neuroscience,* 17:5503–5508.

Briner, R.P., Carlton, S.M., Coggeshall, R.E., and Chung, K. (1988) Evidence for unmyelinated sensory fibres in the posterior columns in man. *Brain,* 111:999–1007.

Buchner, H., Kauert, C., and Radermacher, I. (1995) Short-term changes of finger representation at the somatosensory cortex in humans. *Neuroscience Letters,* 198:57–59.

Calford, M.B., and Tweedale, R. (1991) Immediate expansion of receptive fields of neurons in area 3b of macaque monkeys after digit denervation. *Somatosensory and Motor Research,* 8:249–260.

Cliffer, K.D., Hasegawa, T., and Willis, W.D. (1992) Responses of neurons in the gracile nucleus of cats to innocuous and noxious stimuli: Basic characterization and antidromic activation from the thalamus. *Journal of Neurophysiology,* 68:818–832.

Cliffer, K.D., and Willis, W.D. (1994) Distribution of the postsynaptic dorsal column projection in the cuneate nucleus of monkeys. *Journal of Comparative Neurology,* 345:84–93.

Coderre, T.J., Katz, J., Vaccarino, A.L., and Melzack, R. (1993) Contribution of central neuroplasticity to pathological pain: review of clinical and experimental evidence. *Pain,* 52:259–285.

Darian-Smith, C., and Gilbert, C.D. (1995) Topographic reorganization in the striate cortex of the adult cat and monkey is cortically mediated. *Journal of Neuroscience,* 15:1631–1647.

Dostrovsky, J.O., and Millar, J. (1977) Receptive fields of gracile neurons after transection of the dorsal columns. *Experimental Neurology,* 56:610–621.

Dostrovsky, J.O., Millar, J., and Wall, P.D. (1976) The immediate shift of afferent drive of dorsal column nucleus cells following deafferentation: A comparison of acute and chronic deafferentation in gracile nucleus and spinal cord. *Experimental Neurology,* 52:480–495.

Dubner, R., and Ruda, M.A. (1992) Activity-dependent neuronal plasticity following tissue injury and inflammation. *Trends in Neurosciences,* 15:96–103.

Fabri, M., and Conti, F. (1990) Calcitonin gene-related peptide-positive neurons and fibers in the cat dorsal column nuclei. *Neuroscience,* 35:167–174.

Faggin, B.M., Nguyen K.T., and Nicolelis, M.A.L. (1997) Immediate and simultaneous sensory reorganization at cortical and subcortical levels of the somatosensory system. *Proceedings of the National Academy of Sciences of the USA*, 94:9428–9433.

Ferrington, D.G., Downie, J.W., and Willis, W.D., Jr. (1988) Primate nucleus gracilis neurons: Responses to innocuous and noxious stimuli. *Journal of Neurophysiology*, 59: 886–907.

Flor, H., Elbert, T., Knecht, S., Wienbruch, C., Pantev, C., Birbaumer, N., Larbig, W., and Taub, E. (1995) Phantom-limb pain as a perceptual correlate of cortical reorganization following arm amputation. *Nature*, 375:482–484.

Garraghty, P.E., and Kaas, J.H. (1992) Dynamic features of sensory and motor maps. *Current Opinions in Neurobiology*, 2:522–527.

Garraghty, P.E., LaChica, E.A., and Kaas, J.H. (1991) Injury-induced reorganization of somatosensory cortex is accompanied by reductions in GABA staining. *Somatosensory and Motor Research*, 8:347–354.

Garrett, L., Coggeshall, R.E., Patterson, J.T., and Chung K. (1992) Numbers and proportions of unmyelinated axons at cervical levels in the fasciculus gracilis of monkey and cat. *Anatomical Record*, 232:301–304.

Jones, E.G. (1993) GABAergic neurons and their role in cortical plasticity in primates. *Cerebral Cortex*, 3:361–372.

Kaas, J.H. (1995) The rorganization of sensory and motor maps in adult mammals. In M.S. Gazzaniga, (ed.), *The Cognitive Neurosciences*. Cambridge, MA: MIT Press, pp. 51–71.

Kaas, J.H., Merzenich, M.M., and Killackey, H.P. (1983) The reorganization of somatosensory cortex following peripheral nerve damage in adult and developing mammals. *Annual Review of Neuroscience*, 6:325–356.

Kano, M., Lino, K., and Kano, M. (1991) Functional reorganization of adult cat somatosensory cortex is dependent on NMDA receptors. *NeuroReport*, 2:77–80.

Kolarik, R.C., Rasey, S.K., and Wall, J.T. (1994) The consistency, extent, and locations of early-onset changes in cortical nerve dominance aggregates following injury of nerves to primate hands. *Journal of Neuroscience*, 14:4269–4288.

Lin, Q., Peng, Y.B., and Willis, W.D. (1996) Possible role of protein kinase C in the sensitization of primate spinothalamic tract neurons. *Journal of Neuroscience*, 16:3026–3034.

McMahon, S.B., Lewin, G.R., and Wall, P.D. (1993) Central hyperexcitability triggered by noxious inputs. *Current Opinion in Neurobiology*, 3:602–610.

McMahon, S.B., and Wall, P.D. (1983) Plasticity in the nucleus gracilis of the rat. *Experimental Neurology*, 80:195–207.

Merzenich, M.M. (1987) Dynamic neocortical processes and the origins of higher brain functions. In J.-P. Changeux and M. Konishi, (eds.), *The Neural and Molecular Bases of Learning*. New York: Wiley, pp. 337–358.

Merzenich, M.M., and Jenkins, W.M. (1993) Reorganization of cortical representations of the hand following alterations of skin inputs induced by nerve injury, skin island transfers, and experience. *Journal of Hand Therapy*, 6:89–104.

Merzenich, M.M., Kaas, J.H., Wall, J.T., Sur, M., Nelson, R.J., and Felleman, D.J. (1983) Progression of change following median nerve section in the cortical representation of the hand in areas 3b and 1 in adult owl and squirrel. *Neuroscience*, 10:639–665.

Merzenich, M.M., Recanzone, G., Jenkins, W.M., Allard, T.T., and Nudo, R.J. (1988) Cortical representational plasticity. In P. Rakic and W. Singer, (eds.), *Neurobiology of Neocortex*. New York: Wiley, pp. 41–67.

Millar, J., Basbaum, A.I., and Wall, P.D. (1976) Restructuring of the somatotopic map and appearance of abnormal neuronal activity in the gracile nucleus after partial deafferentation. *Experimental Neurology,* 50:658–672.

Mogilner, A., Grossman, J.A.I., Ribary, U., Joliot, M., Volkmann, J., Rapaport, D., Beasley, R.W., and Llinás, R.R. (1993) Somatosensory cortical plasticity in adult humans revealed by magnetoencephalography. *Proceedings of the National Academy of Sciences of the USA,* 90:3593–3597.

Northgrave, S.A., and Rasmusson, D.D. (1996) The immediate effects of peripheral deafferentation on neurons of the cuneate nucleus in raccoons. *Somatosensory and Motor Research,* 13:103–113.

O'Leary, D.D.M., Ruff, N.L., and Dyck, R.H. (1994) Development, critical period plasticity, and adult reorganizations of mammalian somatosensory systems. *Current Opinion in Neurobiology,* 4:535–544.

Panetsos, F., Nunez, A., and Avendano, C. (1997) Electrophysiological effects of temporary deafferentation on two characterized cell types in the nucleus gracilis of the rat. *European Journal of Neuroscience,* 9:563–572.

Pettit, M.J., and Schwark, H.D. (1993) Receptive field reorganization in dorsal column nuclei during temporary denervation. *Science,* 262:2054–2056.

Pettit, M.J., and Schwark, H.D. (1996) Capsaicin-induced rapid receptive field reorganization in cuneate neurons. *Journal of Neurophysiology,* 75:1117–1125.

Ramachandran, V.S. (1993) Behavioral and magnetoencephalographic correlates of plasticity in the adult human brain. *Proceedings of the National Academy of Sciences of the USA,* 90:10413–10420.

Rausell, E., and Jones, E.G. (1995) Extent of intracortical arborization of thalamocortical axons as a determinant of representational plasticity in monkey somatic sensory cortex. *Journal of Neuroscience,* 15:4270–4288.

Rustioni A., and Weinberg, R.J. (1989) The somatosensory system. In A. Björklund, T. Hökfelt, and L.W. Swanson (eds.), *Handbook of Chemical Neuroanatomy,* Vol. 7. New York: Elsevier, pp. 219–321.

Silva, A.C., Rasey, S.K., Wu, X.-F., and Wall, J.T. (1996) Initial cortical reactions to injury of the median and radial nerves to the hands of adult primates. *Journal of Comparative Neurology,* 366:700–716.

Sivilotti, L., and Woolf, C.J. (1994) The contribution of $GABA_A$ and glycine receptors to central sensitization: Disinhibition and touch-evoked allodynia in the spinal cord. *Journal of Neurophysiology,* 72:169–179.

Turnbull, B.G., and Rasmusson, D.D. (1991) Chronic effects of total or partial digit denervation on raccoon somatosensory cortex. *Somatosensory and Motor Research,* 8:201–213.

Urban, L., Thompson, S.W.N., and Dray, A. (1994) Modulation of spinal excitability: cooperation between neurokinin and excitatory amino acid neurotransmitters. *Trends in Neurosciences,* 17:432–438.

Waite, P.M.E. (1984) Rearrangement of neuronal responses in the trigeminal system of the rat following peripheral nerve section. *Journal of Physiology,* 352:425–445.

Wall, J.T. (1988) Variable organization in cortical maps of the skin as an indication of the lifelong adaptive capacities of circuits in the mammalian brain. *Trends in Neurosciences,* 11:549–557.

Wall, J.T., Huerta, M.F., and Kaas, J.H. (1992) Changes in the cortical map of the hand following postnatal median nerve injury in monkeys: Modification of somatotopic aggregates. *Journal of Neuroscience,* 12:3445–3455.

Wall, J.T., and Kaas, J.H. (1985) Cortical reorganization and sensory recovery following nerve damage and regeneration. In C.W. Cotman (ed.), *Synaptic Plasticity*. New York: Guilford Press, pp. 231–260.

Wall, J.T., Nepomuceno, V., and Rasey, S.K. (1993) Nerve innervation of the hand and associated nerve dominance aggregates in the somatosensory cortex of a primate (squirrel monkey). *Journal of Comparative Neurology*, 337:191–207.

Weinberger, N.M. (1995) Dynamic regulation of receptive fields and maps in the adult sensory cortex. *Annual Review of Neuroscience*, 18:129–158.

Willis, W.D. (1992) *Hyperalgesia and Allodynia*. New York: Raven Press.

Woolf, C.J. (1991) Central mechanisms of acute pain. In M.R. Bond, J.E. Charlton, and C.J. Woolf (eds.), *Proceedings of the VIth World Congress on Pain*. New York: Elsevier, pp. 25–34.

Woolf, C.J., and Doubell, T.P. (1994) The pathophysiology of chronic pain—increased sensitivity to low threshold AB-fibre inputs. *Current Opinion in Neurobiology*, 4:525–534.

Xu, J., and Wall, J.T. (1996) Cutaneous representations of the hand and other body parts in the cuneate nucleus of a primate, and some relationships to previously described cortical representations. *Somatosensory and Motor Research*, 13:187–197.

Xu, J., and Wall, J.T. (1997) Rapid changes in brainstem maps of adult primates after peripheral injury. *Brain Research*, 774:211–215.

Zhang, S.P., and Rowe, M.J. (1997) Quantitative analysis of cuneate neurone responsiveness in the cat in association with reversible, partial deafferentation. *Journal of Physiology*, 505:769–783.

8

Motor Rehabilitation, Use-Related Neural Events, and Reorganization of the Brain After Injury

TIMOTHY SCHALLERT, SONDRA T. BLAND,
J. LEIGH LEASURE, JENNIFER TILLERSON,
RUEBEN GONZALES, LAWRENCE WILLIAMS,
JAROSLAW ARONOWSKI, AND JAMES GROTTA

Traditionally, investigations of functional recovery following brain injury have focused on treatments that can prevent tissue loss by arresting or reversing early events. This view is driven by the assumption that neural changes permit or mediate behavioral outcomes. However, recent research suggests that neural and behavioral events may interact reciprocally to affect recovery of function following some types of brain damage. In designing experimental investigations of potentially useful treatments for brain injury, it is becoming increasingly important to acknowledge this reciprocal brain–behavior relationship.

Mechanisms of both neuroplasticity and neurodegeneration after focal injury to motor and sensorimotor cortex can be influenced by manipulations of motor behavior. These changes can result in alterations in functional as well as neurochemical and anatomical outcomes in animal models. We and others (e.g., Castro-Alamancos et al., 1992, 1995; Chu et al., 1997; Fulton & Kennard, 1934; Freund, 1996; Greenough et al., 1976; Johansson, 1995; Jones & Schallert, 1992, 1994; Kolb, 1995; Kozlowski et al., 1996a, b; Rosenzweig, 1980; Schallert & Jones, 1993; Schallert & Kozlowski, 1998; Schallert et al., 1997; Stroemer et al., 1995; Whishaw et al., 1991) have examined motor behavior, either with experimental manipulations during different time periods after injury or during spontaneous recovery in relation to anatomical or physiological changes. The findings suggest that the intensity of the manipulation, as well as the time point at which it is implemented, can have profound effects on outcome. Furthermore, these effects differ dramatically, depending on the type, size, and location of the injury. This chapter focuses on compensatory changes, including the functional, neurochemical, and structural consequences of extreme manipulations of movement.

Use-Dependent Recovery of Function

As recovery of function progresses in the weeks following experimental brain injury, a variety of events associated with neuronal plasticity occur. These may include "exuberant" dendritic arborization (Schallert & Jones 1993) and the expression of molecular markers correlated with neurite outgrowth, such as GAP-43, and synaptogenesis, as indicated by synaptophysin (Kawamata et al., 1997; Schallert et al., in press; Stroemer et al., 1995, 1998). N-methyl-D-aspartate (NMDA) receptor hyperexcitability, pruning of dendritic overgrowth, and increases in spine density also occur (Schallert et al., 1997; Witte & Stoll, 1997). Each of these phenomena occur during specific, well-defined intervals, suggesting that the brain may be differentially sensitive to manipulations in a time-dependent manner. Neuronal plasticity may be optimized during a period soon after injury, which indicates that surviving tissue may be "primed" by injury during this early sensitive period (Nieto-Sampedro & Cotman, 1985; Schallert & Jones, 1993) to allow changes in the adult brain similar to those normally occurring only in the immature brain. Mechanisms of priming may include the increased expression of neurotrophic factors, cytokines, excitatory and inhibitory receptor subunits, and other factors to levels similar to those in the developing brain.

Some neural events associated with plasticity may require motor experience; that is, they may be use dependent, with this experience necessarily occurring coincidentally with the period of optimal expression of the neural event. Thus, use-dependent recovery of function may also be time dependent. For example, soon after focal electrolytic lesions of the forelimb sensorimotor cortex (FL-SMC), dendritic arborization in the pyramidal neurons of the homotopic (intact) cortex appears to depend on movement of the unimpaired forelimb (Jones & Schallert, 1994). Arborization can be prevented by restricting the use of the unaffected (ipsilateral) forelimb during this period by immobilizing it in a plaster of paris cast. However, restricting one forelimb of sham-lesioned rats, thereby forcing reliance on the other forelimb, does not cause a significant increase in dendritic arborization in the cortex contralateral to the overused limb. The impaired forelimb is often used as a "crutch" during the period of dendritic growth, with gradually increasing use until a fuller range of functionality is attained. The extensive dendritic arborization found after this type of injury appears to be activated by the combination of recent injury and movement. In contrast, learning a skilled reaching task can lead to changes in motor cortex morphology (Withers & Greenough, 1989) and physiology (Kleim et al., 1998) in intact adult rats.

Following FL-SMC lesions, rats show functional impairment of the forelimb contralateral to the lesion, but they continue to use the limb in a limited manner during exploration. In the period immediately after the injury, the contralateral forelimb is used together with the intact forelimb for locomotion along the floor.

However, it is used infrequently for landing after a rear and not at all for vertical exploration along the walls. During these types of movements, the animal relies on the intact forelimb preferentially for landing and for initiating weight-shifting movements on the wall. During the next several weeks, the impaired forelimb is used increasingly to assist the intact forelimb in landing after a rear and independently in vertical exploration and other movements (Schallert & Kozlowski, 1998). If the damage is confined to the FL-SMC, the impaired forelimb is gradually used independently of the intact forelimb for landing and to initiate weight-shifting movements along a vertical surface (Schallert et al., 2000). Thus, although recovery of some forelimb function occurs, certain limb-use functions may not recover, even up to 60 days after injury, depending on the extent of the damage.

Concurrent with and following pruning of dendritic overgrowth, synaptic restructuring occurs in the intact cortex following FL-SMC lesions and experience. Significant increases in perforated synapses and multiple synaptic boutons, which form synapses with two different dendritic spines, are found in layer V pyramidal neurons in the homotopic motor cortex following the time course of spontaneous recovery (Jones et al., 1996). These types of synapses have been associated with the maintenance of long-term potentiation (LTP) in the hippocampus (Desmond & Levy, 1990; Geinisman et al., 1996; Harris, 1995), an activity- and NMDA receptor–dependent experimental model of learning and memory (see Bliss & Collingridge, 1993, for review). Similar morphological changes in synapses have also been found to be induced in the visual cortex by experience in adult rats (Jones et al., 1997) and developing cats (Friedlander et al., 1991). Synaptic restructuring is thought to reflect changes in the functional strength of neural connections and may facilitate spontaneous recovery of function by "rewiring" the brain; this rewiring can, in turn, be facilitated by behavioral demand during recovery.

Spontaneous recovery of such functions as vibrissae-stimulated forelimb placing and limb use asymmetries for vertical exploration and landing may be dependent on the NMDA receptor, which is a subtype of glutamate receptor. Chronic administration of the NMDA receptor antagonist MK-801 (1 mg/kg/day) during the pruning/synaptic restructuring phase (beginning on day 18) resulted in a reinstatement of the severe deficits seen early after the injury (Barth et al., 1990; Kozlowski & Schallert, 1998) as shown schematically in Figure 8-1. Animals are partially recovered at day 18 and continue to recover to near-preinjury levels by day 60 if treated with saline. However, animals treated with MK-801 beginning on day 18 not only fail to recover, but perform at levels comparable to those on day 1. Similar results have been obtained following the oral administration of ethanol (Kozlowski et al., 1997), which also acts at the NMDA receptor. It is important to note that MK-801, when given during the sensitive period immediately following electrolytic lesions (Barth et al., 1990), ischemic stroke (Gill et al., 1987; Park et al., 1988), and traumatic brain injury (McIntosh et al., 1990), has been shown to be neuroprotective. It is of great clinical importance to investigate whether drugs that have neuroprotective effects when given acutely may be deleterious when given at later periods after an injury (Schallert & Hernandez, 1998).

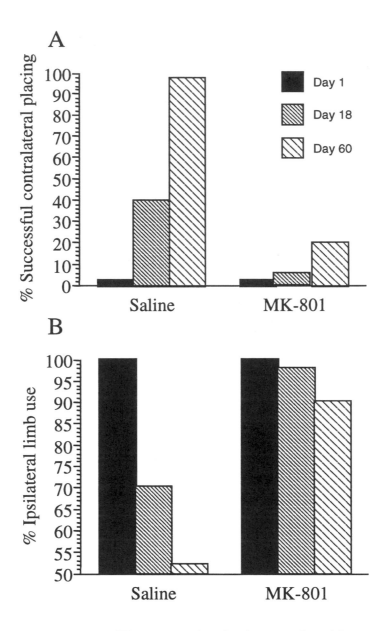

Figure 8-1. Chronic NMDA receptor blockade during the dendritic pruning/synapse restructuring phase reinstates functional deficits following recovery from FL-SMC lesions. Both the contralateral forelimb placing response (A) and symmetrical spontaneous limb use (B) are impaired 1 day after the lesion but recover somewhat by day 18 and attain near-perfect levels by day 60 in saline-treated animals. MK-801 treatment beginning on day 18 results in a long-lasting reversal of recovery of the placing response and symmetrical limb use for postural support. (Adapted from Barth et al., 1990)

Rehabilitation and Use-Related Plasticity

Although spontaneous recovery of function of the contralateral limb following damage to the motor cortex often occurs in humans and other animals, complete recovery is uncommon in humans and, if the test is sensitive enough, in nonhuman animals as well (Aronowski et al., 1996). Functional MRI studies demonstrate that spontaneous recovery of function following stroke in humans may involve the recruitment of the ipsilateral hemisphere (Cramer et al., 1997). There is frequently residual impairment of function. Some of this residual impairment may be due to "learned nonuse" of the affected limb, according to Taub et al. (1994). In order to compensate for dysfunction following injury, alternative strategies involving different motor patterns are often adopted. During the sensitive period soon after injury, the use of these strategies may impede the reestablishment of normal motor patterns. Taub's group has immobilized the good arm of patients several months after disruption of function due to unilateral stroke and found that, in combination with physical therapy, significant functional improvement in the impaired arm occured (Taub et al., 1996; Liepert, 1998; Miltner, 1999).

Immobilizing the good (ipsilateral) forelimb too soon after some types of injury, however, appears to have extremely deleterious effects, as we found in a rodent model. Kozlowski et al. (1996a) immobilized the ipsilateral forelimbs of rats immediately after FL-SMC lesions, forcing *overuse* of the affected limb for 14 days. Rather than enhancing recovery, ipsilateral casting resulted in retardation of functional improvement. Contralateral casting, forcing total *disuse* of the affected limb, also slowed recovery. Moreover, a dramatic expansion of the original injury was found, in ipsilaterally but not contralaterally casted rats, when brain tissue volume was assessed using a stereological analysis.

Representative T_2-weighted magnetic resonance imaging (MRI) brain scans, recently acquired in collaboration with Nicholas van Bruggen, are shown in Figure 8-2. A comparison of lesion size in coronal slices from an uncasted rat and from a rat than had been casted ipsilaterally for 10 days immediately following the lesion, both imaged at 31 days, shows that gross expansion of the lesion can be readily detected in animals that had been forced to overuse the affected forelimb. Lesion expansion can be viewed in the same animals by imaging the brain at various time points after the original insult, as we have shown in collaboration with Neal Rutledge (data not shown).

Recently, Humm et al. (1998) found that use-dependent exacerbation of damage occurs when rats are casted during the first week following an electrolytic lesion. Additional experiments revealed that this damage appears to be mediated by the NMDA receptor (Humm et al., 1999). MK-801, when given during the casting period, improved functional outcome and blocked expansion of the lesion. This suggested that use-dependent enhancement of injury may be similar to the excitotoxicity that causes damage due to ischemic stroke, which is also NMDA receptor mediated (Choi, 1988). However, the level of the excitatory neurotransmitter glutamate, which increases dramatically during ischemia, was not found to increase in the perilesional region of animals with ipsilateral casts. It is possible that the NMDA re-

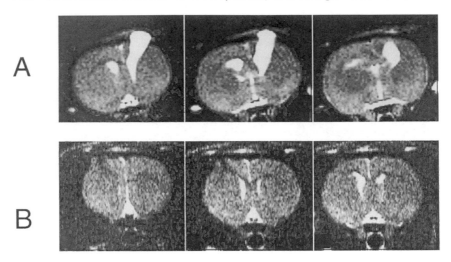

Figure 8-2. MRI images of rat brains with unilateral FL-SMC lesions. T_2-weighted fast spin echo sequences of 1 mm thick coronal slices at the lesion level acquired 31 days after surgery are shown. Overuse of the impaired forelimb by immobilization of the good limb in a plaster cast for 10 days during the early critical period results in gross enlargement of the original lesion (in the hemisphere on the right) and damage to the corpus callosum (A). The hyperintensity reflects cerebral spinal fluid that has filled the remaining cavity. An animal that was not casted did not sustain enlargement of the lesion (in the hemisphere on the left) and has an intact corpus callosum (B).

ceptor may be functionally upregulated in the perilesional area, to allow plasticity to occur with minimal use of the limb, which increases slowly, both quantitatively and qualitatively, during recovery. Indeed, Eysel (1996) found enhanced NMDA-mediated excitatory postsynaptic activity during the acute period in the area surrounding heat lesions in the rat. Glutamate receptors, including NMDA receptors but not dopamine receptors, are upregulated in striatum in a time-dependent manner following cortical ablation (Vargo & Marshall, 1996). Furthermore, Schiene et al. (1996) have demonstrated extensive reductions in inhibitory $GABA_A$ receptor densities in the perilesional region following photothrombotic lesions. Witte (1997) proposes that functional changes such as these not only can lead to cell death, but also can allow "reactive" synaptic plasticity and reorganization to occur. After some types of damage, vulnerable neurons may be pushed beyond the threshold of viability by normal activity. Ischemic hippocampal CA1 neurons were irreversibly depolarized by input stimulation, causing cell death at levels that did not induce cell death in normal neurons (Tsubokawa et al., 1992). It may be argued that interfering with these processes, by either too much activity (overuse) or too little (disuse), can have profoundly negative effects on recovery.

Bland et al. (1999) have observed that in intact rats, forced disuse for 1 week reduces basal levels of neuroactive amino acids in the sensorimotor cortex. Animals were casted and implanted bilaterally with microdialysis probes in the FL-SMC

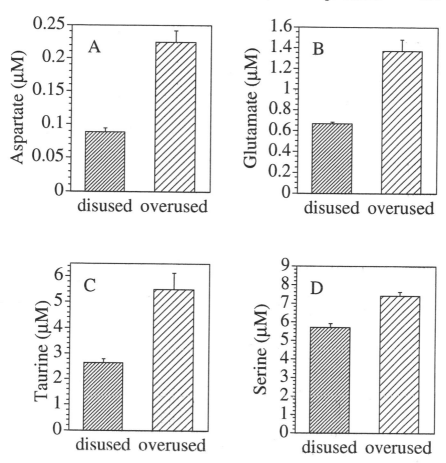

Figure 8-3. Disuse of one forelimb by immobilization in a unilateral one-sleeved cast for 1 week decreases dialysate amino acids in the corresponding FL-SMC in intact rats. Aspartate (A), glutamate (B), and taurine (C) but not serine (D) levels were measured in a within-subjects microdialysis experiment ($n = 5$) comparing hemispheres contralateral to either the disused or the overused limb. Rats were fitted with plaster of paris casts and implanted with bilateral microdialysis probes. One week later, the probes were perfused with artificial cerebro spinal fluid, and dialysates were collected every 10 minutes for 70 minutes after an overnight equilibration period. Samples were analyzed separately and pooled for graphical representation. Amino acid levels (μM) in the FL-SMC contralateral to the overused forelimb are similar to those observed in uncasted animals (Adapted from Bland et al., 1999).

of both hemispheres. One week later, dialysis experiments were performed and the levels of dialysate glutamate, aspartate, taurine, and serine were measured using high-performance liquid chromatography (HPLC) coupled with fluorometric detection. Figure 8-3 shows the levels of dialysate amino acids in the hemisphere contralateral to the disused and overused forelimb. The levels of glutamate and aspartate, both of which interact with the NMDA receptor, were reduced in the hemisphere contralateral to the disused forelimb, while the levels in the hemisphere contralateral to the overused forelimb were similar to those found in uncasted animals. The level of taurine, an inhibitory amino acid, was also reduced, although the serine level were not significantly affected. Although high levels of glutamate and other amino acids inhibit dendritic growth (Mattson, 1988), it is also possible that chronically *reduced* levels of these neurotransmitters due to chronic disuse interfere with recovery of function in lesioned rats.

Behavior-Sensitive Expression of Basic Fibroblast Growth Factor

Neurotrophic factors, including basic fibroblast growth factor (bFGF), are increased after many types of brain injury and appear to contribute to cell survival, maintenance, and plasticity (Finklestein, 1996; Finklestein et al., 1988; Humpel et al., 1994; Kawamata et al., 1997; Mattson & Scheff, 1994; Nieto-Sampedro & Cotman, 1985; Speliotes et al., 1996). The expression of bFGF and its mRNA has been observed in the nuclei and cell bodies of reactive astrocytes surrounding the damage after injury. Following suction ablation of the FL-SMC, Rowntree and Kolb (1997) observed bFGF immunoreactivity in the perilesional area as early as day 2 that peaked on day 7 and was still detectable on day 21. Increases in glial fibrillary acidic protein (GFAP)-positive astrocytes also were found. More recently, Hernandez and her colleagues (Buytaert et al., 1988) found increased bFGF expression following lesions of the anteromedial cortex (AMC) that correlated with recovery of somatosensory function.

In collaboration with Bryan Kolb, we showed that after electrolytic lesions of the FL-SMC, both bFGF-positive and GFAP-positive astrocyte numbers are increased in the region surrounding the injury (Humm et al., 1997). The expression of growth factors such as bFGF may be behavior-sensitive (Gomez-Pinilla et al., 1998) and may prime vulnerable tissue for plasticity-associated events reflected in neuronal structure, organization, and function. These results may explain why casting the impaired forelimb for the first 15 days after injury retards the rate of functional recovery (Kozlowski et al., 1996). Expression of bFGF after injury may promote the integrity of surviving neurons in the perilesion region and appears to be important for functional outcome (Rowntree & Kolb, 1997). Minimal forelimb use, as observed in uncasted animals, may initiate at least partial plasticity, which may provide significant neural protection against later, more aggressive rehabilitative intervention. It is possible that in uncasted rats bFGF-reactive astrocytes in the tissue surrounding the injury may provide a trophic influence that could protect the tissue from later insults.

When the impaired forelimb is immobilized during the first 7 days after injury, a window of vulnerability to forced overuse of the impaired forelimb is extended to later periods. Forced overuse of the impaired forelimb for 7 days beginning immediately after FL-SMC lesions results in expansion of the lesion, while forced

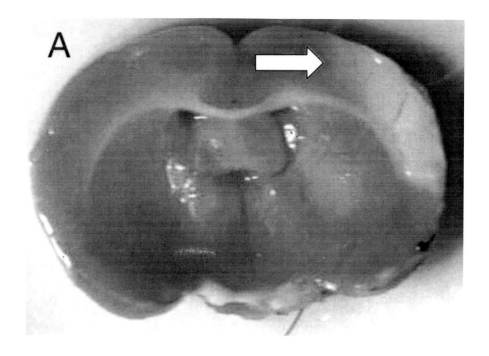

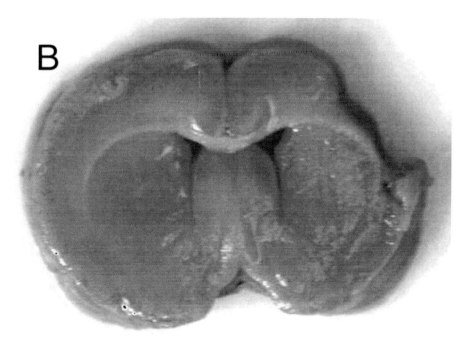

Plate 1. Representative, moderately large infarctions resulting from 30 minutes of unilateral MCA/bilateral CCA occlusion in two casted rats. Two mm thick TTC-stained slices 3 days (A) and 31 days (B) after ischemia are illustrated. The arrow (A) indicates the penumbra, which is adjacent to the FL-SMC.

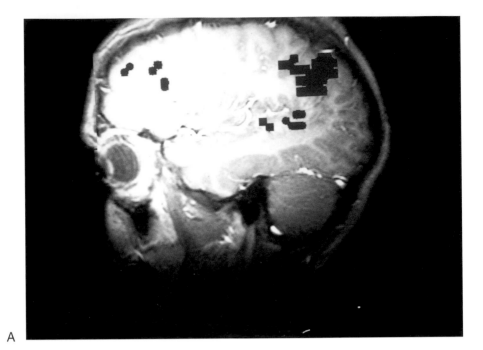

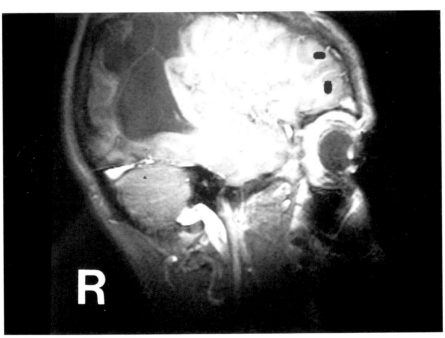

Plate 2. Sagittal fMRI images obtained under the serial subtraction condition indicating activation in the patient's left hemisphere (A) and reduced activation in the right hemisphere (B). In comparison, administration of this task to nine normal subjects produced bilateral activation in the supramarginal gyrus (n = 7) and the angular gyrus (n = 6). Adapted from Levin et al. (1966). Reproduced with permission.

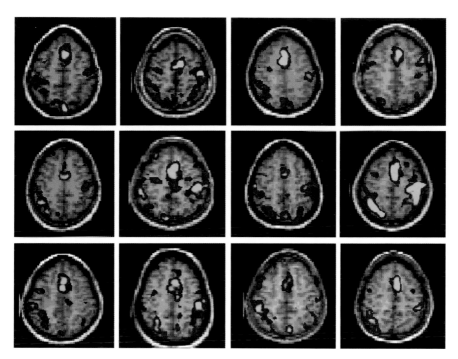

Plate 3. Data from 12 separate individual subjects are shown to illustrate the reliability of fMRI brain imaging techniques. Similar observations have been made using PET. The fMRI images show significant changes in the fMRI signal in a transverse dorsal section from each subject cut through the supplementary motor area (SMA) during a memory task. In all instances, clear activity change is observed in or near the SMA along the midline. Modified from Buckner et al. (1998).

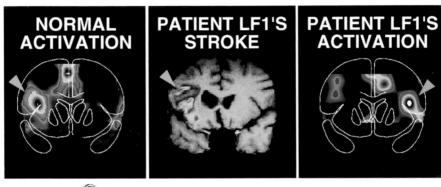

| NORMAL ACTIVATION | PATIENT LF1'S STROKE | PATIENT LF1'S ACTIVATION |

Plate 4. Stroke recovery in patient LF1 (Buckner et al., 1996a) is illustrated. Coronal sections show brain activation patterns in normal subjects that involve robust activation of the left frontal cortex near the operculum during speech production (left image). LF1 suffered a stroke that damaged this region of the cortex (center image), in spite of his ability to perform certain speech production tasks reasonably well. Brain imaging of LF1 demonstrated that he activated a homologous right-lateralized frontal region durng speech production that may represent a compensatory brain pathway (right image).

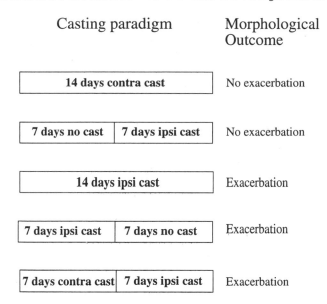

Figure 8-4. Disuse of the impaired forelimb during an early critical period extends the window of vulnerability to overuse. This schematic representation shows the effects of overuse and disuse on lesion volume following FL-SMC lesions. Seven and 14 days of overuse immediately after damage exacerbates the damage, while 7 or 14 days of disuse does not. Seven days of normal use followed by 7 days of overuse also does not exacerbate the damage. However, 7 days of *disuse* followed by 7 days of *overuse* exacerbates the damage.

overuse for 7 days beginning at day 7 does not. However, Humm et al. (1997) found that complete disuse via casting of the impaired limb for the first 7 days, followed by forced overuse via casting of the good limb for the second 7 days, results in expansion of the lesion (see Schallert et al., in press, and Fig. 8-4 for a schematic representation). Thus, complete rest of the affected limb extended the window of vulnerability to damage due to overuse into the formerly safe period, that is, the second 7 days postlesion.

Mild or delayed physical therapy has not been shown to be harmful and can improve functional outcome following some types of brain damage (Hart et al., 1997; Taub et al., 1994, 1996, 1998, 1999; Xerri et al., 1998). Our results imply that in the early period after injury, there may be a window of opportunity during which the beneficial effects of physical rehabilitation may be potentiated by the increased expression of endogenous trophic factors. However, Risedal et al. (1999) found that moderate motor "training" in uncasted rats exaggerated the size of the infarct if it occurred during the first week after middle cerebral artery occlusion (MCAO), but not if it occurred during the second week. The adverse training began 24 hours after MCA ligation distal to the striatal branches in spontaneously hypertensive rats. The training regimen consisted of an enriched environment plus motor challenges three times during the week, including traversing a rotating pole, hanging on to a rope, and maintaining balance on an inclined plane. These data raise further concerns about what the most appropriate rehabilitation regimen should be, both preclinically and in patients with brain injury.

Interaction of Amphetamine and Experience to Enhance Recovery of Function

Establishing that an animal's motor response to the injury can influence neuro-trophic expression and related events has implications for studies of recovery of function in which motor behavior might be changed directly by pharmacological interventions (Schallert & Hernandez, 1998). For example, there is ample evidence that the postlesion functional outcome is improved by the administration of am-phetamine (Feeney et al., 1982; Goldstein & Hulseboch, 1999; Hovda & Feeney, 1984; Hurwitz et al., 1991; Schmanke et al., 1996; Walker-Batson et al., 1995), which raises extracellular dopamine and norepinephrine levels and increases the ex-pression of bFGF in astrocytes (Flores et al., 1998). In a discussion of use-related events, it is essential to note that this facilitatory effect of amphetamine is opti-mum when it is combined with task-specific practice. For example, Feeney et al. (1982) administered amphetamine to rats after suction ablation of motor cortex and found that beam-walking performance was significantly improved only when the animals were allowed practice trials on the beam after administration of the drug. Animals given amphetamine and restraint performed no better than controls. Schmanke et al. (1996) extended this result by demonstrating that amphetamine facilitates recovery when the task produces a deficit in the initiation of locomo-tion but not when the task requires somatosensory or proprioceptive cues. Thus, performance on the forelimb-placing task, but not the bilateral-tactile stimulation task, was enhanced when amphetamine was administered prior to testing. In a study of human stroke patients, Walker-Batson et al. (1995) found that amphetamine paired with physical therapy led to enduring increases in motor function as-sessed by the Fugl-Meyer Scale. Goldstein and Hulsebosch (1999) suggested that the effects of amphetamine are due to enhanced noradrenergic activity in the in-tact homotopic cortex. This is consistent with the findings of earlier studies indi-cating that increased arborization, synaptogenesis, and other growth-associated markers are elicited and shaped by motor experience and may provide a basis for improved outcome in tests that depend on experience (reviewed in Kolb, 1995, and Schallert et al., in press).

Amphetamine has been shown to increase the expression of gene products and proteins associated with plasticity. For example, a single dose of amphetamine upregulated the transcription factor zif/268 mRNA in rat cortex in an NMDA receptor–dependent manner (Wang et al., 1994). The expression of GAP-43, a protein found in the growth cone of sprouting neurons, and synaptophysin, a presynaptic vesicle protein, are increased in the perilesion area following MCAO in a time course that correlates with recovery, and this increase is enhanced by an amphetamine regimen (Stroemer et al., 1998). Gnegy et al. (1993) showed that amphetamine increased GAP-43 (neuromodulin) phosphorylation. Robinson and Kolb (1997) reported structural changes (increased arborization and multiple spine heads), in both prefrontal cortex and nucleus accumbens, in the dendrites of intact rats given repeated (sensitizing) doses of amphetamine. They interpreted these results to indicate that sensitization is a form of experience-dependent plasticity. In light of the observation that the neuroprotective drug clenbuterol, an agonist of the beta 2-adrenergic receptor, increases nerve growth factor (NGF) (Semkova et al., 1996), it is tempting to speculate that amphetamine's effects may involve use-dependent increases in activity-dependent substrates, including the expression of bFGF, in perilesion areas as well as homotopic areas in the intact hemisphere.

Forced Use and Focal Ischemic Stroke

Following focal ischemia, a reduction in energy availability triggers a complex cascade of events that can lead to cell death. The MCA, along with its branches, supplies the main part of the cerebral hemispheres, including motor cortex and somatosensory cortex, and is the cerebral artery most often affected by cerebrovascular accidents leading to ischemic stroke. Middle cerebral artery occlusion results in a variety of neurological deficits, including aphasia, neglect, and contralateral hemiplegia. Although some spontaneous recovery often occurs, rehabilitation may hasten or improve the outcome. However, the optimal rehabilitation program has not been established. Animal models of physical therapy and its effects on functional recovery following MCAO may prove useful when applied in the clinic.

We are investigating the effects of forced overuse of the affected forelimb in experimentally induced MCAO in the rat using graded "doses" of ischemia. To investigate the effects of overuse following a subthreshold ischemic event, rats were either casted or left uncasted immediately following 30 minutes of tandem unilateral MCA/bilateral common carotid artery (CCA) occlusion or sham surgery. This duration of ischemia has been shown to result in minimal damage. Forced overuse via casting was implemented for 10 days, and the animals were sacrificed at 31 days. Consistent with the results obtained following electrolytic lesions, Bland et al. (1998a) demonstrated that forced overuse results in an increased infarct volume in this model of focal ischemic stroke. Figure 8-5 shows the infarct volume in ipsilaterally casted, uncasted, and sham-operated rats (because there was no difference between the groups, the data from casted and uncasted shams were pooled).

Examples of triphenyl tetrazolium chloride (TTC)–stained 2 mm brain slices can be seen in Plate 1. Plate 1A shows a moderately large infarction 3 days following 30 minutes of 3 vellel occlusion (3VO) in an ipsilaterally casted rat. Note that the penumbra of the infarction (arrow) is adjacent to the FL-SMC, and that there is little direct damage to the FL-SMC and no perceptible subcortical damage. Plate 1B also shows a moderately large infarction in a rat that was ipsilaterally casted for 10 days and then sacrificed 31 days following 3VO. At this endpoint a cavity is all that remains, allowing only indirect measurements of infarct volume.

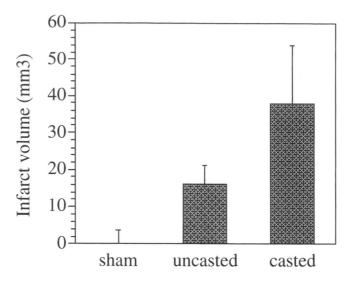

Figure 8-5. Overuse of the affected forelimb following 30 minutes of unilateral MCA/ bilateral CCA occlusion increases infarct volume. Infarct volume was measured 30 days after the ischemic insult by subtracting the remaining ipsilateral cortex from the intact contralateral cortex and using the thickness of the slice to derive the volume. Forced overuse via ipsilateral forelimb immobilization for 10 days resulted in infarctions that were 230% larger than those of uncasted animals. Sham surgery resulted in no difference in hemisphere volumes. (Bland et al., 1998a)

We then increased the duration of ischemia to 45 minutes of tandem MCA/ CCA occlusion followed by casting, again for 10 days. Behavioral testing was begun 7 days after removal of the cast. Animals that had been casted were significantly less able to place their contralateral forelimbs on a tabletop in response to vibrissae stimulation, a normal response in intact animals. Overuse also resulted in increased asymmetry on the footfault task, in which animals are placed on an elevated grid and scored for the number of times the contralateral paw slips through a grid opening (a fault) as they traverse the grid surface relative to the number of ipsilateral faults and corrected for the total number of steps taken (see Fig. 8-6). There was no effect of overuse in the acquisition of a cognitive task, the Morris water maze (data not shown).

It is important to note that in a more exteme model of focal ischemia, forced overuse for 14 days did not exacerbate either infarct volume or functional deficits 30 days following the insult (see Fig. 8-7). Overuse did not increase tissue damage, as assessed using hematoxylin and eosin staining (A), nor did it increase secondary degeneration (B). Spontaneous limb use, observed while animals engaged in exploratory behavior in a clear glass cylinder, was severely affected but was not different between casted and uncasted animals (C). Furthermore, asymmetry in the footfault test was the same between the groups (D). We observed that 90 minute 3VO caused large infarctions that involved the motor cortex as well as subcortical

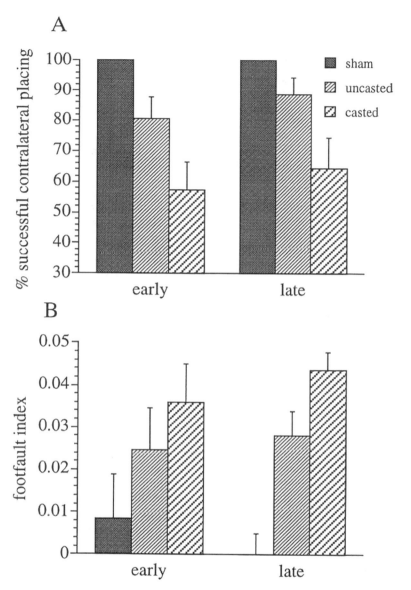

Figure 8-6. Overuse of the affected forelimb results in enduring exaggeration of functional deficits following unilateral MCA/bilateral CCA occlusion for 45 minutes. Rats were casted for 10 days immediately after ischemia, and testing began 1 week after removal of the cast and occurred once a week for 4 weeks. Data are pooled into the early (one and 2 weeks following cast removal) and late (3 and 4 weeks after cast removal) periods. Early overuse resulted in fewer successful vibrissae-stimulated contralateral forelimb placing responses (A). Early overuse resulted in more contralateral forepaw slips (faults) when rats explored an elevated grid, as indicated by footfault index scores [(contra faults − ipsi faults) / total steps] (B). (Adapted from Bland et al., in press)

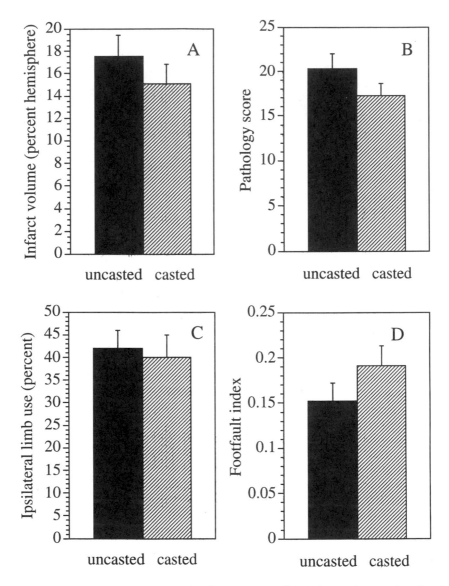

Figure 8-7. Overuse of the affected forelimb does not affect infarct volume or functional outcome following a *severe* focal ischemic stroke. Animals were casted for 14 days after unilateral MCA/bilateral CCA occlusion for 90 minutes. Following testing, the animals were sacrificed on day 30. There were no significant differences in cortical infarct volume, expressed as a percentage of the contralateral hemisphere (A), or in morphological pathology scores indicating secondary degeneration in the striatum, thalamus, and corpus callosum (B). Ipsilateral (unaffected) limb use, expressed as a percentage of total limb use, was not increased during exploratory behavior (C). Contralateral forepaw slips (faults) while traversing an elevated grid, expressed as an index [(contra faults − ipsi faults) / total steps], were not significantly different between the groups (D). (Bland et al., 1998a)

regions including the striatum and thalamus. Damage appears to have been maximal in this model, suggesting that a "penumbra" of vulnerable yet potentially salvagable tissue surrounding the core of the infarct must be present and is being pushed beyond the threshold of viability by forced overuse in the milder MCAO models. An alternative explanation is that lesions involving subcortical damage are not vulnerable to the damaging effects of forced overuse. Secondary and tertiary cell death resulting from forced overuse in a purely cortical model may already be a part of the cascade of damage in a more severe occlusion model. These data indicate that the adverse effcts of early motor rehabilitation are not inevitable and depend on many factors (Forgie et al., 1996; Schallert et al., 1997).

Colbourne et al. (1998) sought to determine whether increased use of the hippocampus would result in increased damage to neurons in the CA1 subfield following borderline damage due to global ischemia in gerbils. Multiple behavioral tests involving hippocampal-dependent tasks failed to exacerbate the damage. It is possible that, in contrast to cortical injury due to moderate to severe physical training (Kozloswki et al., 1996a; Risedal et al., 1999) hippocampal neurons may not be vulnerable to overuse effects. However, it should be noted that behavioral pressure was very mild and was not implemented until 4 days following the insult in this experiment. It is likely that behavioral pressure at this time point was too late to cause any additional damage to vulnerable neurons. However, Humm et al. (unpublished data) have shown that 5 minutes of swimming each day following an FL-SMC lesion does not exaggerate the extent of the lesion and has no adverse effect on functional outcome.

Holland et al. (1993) conducted one of the few studies involving systematic manipulations of early rehabilitation intensity in human brain-damaged patients. In this investigation of thrombolytic stroke, performance on Kertesz's Western Aphasia Battery was worse when patients received several weeks of extreme didactic training (pushing them to the limit) than when they were allowed to simply engage in brief (15 minutc) conversation. The adverse effect was not permanent, however, which suggests that the therapy either did not exaggerate tissue loss or that tissue loss expansion did not extend into relevant speech areas.

Amelioration of Parkinsonian Symptoms with Forced Use

We have recently investigated the effects of behavioral pressure in a rat model of Parkinson's disease (PD). Parkinson's disease is a progressive neurodegenerative disorder of the basal ganglia, and is functionally characterized by tremor, muscle rigidity, and difficulty in initiating motor activity. Neurochemically, it is characterized by a loss of dopaminergic neurons in the nigrostriatal system. Parkinsonism can be induced experimentally in the rat by the infusion of 6-hydroxydopamine (6-OHDA) into the medial forebrain bundle, which preferentially destroys neurons containing the neurotransmitter dopamine (DA). Unilateral 6-OHDA infusion creates a useful model in which movement asymmetries resulting from DA depletion can be detected and in which therapeutic treatments can be assessed by measuring the magnitude of these asymmetries.

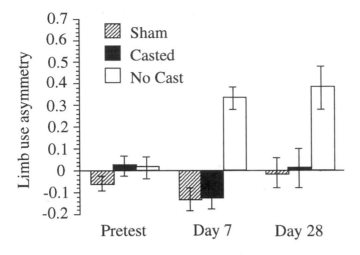

Day Post 6-OHDA

Figure 8-8. Overuse of the impaired forelimb protects against ipsilateral forelimb bias during spontaneous movements following 6-OHDA infusion. Ipsilateral asymmetry was analyzed by calculating the number of times the animal placed the left, right, or both forepaws against the wall of a clear cylinder while rearing and during exploration of the wall, and the number of times the animal landed on either its ipsilateral, contra lateral, or both paws. Asymmetry scores were calculated using the following equation: [(ipsi wall / total wall) + (ipsi land / total land) / 2]. Early overuse significantly protected against ipsilateral limb use bias in the casted group.

When rats with unilateral 6-OHDA lesions were forced to overuse the affected limb immediately following the infusion, the results were surprising in light of the effects of forced use on electrolytic cortical lesions and focal cortical ischemia. Tillerson et al. (1998) observed that, in contrast to the enhanced damage and decrements in motor performance found in previous studies with cortical lesions, 7 days of forced overuse via ipsilateral casting *improved* the functional outcome following 6-OHDA infusion. Figure 8-8 shows that casted animals demonstrated decreased limb use asymmetries during exploratory behavior at both early and late time points after the insult. Decreases in apomorphine-induced rotation were also observed as a result of the casting regimen, as seen in Table 8-1. Futhermore, casted animals showed increased expression of dopamine in the striatum compared to non-casted animals (data not shown). Congruent with the "ceiling effect" of severe ischemia, animals with severe damage, reflected in high levels of DA depletion, were not affected by the casting regimen (Bland et al., 1998b).

A behavioral manipulation has previously been shown to reverse the symptoms of parkinsonian. A recent study by van Keuren et al. (1998) revealed that fixed-ratio lever pressing eliminated the hyperresponsiveness of 6-OHDA-treated rats to

Table 8-1. Overuse of the Affected
Forelimb Following 6-OHDA Infusion
Protects Against Apomorphine-Induced
Contralateral Rotation

Treatment Group	Rotations
6-OHDA not casted	535 ± 133*
6-OHDA casted	105 ± 72
Sham	25 ± 6

Overuse of the affected forelimb was forced by immobilizing the unaffected forelimb in a plaster cast for 7 days. The
DA agonist apomorphine (0.25 mg/kg subcutaneous) was
injected on day 14 and rotations were recorded for 90 minutes. The number of rotations was significantly reduced in
the casted group.

*$p < .05$, different from casted and sham. Values are means
± SEMs.

apomorphine; however, it did not result in changes in nigrostriatal DA. The study
of Tillerson et al. (1998) was the first to show changes in DA status, as well as the
first to show improvements in spontaneous motor behavior resulting from physical therapy in a PD model.

The mechanism for the divergent results found in the PD model compared to
focal cortical models remains unclear. It is possible that overuse is beneficial in a
slowly evolving type of neurodegenerative disorder such as PD (Sasco et al., 1992).
However, it should be noted that some groups have reported delayed degeneration
following low-dose ischemia (Du et al., 1996), although we have not characterized
the time course of infarct evolution in our ischemia model. It is also possible that
overuse specifically benefits some types of neurons, such as DA neurons. Regular
physical exercise in college and adulthood may be associated with a lower risk of
PD (Sasco et al., 1992). Finally, overuse could be beneficial in lesions involving
primarily subcortical regions such as the basal ganglia. In this context, the observation that the anatomical damage resulting from the high dose of ischemia used
in our studies, which included some subcortical damage, was not exacerbated by
casting becomes of interest.

Summary

Spontaneous and evoked motor behaviors are significantly altered in adult rats
following many types of injury to the central nervous system. Although standard
vivariums use individual housing and isolation of experimental animals, these
conditions are not analogous to the conditions experienced by human patients following injury. Moderate forms of exercise, taming, and enrichment may prime the
brain for an improved outcome after brain injury and may activate neural events

associated with plasticity. However, extreme forms of physical therapy may be harmful after some types of brain damage, especially if implemented too soon after the insult. The observation that neural events are modifiable by disuse, use, or overuse could have profound implications for understanding the molecular events associated with neuroplasticity, treatment, and preventive behavioral medicine.

References

Aronowski, J., Samways, E., Strong, R., Rhoades, H.M., and Grotta, J.C. (1996) An alternative method for the quantitation of neuronal damage after experimental middle cerebral artery occlusion in rats: Analysis of behavioral deficit. *Journal of Cerebral Blood Flow Metabolism,* 16:705–713.

Barth, T.M., Grant, M.L., and Schallert, T. (1990) Effects of MK-801 on recovery from sensorimotor cortex lesions. *Stroke,* 21(suppl III):153–157.

Bland, S.T., Gonzales, R.A., & Schallert, T. (1999). Movement-related glutamate levels in rat hippocampus, striatum, and sensorimotor cortes. *Neuroscience Letters,* 227:119–122.

Bland, S.T., Humm, J.L., Kozlowski, D.A., Williams, L., Strong, R., Aronowski, J., Grotta, J., and Schallert, T. (1998a) Forced overuse of the contralateral forelimb increases infarct volume following a mild, but not a severe, transient cerebral ischemic insult. *Society for Neuroscience Abstracts, 774.14*:1955.

Bland S.T., Strong R., Aronowski J., Grotta J., and Schallert T. (in press). Early overuse of the affected forelimb following moderate transient focal ischemia in rats: Functional and anatomical outcome. *Stroke.*

Bland, S.T., Tillerson, J.L., Humm, J.L., Morin, S., Aronowski, J., Grotta, J., and Schallert, T. (1998b) Extreme forced motor therapy has an adverse effect on outcome in a cerebral ischemia model but a beneficial effect in a parkinsonian model. *National Neurotrauma Society Abstracts,* 15:28.

Bliss, T.V.P., and Collingridge, G.L. (1993) A synaptic model of memory: Long-term potentiation in the hippocampus. *Nature,* 361:31–39.

Bury S.D., Eichorn A.C., Kotzer C.M., and Jones T.A. (in press). Reactive astrocytic responses to denervation in the motor cortex of adult rats are sensitive to manipulations of behavioral experience. *Neuropharmacology.*

Buytaert, K.A., Kline, A.E., Montanez, S., Likler, E.L., Bowie, V., and Hernandez, T.D. (1998) Upregulation of basic fibroblast growth factor expression during the critical period following anteromedial cortex lesions. *Society for Neuroscience Abstracts,* 288.8:737.

Castro-Alamancos, M.A., and Borrell, J. (1995) Functional recovery of forelimb response capacity after forelimb primary motor cortex damage in the rat is due to the reorganization of adjacent areas of cortex. *Neuroscience,* 68:793–805.

Castro-Alamancos, M.A., Garcia-Segura, L.M., and Borrell, J. (1992) Transfer of function to a specific area of the cortex after induced recovery from brain damage. *European Journal of Neuroscience,* 4:853–863.

Choi, D. (1998) Glutamate neurotoxicity and diseases of the nervous system. *Neuron,* 1:623–634.

Chu, C., Gregory, A., Grande, L., Kim, J.H., and Jones, T.A. (1997) Motor skills training effects on behavioral and neocortical structural plasticity following unilateral sensorimotor cortex lesions in adult rats. *Society for Neuroscience Abstracts,* 23:95.18.

Colbourne, F., Auer, R.N., and Sutherland, G.R. (1998) Behavioral testing does not exacerbate ischemic CA1 damage in gerbils. *Stroke*, 29:1967–1971.

Cramer, S.C., Nelles, G., Benson, R.R., Kaplan, J.D., Parker, R.A., Kwong, K.K., Kennedy, D.N., Finklestein, S.P., and Rosen, B.R. (1997) A functional MRI study of subjects recovered from hemiparetic stroke. *Stroke*, 28:2518–2527.

Desmond, N.L., and Levy, W.B. (1990) Morphological correlates of long-term potentiation imply the modification of existing synapses, not synaptogenesis, in the hippocampal dentate gyrus. *Synapse*, 5:139–143.

Du, C., Hu, R., Csernansky, C.A., Hsu, C.Y., and Choi, D.W. (1996) Very delayed infarction after mild focal cerebral ischemia: A role for apoptosis? *Journal of Cerebral Blood Flow Metabolism*, 16:195–201.

Eysel, U.T. (1996) Perilesional cortical dysfunction and reorganization. In H.-J. Freund, B.A. Sabel, and O.W. Witte (eds.): *Brain Plasticity: Advances in Neurology*. Philadelphia: Lippincott-Raven, pp. 195–206.

Feeney, D.M., Gonzalez, A., and Law, W.A. (1982) Amphetamine, haloperidol, and experience interact to affect rate of recovery after motor cortex injury. *Science*, 217:855–857.

Finklestein, S.P. (1996) The potential use of neurotrophic factors in the treatment of cerebral ischemia. *Advances in Neurology*, 71:413–417.

Finklestein, S.P., Apostolides, P.J., Caday, C.G., Prosser, J., Philips, M.F., and Klagsbrun, M. (1988) Increased basic fibroblast growth factor (bFGF) immunoreactivity at the site of focal brain wounds. *Brain Research*, 460:23–29.

Flores, C., Rodaros, D., and Stewart, J. (1998) Long-lasting induction of astrocytic basic fibroblast growth factor by repeated injections of amphetamine: blockade by concurrent treatment with a glutamate agonist. *Journal of Neuroscience*, 18:9547–9555.

Forgie, M.L., Gibb, R., and Kolb, B. (1996) Unilateral lesions of the forelimb area of rat motor cortex: Lack of evidence for use-dependent neural growth in the undamaged hemisphere. *Brain Research*, 710:249–259.

Freund, H.J. (1996) Remapping the brain. *Science*, 272:1754.

Friedlander, M.J., Martin, K.A., and Wassenhove-McCarthy, D. (1991) Effects of monocular visual deprivation on geniculo-cortical innervation of area 18 in cat. *Journal of Neuroscience*, 11:3268–3288.

Fulton, J.F., and Kennard, M.A. (1934) A study of flaccid and spastic paralysis produced by lesions of the cerebral cortex in primates. *Research Pubublication of the Association of Mental Disease*, 13:158–210.

Geinisman, Y., Detoledo-Morrell, L., Morrell, F., Persina, I.S., and Beatty, M.A. (1996) Synapse restructuring associated with the maintenance phase of hippocampal long-term potentiation. *Journal of Comparative Neurology*, 368:413–423.

Gill, R., Foster, A.C., and Woodruff, G.N. (1987) Systemic administration of MK-801 protects against ischaemia-induced hippocampal neurodegeneration in the gerbil. *Journal of Neuroscience*, 7:3343–3349.

Gnegy, M.E., Hong, P., and Ferrell, S.T. (1993) Phosphorylation of neuromodulin in rat striatum after acute and repeated, intermittent, amphetamine. *Molecular Brain Research*, 20:289–298.

Goldstein, L.B., and Hulsebosch, C.E. (1999) Amphetamine-facilitated post-stroke recovery. *Stroke*, 30:696–698.

Gomez-Pinilla F., So V., and Kesslak J.P. (1998). Spatial learning and physical activity contribute to the induction of fibroblast growth factor: Neural substrates for increased cognition associated with excercise. *Neuroscience*, 85:53–61.

Greenough, W.T., Fass, B., and DeVoogd, T. (1976) The influence of experience on recovery following brain damage in rodents: Hypotheses based on developmental research. In R. Walsh and W.T. Greenough (eds.): *Environments as Therapy for Brain Dysfunction.* New York: Plenum Press, pp. 10–50.

Harris, K.M. (1995) How multiple-synapse boutons could preserve input specificity during an interneuronal spread of LTP. *Trends in Neurosciences,* 18:365–369.

Hart, C.L., Davis, G.W., and Barth, T.M. (1997) Forced activity facilitates recovery of function following cortical lesions in rats. *National Neurotrauma Society Abstracts,* 101.

Holland, A.L. (1993) In R.K. Brookshire (ed.): *Clinical Aphasiology Conference Proceedings.* Minneapolis: BRK Publishers, pp. 44–48.

Hovda, D.A., and Feeney, D.M. (1984) Amphetamine with experience promotes recovery of locomotor function after unilateral frontal cortex injury in the cat. *Brain Research,* 298:358–361.

Humm, J.L., Kozlowski, D.A., Bland, S.T., James, D.C., and Schallert, T. (1999) Use-dependent exaggeration of brain damage: Is glutamate involved? *Experimental Neurology.* 157:349–358.

Humm, J.L., Kozlowski, D.A., James, D.C., Gotts, J.E., and Schallert, T. (1998) Use-dependent exacerbation of brain damage occurs during an early post-lesion vulnerable period. *Brain Research,* 783:286–292.

Humpel, C., Chadi, G., Lippoldt, A., Ganten, D., Fuxe, K., and Olson, L. (1994) Increase in basic fibroblast growth factor (bFGF, FGF-2) messenger RNA and protein following implantation of a microdialysis probe into rat hippocampus. *Experimental Brain Research,* 98:229–237.

Hurwitz, B.E., Dietrich, W.D., McCabe, P.M., Alonso, O., Watson, B.D., Ginsberg, M.D., and Schneiderman, N. (1991) Amphetamine promotes recovery from sensory-motor integration deficit after thrombotic infarction of the primary somatosensory rat cortex. *Stroke,* 22:648–654.

Johansson, B.B. (1995) Functional recovery after brain infarction. *Cerebrovascular Disease,* 5:278–271.

Jones, T.A., Kleim, J.A., and Greenough, W.T. (1996) Synaptogenesis and dendritic growth in the cortex opposite unilateral sensorimotor cortex damage in adult rats: A quantitative electron microscopic examination. *Brain Research,* 733:142–148.

Jones, T.A., Klintsova, A.Y., Kilman, V.L., Sirevaag, A.M., and Greenough, W.T. (1997) Induction of multiple synapses by experience in the visual cortex of adult rats. *Neurobiology of Learning and Memory,* 68:13–20.

Jones, T.A., and Schallert, T. (1992) Overgrowth and pruning of dendrites in adult rats recovering from neocortical damage. *Brain Research,* 581:156–160.

Jones, T.A., and Schallert, T. (1994) Use-dependent growth of pyramidal neurons after neocortical damage. *Journal of Neuroscience,* 14:2140–2152.

Kawamata, T., Dietrich, W.D., Schallert, T., Gotts, J.E., Cocke, R.R., Benowitz, L.I., and Finklestein, S.P. (1997) Intracisternal basic fibroblast growth factor (bFGF) enhances functional recovery and upregulates the expression of a molecular marker of neuronal sprouting following focal cerebral infarction. *Proceedings of the National Academy of Sciences of the USA,* 94:8179–8184.

Kleim, J.A., Barbray, S., and Nudo, R.J. (1998) Functional reorganization of the rat motor cortex following motor skill learning. *Journal of Neurophysiology,* 80:3321–3325.

Kolb, B. (1995) *Brain Plasticity and Behavior.* New York: Erlbaum.

Kozlowski, D.A., Hilliard, S., and Schallert, T. (1997) Ethanol consumption following recovery from unilateral damage to the forelimb area of the sensorimotor cortex: Reinstatement of deficits and prevention of dendritic pruning. *Brain Research,* 763:159–166.

Kozlowski, D.A., James, D.C., and Schallert, T. (1996a) Use-dependent exaggeration of neuronal injury following unilateral sensorimotor cortex lesions. *Journal of Neuroscience,* 16:4776–4786.

Kozloswki, D.A., and Schallert, T. (1998) Relationship between dendritic pruning and behavioral recovery following sensorimotor cortex lesions. *Behavioural Brain Research,* 97:89–98.

Kozlowski, D.A., von Stuck, S.L., Lee, S.M., et al. (1996b) Behaviorally-induced contusions following traumatic brain injury: Use-dependent secondary insults. *Society for Neuroscience Abstracts,* 744.17.

Liepert, J., Miltner, W.H.R., Bauder, H., Sommer, M., Dettmers, C., Taub, E., and Weiller, C. (1998) Motor cortex plasticity during constraint-induced movement therapy in stroke patients. *Neuroscience Letters,* 259:5–8.

Mattson, M.P. (1988) Neurotransmitters in the regulation of neuronal architecture. *Brain Research,* 472:179–212.

Mattson, M.P., and Scheff, S. (1994) Endogenous neuroprotection factors and traumatic brain injury: Mechanisms of action and implications for therapy. *Journal of Neurotrauma,* 11:3–33.

McIntosh, T.K., Vink, R., Soares, H., Hayes, R., and Simon, R. (1990) Effect of noncompetitive blockade of *N*-methyl-D-aspartate receptors on the neurochemical sequelae of experimental brain injury. *Journal of Neurochemistry,* 55:1170–1179.

Miltner, W.H.R., Bauder, H., Sommer, M., Dettmers, C., and Taub, E. (1999) Effects of constraint-induced movement therapy on patients with chronic motor deficits after stroke: A replication. *Stroke,* 30:586–592.

Nieto-Sampedro, M., and Cotman, C.W. (1985) Growth factor induction and temporal order in central nervous system repair. In C.W. Cotman (ed.): *Synaptic Plasticity.* New York: Guilford Press, pp. 407–456.

Nudo, R.J., Wise, B.M., and SiFuentes, F. (1996) Neural substrates for the effects of rehabilitative training on motor recovery after ischemic infarct. *Science,* 272:1791–1794.

Park, C.K., Nehls, D.G., Graham, D.I., Teasdale, G.M., and McCulloch, J. (1988) The glutamate antagonist MK-801 reduces focal ischemic brain damage in the rat. *Annals of Neurology,* 24:543–551.

Risedal, A., Zheng, J., and Johansson, B.B. (1999) Early training may exacerbate brain damage after focal brain ischemia in the rat. *Journal of Cerebral Blood Flow and Metabolism,* 19:997–1003.

Robinson, T.E., and Kolb, B. (1997) Persistent structural modifications in nucleus accumbens and prefrontal cortex neurons produced by previous experience with amphetamine. *Journal of Neuroscience,* 17:8491–8497.

Rosenzweig, M.R. (1980) Animal models for effects of brain lesions and for rehabilitation. In P. Bach-y-Rita (ed.): *Recovery of Function: The oretical Considerations For Brain Injury Rehabilitation.* Baltimore: University Park Press.

Rowntree, S., and Kolb, B. (1997) Blockade of basic fibroblast growth factor retards recovery from motor cortex injury. *European Journal of Neuroscience,* 9:2432–2441.

Sasco, A.J., Paffenbarger, R.S., Gendre, I., & Wing, A.L. (1992). The role of physical exercise in the occurrence of Parkinson's disease. *Archives of Neurology,* 49:360–365.

Schallert T., Fleming S., Leasure J.L., Tillerson J.L., and Bland S.T. (in press). Assessment of forelimb sensorimotor outcome in unilateral rat models of stroke, trauma, parkinsonism and spinal cord injury. *Neuropharmacology.*

Schallert, T., and Hernandez, T.D. (1998) GABAergic drugs and neuroplasticity after brain injury: Impact of functional recovery. In L. Goldstein (ed.), *Restorative Neurology: Advances in the Pharmacotherapy of Recovery after Stroke.* Armonk, NY: Futura Press, pp. 91–120.

Schallert, T., and Jones, T.A. (1993) "Exuberant" neuronal growth after brain damage in adult rats: The essential role of behavioral experience. *Journal of Neural Transplantation and Plasticity,* 4:193–198.

Schallert, T., and Kozlowski, D.A. (1998) Brain damage and plasticity: Use-related neural growth and overuse-related exaggeration of injury. In M.D. Ginsberg and J. Bogousslavsky (eds.): *Cerebrovascular Disease: Pathology, Diagnosis, and Management.* Cambridge, MA: Blackwell Science, pp. 611–619.

Schallert, T., Kozlowski, D.A., Humm, J.L., and Cocke, R. (1997) Use-dependent events in recovery of function. In: H.-J. Freund, B.A. Sabel, and O.W. Witte (eds.), *Brain Plasticity, Advances in Neurology.* Philadelphia: Lippincott-Raven, pp. 229–238.

Schiene, K., Bruehl, C., Zilles, K., Qu, M., Hagemann, G., Kraemer, M., and Witte, O.W. (1996) Neuronal hyperexcitability and reduction of GABA receptor expression in the surround of cerebral thrombosis. *Journal of Cerebral Blood Flow and Metabolism,* 16: 906–914.

Schmanke, T.D., Avery, R.A., and Barth, T.M. (1996) The effects of amphetamine on recovery of function after cortical damage in the rat depend on the behavioral requirements of the task. *Journal of Neurotrauma,* 13:293–307.

Semkova, I., Schilling, M., Henrich-Noack, P., Rami, A., and Krieglstein, J. (1996) Clenbuterol protects mouse cerebral cortex and rat hippocampus from ischemic damage and attenuates glutamate neurotoxicity in cultured hippocampal neurons by induction of NGF. *Brain Research,* 717:44–54.

Speliotes, E.K., Caday, C.G., Do, T., Weise, J., Kowall, N.W., and Finklestein, SP. (1996) Increased expression of basic fibroblast growth factor (bFGF) following focal cerebral infarction in the rat. *Molecular Brain Research,* 39:31–42.

Stroemer, R.P., Kent, T.A., and Hulsebosch, C.E. (1995) Neocortical neural sprouting, synaptogenesis, and behavioral recovery after neocortical infarction in rats. *Stroke,* 26: 2135–2144.

Stroemer, R.P., Kent, T.A., and Hulsebosch, C.E. (1998) Enhanced nerocortical neural sprouting, synaptogenesis, and behavioral recovery with D-amphetamine therapy after neocortical infarction in rats. *Stroke,* 29:2381–2395.

Taub, E., Crago, J.E., Burgio, L.D., Groomes, T.E., Cook, E.W., DeLuca, S.C., and Miller, N.E. (1994) An operant approach to rehabilitation medicine: Overcoming learned nonuse by shaping. *Journal of Experimental Analysis of Behavior,* 61:281–293.

Taub, E., Pidikiti, D., DeLuca, S.C., et al. (1996) Effects of motor restriction of an unimpaired upper extremity and training on improving functional tasks and altering brain/ behaviors. In J.F. Toole and D.C. Good (eds.): *Imaging in Neurologic Rehabilitation.* New York: Demos Vermande, pp. 133–154.

Tillerson, J.L., Castro, S.L., Zigmond, M.J., and Schallert, T. (1998) Motor rehabilitation of forelimb use in a unilateral 6-hydroxydopamine (6-OHDA) rat model of Parkinson's disease. *Society for Neuroscience Abstracts,* 672.18:1720.

Tsubokawa, H., Oguro, K., Robinson, H.P.C., Masazawa, T., Kirino, T., and Kawai, N. (1992) Abnormal Ca^{2+} homeostasis before cell death revealed by whole cell recording of ischemic CA1 hippocampal neurons. *Neuroscience,* 49:807–817.

van Keuren, K.L., Stodgell, C.J., Schroeder, S.R., and Tessel, R.E. (1998) Fixed-ratio discrimination training as replacement therapy in Parkinson's disease: Studies in a 6-hydroxydopamine-treated rat model. *Brain Research,* 780:56–66.

Vargo, J., and Marshall, J.F. (1996) Unilateral frontal cortex ablation producing neglect causes time-dependent changes in striatal glutamate receptors. *Behavioural Brain Research,* 77:189–199.

Walker-Batson, D., Smith, P., and Curtis, S. (1995) Amphetamine paired with physical therapy accelerates motor recovery after stroke: Further evidence. *Stroke,* 26:2254–2259.

Wang, J.Q., Daunais, J.B., and McGinty, J.F. (1994) NMDA receptors mediate amphetamine-induced upregulation of zif/268 and preprodynorphin mRNA expression in rat striatum. *Synapse,* 18:343–353.

Whishaw, I.Q., Pellis, S.M., Gorny, B.P., and Pellis, V.C. (1991) The impairments in reaching and the movements of compensation in rats with motor cortex lesions: An endpoint, videorecording, and movement notation analysis. *Behavioural Brain Research,* 42: 77–91.

Withers, G.S., and Greenough, W.T. (1989) Reach training selectively alters dendritic branching in subpopulations of layer II-III pyramidals in rat motor-somatosensory forelimb cortex. *Neuropsychologia,* 27:61–69.

Witte, O.W., and Stoll, G. (1997) Delayed and remote effects of focal cortical infarctions: secondary damage and reactive plasticity. In H.J. Freund, B.A. Sabel, and O.W. Witte (eds.): *Brain Plasticity: Advances in Neurology.* Philadelphia: Lippincott-Raven, pp. 207–227.

Xerri, C., Merzenich, M.M., Peterson, B.E., and Jenkins, W. (1998) Plasticity of primary somatosensory cortex paralleling sensorimotor skill recovery from stroke in adult monkeys. *Journal of Neurophysiology,* 79:2119–2148.

9

Role of Neuroplasticity in Functional Recovery After Stroke

RANDOLPH J. NUDO, SCOTT BARBAY,
AND JEFFREY A. KLEIM

Clinical stroke is frequently characterized by hemiparesis immediately after the is-chemic event and by substantial functional recovery over the ensuing weeks to months. While the most dramatic recovery occurs within the first 30 days after stroke, in many cases of severe stroke recovery can be protracted, reaching a plateau at 6 months or more after injury (Duncan & Lai, 1997; Wade et al., 1985). In these cases, recovery is usually more limited, and chronic impairments are common. The phenomenon of motor recovery after stroke, its underlying causes, and therapeutic techniques for modifying the extent and time course of recovery have been under intense investigation for well over a century. However, many of the most fundamental questions about motor recovery after stroke remain unanswered. While several studies have shown that stroke patients improve during rehabilitative therapy, for example, it has been much more difficult to demonstrate the efficacy of rehabilitation over and above what might be expected to occur spontaneously. Further, the superiority of one type of exercise program over others has not been adequately established.

Neurologic models have suggested that recovery involves at least three separate but interactive processes: resolution of diaschisis (and other acute events following cerebral infarction), behavioral compensation, and neuroplasticity (for a more complete discussion, see the review by Stein, 1998, and see Chapter 1). Neuroplasticity processes (including unmasking, vicariation, synaptogenesis, etc.) are particularly intriguing in light of the wealth of recent studies demonstrating functional remodeling of cortical sensory and motor areas as a result of peripheral injury, central injury, or behavioral experience (Jenkins et al., 1990; Kaas et al., 1990; Recanzone et al., 1993; Wall et al., 1992; Xerri et al., 1998). While some short-term recovery (hours to days) may be explained at least partially by resolution of stroke-related pathology in the acute stages, it now appears likely that long-

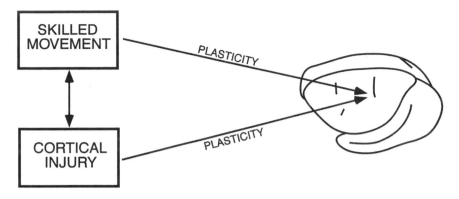

Figure 9-1. Interactive effects of use and injury on cortical organization.

term recovery (weeks to months) involves neuroplastic changes in the anatomy and physiology of intact cortical (and subcortical) tissue. Thus, studies of plastic changes in cerebral cortex may offer unique insights into the neural substrates for recovery, and could suggest novel behavioral and pharmacologic approaches to improving the outcome in stroke patients.

This chapter will focus on one aspect of neuroplasticity: reorganization of functional maps after stroke. It has been suggested that representational substitution, or vicariation in cortical maps, can mediate behavioral restitution of function after cortical stroke (Xerri et al., 1998). By examining the changes that take place in representational maps in the motor cortex after cerebral infarction, it may be possible to determine the neurophysiologic correlates of motor recovery. A thorough understanding of these neurophysiologic events is essential to understanding the functional role of the motor cortex in the recovery process and, ultimately, to improving the effectiveness of stroke rehabilitation strategies.

The conceptual framework for these studies is outlined in Figure 9-1. This model proposes that the learning of new motor skills results in predictable and adaptive neurophysiologic changes in the functional organization of motor cortex. The model proposes that cortical injury results in inevitable changes in cortical organization due to *(1)* neuronal degeneration at the site of injury and *(2)* disruption of neuronal networks in undamaged brain regions that are reciprocally connected with neurons in the damaged region. These undamaged brain regions may be adjacent to the site of injury, interconnected with damaged neurons by local (intrinsic) circuitry, or more remote (e.g., other cortical motor areas, contralateral motor cortex, subcortical motor structures), interconnected with damaged neurons by extrinsic circuitry. Finally, the model proposes that skilled movement and cortical injury interact, to the extent that use of the affected musculature after injury can have a profound effect on the subsequent reorganization that inevitably occurs in spared neuronal networks.

First, we will briefly review some of the early history of the study of motor recovery after cortical injury, highlighting a few of the seminal papers in this area.

Then we will examine more recent studies of the effects of use and injury on the functional organization of cerebral cortex. These studies demonstrate that the functional organization of motor maps adjacent to microlesions is predictably altered, as outlined in the above model. Finally, we will discuss some of the neurophysiologic mechanisms underlying plastic change in the cerebral cortex.

Motor Reeducation

Experimental examination of the effects of use on motor recovery from brain injury dates to at least the beginning of the twentieth century with the studies of Shepherd Ivory Franz (Franz, 1915; Franz et al., 1915; Ogden & Franz, 1917). In his capacity as Scientific Director at the Government Hospital for the Insane (St. Elizabeth's Hospital, Washington, DC), Franz published data from a large number of clinical observations and treatments of patients with cerebral lesions. From casual observations of recovery of function in patients with chronic hemiplegia, Franz suggested that, to a large extent, motor disabilities were the result of disuse. He implied that there was a latent ability to produce movements given the proper conditions. Using a variety of therapeutic techniques (such as massage, vibration, mechanical stimulation, and passive movement of extensors) Franz and his colleagues claimed to provide conditions under which voluntary movement could be obtained. In 1915, Franz wrote:

> The facts which we have already collected indicate that lesions of the motor cortex or of the upper part of the pyramidal tract in man do not abolish function, but put the function in abeyance until such time as the appropriate condition is present for the production of movement. We should probably not speak of permanent paralyses, or of residual paralyses, but of uncared-for paralyses. This we say because many of the conditions which we have met appear to resemble, if they are not real, phenomena of disuse, rather than actual inabilities.
>
> Franz et al., 1915, p. 2154

This theory is remarkably similar to the model recently formalized by Taub (Taub, 1994; Taub & Wolf, 1997; and see LeVere, 1980). Taub's model is based on earlier studies of nonuse of deafferented forelimbs in monkeys. Taub hypothesized that after an initial period of spinal shock, sometimes lasting several months, monkeys fail to use the deafferented limb not because they cannot do so, but because of a phenomenon known as learned nonuse. Learned nonuse is entirely predictable from established principles of behavioral conditioning. According to the model, during the initial period of spinal shock, the monkey is not rewarded for using the deafferented limb because the movements are unsuccessful and thus nonrewarded. Clumsy movements often result in painful consequences. Instead, the monkey develops compensatory strategies for executing daily activities, such as using the intact limb. While movements of the intact limb may not be as effective, they are positively reinforced. In chronic stages, the deafferented limb may possess some latent abilities. However, because the learned nonuse of the limb is so effectively

Table 9-1. Effect of Use on Motor Recovery After Cortical Injury

Exp No.	Monkey	Lesion	Restraint	Passive Treatment	Active Treatment	Recovery at 1 mo[1]
1	1	Left motor cortex	Yes	No	Yes	++
2	1	Right motor cortex in same monkey	No	No	No	0
3	2	Left motor cortex	No	Yes	No	+
4	2	Right motor cortex in same monkey	Yes	Yes	Yes	++
5a[2]	3	Left motor cortex	Yes	No	No	+
5b	3	Same monkey; no additional lesion	Yes	Yes	Yes	++
6	3	Right motor cortex in same monkey	No	Yes	No	+
7	4	Left motor cortex	Yes	Yes	Yes	++

[1]0 = no recovery; + = limited recovery; ++ = full recovery.

[2]In experiment 5a, restraint alone wa sused for 1 month. In the subsequent experiment, 5b (same monkey), active and passive treatments in addition to restraint were used for 1 month.

Source: Adapted from Ogden and Franz (1917).

conditioned, its abilities are masked. Taub and his colleagues suggest that this same phenomenon of learned nonuse may apply equally well to motor impairments following cortical injury.

If the learned nonuse hypothesis is valid, it should be possible to overcome nonuse by retraining the impaired limb, as suggested by Taub and Wolf (Taub, 1994; Taub & Wolf, 1997). Formal studies of increased use of the impaired limb after cortical injury first were conducted early in the twentieth century. Over 80 years ago, Ogden & Franz published experimental studies on recovery from motor cortical injury in monkeys (Ogden & Franz, 1917). Because the results of that study parallel so remarkably those of similar modern experiments, they are related here in detail. Using that era's state-of-the-art techniques, Ogden and Franz destroyed the motor cortex and then verified the extent of the lesion by using electrical stimulation to identify any remaining tissue where movements could be evoked. In each of the experiments, most if not all of the precentral gyrus was removed in the left hemisphere by electrocautery. By the authors' accounts, it is likely that this procedure rendered some damage to the postcentral gyrus as well. The lesions resulted in hemiplegia of the face, arm, and leg on the contralateral side. Then one or another treatment was instituted for approximately 1 month, and the monkey's motor behavior was examined. Next, the precentral gyrus of the right hemisphere was removed and another treatment regimen instituted. In most cases, these monkeys were then followed for 6 months.

Although only four monkeys were examined, the results are entirely what would be expected from the learned nonuse model. We have summarized the individual case results in Table 9-1. The designations of specific treatments and their effects on recovery are not those of Ogden and Franz but our own interpretations based on the original case accounts. Our designations for recovery are as follows. "No recovery" was designated for cases in which the monkey was described as hemiplegic, displaying extreme weakness, and so on. "Limited recovery" was designated for cases in which there was some evidence of returning function but not normal function. "Full recovery" was designated for cases in which the monkey's behavior was indistinguishable from normal behavior.

The treatments were as follows: "Restraint" consisted in strapping the monkey's unimpaired upper limb (i.e., ipsilateral to the lesion) to its trunk by the use of a custom jacket. Thus, the animal was forced to use its impaired upper limb for climbing, food retrieval, and other activities. "Passive treatment" consisted of general massage of the affected limbs, usually with special emphasis on the extensors. "Active treatment" consisted of mechanical stimulation of the affected limbs in order to encourage both reflexive and voluntary movements. In some cases, the monkey was led by a strap to encourage walking with the impaired leg. The results show that in the absence of treatment, no recovery was observed. Limited recovery was found when passive treatment or restraint was employed. However, when active treatment (encouragement of movement) was employed in combination with restraint (experiment 1), or in combination with restraint and passive treatment (experiments 4, 5b, and 7), the monkeys were reported to have recovered fully. One of the most remarkable aspects of this early study is the author's interpretation. Ogden and Franz suggested that the recovery may have been the result of substitution of other brain regions for the damaged function. They wrote:

> The results are of interest in another direction, in that they place in the hands of the experimenter the means for the rapid recovery of motor function so that the 'vicarious' functions of other cerebral parts may be investigated.
>
> 1917, p. 46

Other animal studies in the first half of the twentieth century also suggested that postinjury training may promote recovery of sensorimotor functions (Graham Brown & Steward, 1916; Lashley, 1924; Tower, 1940). More recently, systematic studies of the effects of use of the impaired limb in human stroke patients were conducted by Wolf and his colleagues (Ostendorf & Wolf, 1981; Wolf et al., 1989). Patients with limited movement were required to wear a sling during waking hours for 2 weeks. These patients showed significant improvement in several motor tasks. This approach has been combined with shaping and task practice with the impaired hand and is now usually referred to as *constraint-induced (CI) movement therapy* (Taub & Wolf, 1997). These studies provide strong evidence for the hypothesis of learned nonuse and suggest that recovery of function can occur in the impaired limb by overcoming learned nonuse.

With this compelling evidence that use of the impaired limb is important to functional recovery, it is reasonable to ask whether the suggestions of Franz are correct. What is the evidence for vicariation of function? Does the brain have the capacity to be functionally altered, and can such plasticity allow new circuitry to produce movements that are abandoned after cortical injury? In other words, can brain reorganization account for motor reeducation?

Anatomic and Physiologic Organization
of Primary Motor Cortex

To understand the neurophysiologic and neuroanatomic changes that have been demonstrated in cerebral cortex in response to use and injury, it is helpful to review the normal organization of motor cortex and the methods used to study these phenomena. Primary motor cortex can be identified anatomically by the presence of a high density of large corticospinal (or pyramidal tract) neurons. In addition, this area is characterized by relatively low current thresholds for eliciting movements by electrical stimulation. This electrophysiologic characteristic has been the basis for a large number of studies examining the functional topography of the primary motor cortex (Asanuma & Rosén, 1972; Donoghue & Sanes, 1998; Gould et al., 1986; Neafsey et al., 1986). The results described in this chapter are based on cortical stimulation techniques not unlike those used to derive maps of the motor homunculus in the human motor cortex by Wilder Penfield over half a century ago and still illustrated in many neurology textbooks (Penfield & Boldrey, 1937). The technique used in our laboratory to stimulate the motor cortex electrically in adult primates is similar to this method in many respects, except that the tip of the stimulating electrode is very fine (10–15 μm) and is introduced into deep laminae of the cortex (about 1.8 mm below the surface). Typically, a fine microelectrode is introduced into the cortex in anesthetized animals. Then a train of low-intensity current pulses is delivered. At each site within the primary motor cortex (M1), contraction of a small group of muscles can be elicited. At threshold current levels in monkeys (typically 10–15 μA), these movements are typically limited to a single joint (or joint category, such as the fingers), although movements of multiple joints are sometimes observed.

Using these microelectrode stimulation techniques, it has been repeatedly demonstrated that M1 is somatotopically organized with the legs medial and the hands lateral. However, on a more local scale, muscle representations are highly overlapping (Nudo et al., 1997; Sanes et al., 1995). By defining movements evoked by microstimulation, representations are said to be fractionated (Gould et al., 1986; Nudo et al., 1992). In other words, within a local area of M1 (such as the hand area), there is no strict topographic and orderly projection from cortical module to motor neuron pool. Rather, there is considerable convergence and divergence even at the level of the individual projection neuron (Cheney & Fetz, 1985). This overlap in anatomic organization may contribute to the ability of the system to reorganize functionally after injury (Figure 9-2).

Local intrinsic connections allow communication among the various parts of M1—for example, between different movement representations within the M1 hand area (Huntley & Jones, 1991; Keller, 1993). Because local connections also appear to be highly overlapping within a specific portion of the motor map (e.g., the hand

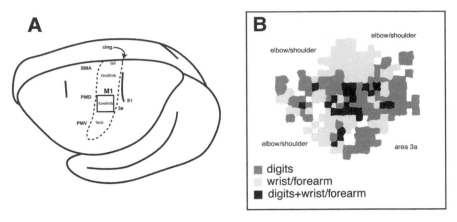

Figure 9-2. Location and somatotopic organization of the primary motor cortex (M1) in a squirrel monkey. (A) The distal forelimb, or hand area of M1, is located anterior to the central sulcus, near its lateral edge. In addition to M1, other motor areas include the dorsal premotor cortex (PMD), ventral premotor cortex (PMV), the supplementary motor area (SMA), and cingulate motor areas (cing.; hidden from view on the medial wall of the cerebral cortex). The locations of the primary somatosensory areas (S1) and area 3a are also shown. (B) Representations of movements in the hand area of M1. Movement representations were derived using microelectrode stimulation techniques in an anesthetized monkey.

area), they may also constitute an anatomic substrate for functional plasticity. In addition, corticocortical connections allow communication between M1 and ipsilateral premotor cortex, ipsilateral supplementary motor areas, and contralateral motor cortex.

Neurophysiologic Correlates of Motor Skill Learning

There is a great deal of individual variation in cortical motor topography. This has been demonstrated in a number of studies dating to the early work of Franz. At least some of the variation can be attributed to the hand preference of the animal. That is, the motor map contralateral to the animal's preferred hand is somewhat larger and spatially more complex (Nudo et al., 1992). This finding, demonstrating a correlation between the functional organization of motor cortex and handedness, is in agreement with the findings of human studies using magnetoencephalography and transcranial magnetic stimulation (Triggs et al., 1994; Volkmann et al., 1998; Wassermann et al., 1992). Because of this individual variation, it is often necessary to derive maps at different points in time in the same animal, i.e., before and after a manipulation, rather than compare the maps of different experimental groups. These so-called map/remap experiments are very important for addressing issues of use-dependent and injury-dependent changes.

To examine the dynamic features of motor cortex representations, we studied stimulation maps in squirrel monkeys before and after training on a task requiring skilled use of the digits. In this task, food pellets were placed in different-sized wells in a Plexiglas board, and the animals were required to retrieve them. The largest well was large enough for insertion of the entire hand. The smallest well required the insertion of one or two fingers to retrieve the pellet. Motor skill increased over several days of training, as evidenced by a decrease in the number of finger flexions required to extract the pellet. In addition, monkeys retrieved pellets in a highly stereotypic manner by flexing the fingers and extending the wrist. While this digit flexion/wrist extension combination can be said to be an obligatory synergistic pattern, the overt expression of this combination increased during the course of training.

Following training on the reach and retrieval task, representations of the fingers expanded significantly. In addition, there was a striking parallel between the specific multijoint movement representations that expanded in the posttraining maps and the actual multijoint movements (digit flexion/wrist extension) that were used in combination during the motor learning task. Thus, temporal contiguity of motor outputs (and temporal contiguity of proprioceptive and cutaneous inputs as well) may contribute to dynamic processes in the motor cortex during motor learning (Karni et al., 1998). This hypothesis is similar to one proposed for somatosensory cortex to explain map changes induced by experimental digital syndactyly (Clark et al., 1988).

More recent studies in our laboratory suggest that changes in motor cortex are driven by acquisition of new motor skills and not simply by motor use. When monkeys are required to retrieve pellets repetitively out of a large well in the reach and retrieval task, no systematic changes are observed in motor maps (Nudo et al., 1997; Plautz et al., 1995).. This result occurs even when the motor activity of the large-well and small-well groups are matched (based on cumulative finger flexions). We have concluded from these studies that adaptive change in motor cortex is skill dependent rather than use dependent.

Studies using a variety of other techniques have suggested this same conclusion. Using positron emission tomography (PET), transcranial magnetic stimulation (TMS), and functional magnetic resonance imaging (FMRI) techniques, several investigators have now shown that the area of activation for the hand representation in M1 increases as subjects practice complex finger movement tasks (Elbert et al., 1995; Grafton et al., 1992; Jenkins et al., 1994; Karni et al., 1995, 1998; Pascual-Leone et al., 1994, 1995; Schlaug et al., 1994; Seitz et al., 1990). Aside from the theoretical importance of these results for understanding the role of motor cortex in motor learning, these results may also be relevant for developing optimum rehabilitation strategies after stroke. If physiologic plasticity in cortical maps is critical for functional recovery, then it follows that tasks requiring progressively increasing motor skill are more important than tasks that simply require the patient to move the limb repetitively in the absence of skill acquisition (Figure 9-3).

Neuropsychologic Consequences of Cortical Injury: Investigations into Vicarious Functioning of Intact Motor Areas

If motor maps are alterable, it seems reasonable to ask whether alteration in functional motor topography can account for recovery of function after injury to M1. In their pioneering studies of functional localization in the cerebral cortex, Fritsch

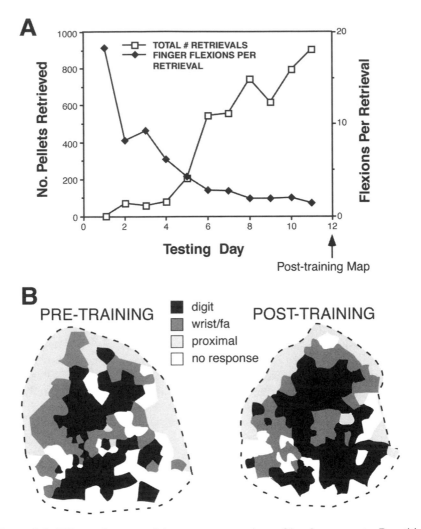

Figure 9-3. Effects of motor training on representations of hand movements. Repetitive training on a task requiring manual skill results in enlargement of digit representations in the motor cortex. Representations of the digits expand, while representations of the wrist and forearm contract (Nudo et al., 1996). (A) Performance of a squirrel monkey on a pellet retrieval task requiring skilled use of the fingers. The graph shows the total number of successful retrievals per day (open squares) and the average number of finger flexions per retrieval (filled diamonds). (B) Representation of hand movements before and after training on the retrieval task. The dotted line indicates the limits of map exploration.

176

and Hitzig (1870) proposed the theory of vicarious function to account for motor recovery after unilateral removal of motor cortex in dogs. Direct investigation of this issue using cortical stimulation techniques has been undertaken since the early twentieth century. In 1917, Leyton and Sherrington published the findings of a study involving ablation of the arm area in chimpanzees (Leyton & Sherrington, 1917). The M1 arm area was first identified using surface stimulation techniques. Then the area-yielding movements of the thumb, fingers, wrist, and elbow were excised. Significant paresis was observed in the hand contralateral to the lesion during the initial week after the lesion. However, after 1 month, significant recovery of movement was observed in the affected hand. When the motor cortex was reexamined using stimulation techniques, no hand movements could be obtained by stimulation of the adjacent, intact cortical tissue. Leyton and Sherrington concluded that "neither the ablation [n]or excitation methods gave any evidence that the remaining part of the arm area had taken on the functions of the ablated hand area."

During the next 30 years, several investigators examined the behavioral consequences of lesions in motor cortex of a variety of mammals, including primates. However, no direct evidence of vicarious function by intact cortical areas was reported despite a number of ablation-behavior experiments that used stimulation mapping techniques (e.g., Lashley, 1938). However, in a landmark experiment in 1950, Glees and Cole reported physiologic results indicating substitution of motor function (Glees & Cole, 1950). Glees and Cole made repeated small lesions in the motor cortex thumb representation in macaques. Using surface stimulation techniques, these investigators reported that the thumb representation reappeared in the intact motor cortex.

There are at least two possible reasons why so many prior researchers (including some of the icons of physiology and psychology such as Franz, Sherrington, and Lashley) failed to observe any evidence of vicariation. First, in many cases, the lesions were quite large. For example, in Lashley's (1924) study, the entire precentral gyrus of both hemispheres was destroyed to within 2 mm of the longitudinal fissure. A large portion of the premotor cortex was also destroyed, although the supplementary motor area was probably still intact. In contrast, Glees and Cole (1950) destroyed only a small part of the motor cortex, limiting the lesions to the electrophysiologically defined thumb area. It is quite possible that there are anatomic limits on vicariation of motor function, so that if a large proportion of the motor cortex is destroyed, no substitution is possible. Lashley subscribed to this view stating that

> restitution of function by reëducation depends in every case upon the preservation of some part of a limited system which is normally concerned in the same function. There is not an unlimited capacity for vicarious function but a limitation to the system which is more or less directly concerned with the function under normal conditions.
>
> (1938), p. 741

Second, except for the study of the effects of large lesions by Lashley in 1924, specific training procedures were not employed. Only anecdotal observations of spontaneous recovery were reported. Glees and Cole trained monkeys before and after lesions on a puzzle box task. This relatively complex task may have contributed to restitution of both behavioral and physiologic function.

Because modern microelectrode stimulation techniques for motor mapping provide substantially greater spatial resolution, it is now possible to readdress these questions, but in more detail. Recently, we have used microelectrode stimulation techniques to isolate the effects of cortical injury and postinjury use on the function of intact cortical areas (Friel & Nudo, 1998a; Nudo & Milliken, 1996; Nudo et al., 1996b, 1997). In these studies, the injury is created by bipolar electrocoagulation of a vascular bed over the physiologically identified motor cortex. The procedure is not intended to mimic stroke per se, but rather to create a focal ischemic lesion in a physiologically identified cortical region without damaging the surrounding tissue. The injury differs from one produced by a stroke in that it involves primarily venous drainage and, to a lesser extent, small end arteries supplying the targeted tissue. The lesions are relatively small, about 2–4 mm^2, or about 25%–30% of the monkey's hand representation. Each of the lesions was focused on the digit representations, but because of the mosaic composition of the maps, some wrist/forearm representations necessarily were also destroyed.

After electrophysiologic mapping and creation of the microlesions, monkeys were assigned to one of two experimental conditions: *(1)* spontaneous recovery or *(2)* rehabilitative training. After an interval ranging from several weeks to a few months, the motor maps were reexamined. In the initial 1–2 days after the microlesion, the affected forelimb typically was somewhat limp and was moved only sporadically, although it was sometimes used for support. The unaffected limb was used for prehension of food. Over the next several days to weeks, the affected limb was used more frequently. Deficits in motor efficiency on the pellet retrieval task were usually demonstrable. However, after several weeks, the monkeys recovered skilled use of the hand and were indistinguishable from normal, surgically unaltered monkeys on the pellet retrieval task.

There is some indication that the spontaneously recovering monkeys achieved normal performance somewhat more slowly, but these data are complicated by two factors. First, in our initial studies of spontaneous recovery, we did not introduce any training effects whatsoever (Nudo & Milliken, 1996). Therefore, performance was assessed only periodically. Thus, we do not yet have a complete and detailed time course of behavioral recovery in these animals. Second, the magnitude of the deficits resulting from the microlesions was quite variable across individuals. Despite the consistency in lesion volume and functional location, in some monkeys the deficits persisted for several weeks, while others displayed little if any behavioral effects even a few days after the lesion. While we speculate that this variability may be due to idiosyncrasies in the microtopography of motor maps, in local network connectivity, or possibly in prelesion experience, we have no definitive answer.

In contrast, the physiologic effects were consistent and predictable. Several weeks after the microlesion, the intact hand area surrounding the infarct underwent significant alteration. In contrast to the results of Glees and Cole (1950), after spontaneous recovery the remaining hand area in M1 was reduced in representational extent (Fig. 9-4). Sites that formerly were associated with digit movements became

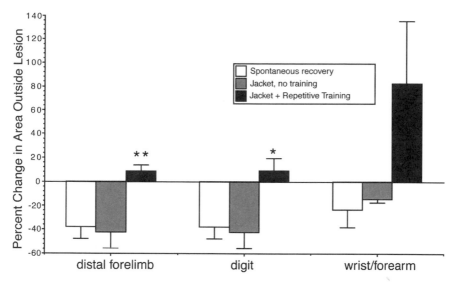

Figure 9-4. Changes in spared motor representations after microlesions in area M1 of squirrel monkeys. After spontaneous recovery of motor function, spared hand representations adjacent to the lesion are further reduced in areal extent. Forced use of the impaired limb by a restrictive jacket has no effect on reorganizational plasticity. However, when forced use is combined with a daily regimen of manual skill training after the microlesion, spared hand representations are retained (Friel & Nudo, 1998; Nudo & Milliken, 1996; Nudo et al., 1996b).

associated with elbow and shoulder movements. In cases in which the lesion was made larger, destroying over 50% of the hand area, the effects were more pronounced (Nudo & Milliken, 1996). Digit and wrist/forearm movements could not be evoked at any sites within the former hand area that was still intact after the lesion, except in a few locations at very high current levels. Instead, stimulation at threshold current levels evoked proximal (elbow and shoulder) movements. It should be emphasized that proximal movements could not be evoked prior to the infarct except at high current levels at only a few sites. Thus, spontaneous recovery, i.e., in the absence of postinfarct training, results in degenerative changes in the physiology of the remaining hand area. These findings are in general agreement with those of Leyton and Sherrington, and lead to the conclusion that spontaneous motor recovery cannot be explained by substitution of function in the spared motor cortex immediately adjacent to the lesion.

The monkeys undergoing spontaneous recovery, as described above, tend to use their unimpaired hand to perform tasks requiring manual dexterity, at least for the first few weeks. Therefore, to study the effects of use of the impaired hand after injury, it is necessary to restrict the movement of the unimpaired hand. This was accomplished by placing each monkey in a jacket with a long sleeve extending the length of the unimpaired limb. The sleeve ended in a mitten that covered the unimpaired hand. Monkeys wearing these jackets could still climb the cage bars, support themselves with the unimpaired hand, and even pick up large pieces of monkey chow. However, they had to use their impaired hand for dexterous tasks, such as small pellet retrieval. Because we specifically examined the effects of repetitive use after injury, it was possible to track motor performance daily throughout the recovery period. After a small ischemic injury to the motor cortex, motor performance on the pellet retrieval task declined. Eventually the motor performance of these animals returned to the normal range and remained within this range until the postinfarct mapping procedure was conducted. When the physiology of these monkeys was examined after recovery (a few weeks after infarction), it was found that the spared hand representation was retained. In some cases, the digit representation expanded into former elbow and shoulder territories. This finding is in contrast to that of the spontaneous recovery group, in which the spared hand area contracted (Fig. 9-4). Increased use of the impaired hand after injury appears to modulate plasticity in the surrounding tissue.

Finally, in a more recent study, we attempted to determine whether restraint of the unimpaired hand alone was sufficient to retain the spared hand area after cortical injury or if retention of the spared hand representation required repetitive use of the impaired limb (Friel & Nudo, 1998b). After a microlesion in the hand area of M1 in adult squirrel monkeys, the unimpaired hand was restrained but the monkeys did not receive additional rehabilitative training. Motor maps were derived using microelectrode stimulation techniques in anesthetized monkeys before and 1 month after the microlesion. One month after the lesion, the size of the hand representation and the sizes of component finger and wrist/forearm representations had decreased. The magnitude of the decrease was no different from that of animals undergoing spontaneous recovery. Hand areas were significantly smaller than those in animals that had received daily repetitive training after infarction (Fig. 9-4). Taken together with previous findings, these findings suggest that retention of hand representations within M1 after cortical injury requires repetitive use of the impaired hand after injury.

Taub's learned nonuse hypothesis describing the behavior deficits that occur after stroke, described earlier in this chapter, is quite applicable to these findings in monkeys. That is, after injury the monkey makes many unsuccessful motor attempts with its impaired hand. These attempts are negatively reinforced, so movements of that hand are suppressed. Compensatory motor patterns develop in the unimpaired hand. After recovery from microlesions, the impaired limb may again be used for skilled tasks, but compensatory patterns are used for retrieval of small objects. The demonstration that the adjacent cortical tissue can display vicarious function suggests that when human patients overcome learned nonuse by restraint-induced movement therapy, the intact motor cortex may play some role in the relearning process. Recently, this hypothesis has gained further support from the demonstration in human stroke patients that constraint-induced movement therapy results in enlargement of the motor representation of the affected and trained limb (Liepert et al., 1998).

Despite the apparent benefits that may accompany repetitive skill training after cortical injury, recent studies in rats suggest that overuse after cortical injury may cause dysfunctional alterations in cortical morphology (see Chapter 8). As overuse of the impaired limb after injury results in exaggeration of neuronal injury, some concerns have been raised regarding the safety of forced-use paradigms after stroke. On the surface, this would seem to contradict the findings in monkeys and humans about the benefits of forced use after stroke. However, it is important to note that the rat and monkey models have at least one notable difference. Since rats are quadrupeds, the effects of a body cast (as in the studies of Schallert and colleagues) and restriction of all movements of the unimpaired limb are much more severe. The casted rat is forced to rely on its impaired limb not only for grasping and manipulation, but also for locomotion and balance. This involves a more exaggerated level of use that is qualitatively different from the increased use we see in a monkey or human with a sling-type restraint. However, the use-dependent exaggeration of injury is an important phenomenon that needs extensive further study.

Short-Term Versus Long-Term Mechanisms of Cortical Plasticity

As mentioned at the beginning of this chapter, recovery after cortical injury involves an interplay of acute (e.g., diaschisis), and chronic (e.g., behavioral compensation and neuroplasticity) processes. While the complex interaction of these processes needs further study, it is clear that functional plasticity in intact cortex is initiated immediately after injury, and subsequent events must shape its eventual functional organization.

To determine the cortical mechanisms that may contribute to short-term versus long-term changes in cerebral cortex, we have initiated a series of studies in the somatosensory cortex of rats. Although much is known about functional reorganization of movement representations in the motor cortex, the underlying neural mechanisms of functional reorganization have been more thoroughly described for the somatosensory cortex (Buonomano & Merzenich, 1998; Florence et al., 1994; Garraghty & Kaas, 1991; Kaas, 1991; Merzenich et al., 1984; Xerri et al., 1998). Since certain aspects of neural plasticity are generalizable across cortical areas (Classen et al., 1998; Karni et al., 1998; Nudo et al., 1996a; Schieber & Deuel; 1997), we believe that an understanding of these fundamental processes of cortical reorganization will further our understanding of how behavioral rehabilitation following partial or subtotal damage to the motor cortex facilitates recovery of function.

As in the motor cortex, functional reorganization in the somatosensory cortex has been described in many mammalian species in response to behavioral experience as well as deafferentation (Buonomano & Merzenich, 1998; Weinberger, 1995). These differing experiences have similar effects on cortical organization in that particular receptive field representations expand tangentially within the somatosensory cortex at the expense of adjacent representations. For example, training monkeys on a task requiring cutaneous discriminations increases the area of cortical representation of the specific digits used in the task while diminishing the areal extent of adjacent representations (Jenkins et al., 1990). Similarly, deafferentation of the median nerve, a peripheral nerve innervating a monkey's hand, results in expansion of an adjacent cortical representation of other nerves that innervate the monkey's hand (the ulnar and radial nerves) into the former median nerve representational territory (Merzenich et al., 1983). In both cases, cortical reorganization occurs in response to altering patterns of afferent input. It is believed that the mechanisms underlying this reorganizational phenomenon are similar to those associated with the facilitative effect that behavioral rehabilitation has on recovery of function after cortical damage (Nudo et al., 1996b; Xerri et al., 1998).

There are two distinct components of functional reorganization that occur in somatosensory cortex (see Karni et al., 1998, for a discussion of similar processes in motor cortex). These components are distinguished temporally and spatially. In terms of temporal characteristics, short-term plasticity is characterized by an immediate reorganization in response to altered afferent inputs, whereas long-term plasticity is characterized by a process of slowly progressing reorganization. In terms of spatial characteristics, reorganization associated with short-term plasticity is limited by existing anatomic constraints, whereas reorganization associated with long-term plasticity can extend beyond preexisting anatomic boundaries, at least as defined by thalamocortical afferents (Cusick et al., 1990; Pons et al., 1991).

It appears that the neural mechanisms that contribute to these two components of cortical plasticity reflect changes in synaptic efficacy, although axonal sprouting may contribute to some of the changes contributing to long-term plasticity (Buonomano & Merzenich, 1998). Current evidence suggests that during short-term plasticity, cortical areas that gain novel receptive field representations do so by the disinhibition of preexisting input within the novel receptive fields. Under normal conditions, such shifts between various possible representations are thought to occur in response to changing environmental conditions and are thought to account for individual differences between animals within the same species (Merzenich, 1985). Long-term plasticity is induced by environmental changes that persist and is thought to be mediated by glutaminergic excitation that leads to long-term potentiation (LTP) or long-term depression (LTD). Thus, short-term plasticity reflects immediate adaptation to temporary changes in environmental conditions (i.e., working memory), while long-term plasticity reflects a more permanent response to persistent changes in environmental conditions (Karni et al., 1998). It is believed that the benefits of behavioral rehabilitation are realized during the long-term process of cortical plasticity, which leads to the consolidation of new or "relearned" skills into procedural memory (Karni et al., 1998). However, it is also believed that long-term plasticity is contingent on the immediate shift in the inhibitory/excitatory balance during the short-term phase of cortical plasticity (Buonomano & Merzenich, 1998; Cusick et al., 1990).

The reorganizational capacity characterized by these temporal and spatial changes in synaptic efficacy seems to rely on a diffuse overlap of "competing" sensory afferents from neighboring receptive fields. The mutability of functional borders between receptive field representations seems to depend on changes in inhibition by gamma-aminobutyric acid (GABA) (Edelman, 1993). Evidence for the inhibitory control of cortical representations has been reported in pharmacologic studies using single-unit recording techniques in the somatosensory cortex (Alloway et al., 1989; Dykes et al., 1984; Hicks & Dykes, 1983). In these studies a GABAergic antagonist, bicuculline, was locally applied iontophoretically to somatosensory neurons in cats after each neuron's peripheral receptive field was identified. Immediately after bicuculline was administered, the receptive fields expanded to include evoked responses from stimulation of skin surfaces that did not elicit a response before the bicuculline treatment. These studies indicate that individual somatosensory neurons in the cortex have the potential to respond to a wide array of inputs from widespread surfaces on the skin. However, under normal circumstances, overlapping input from various receptive fields are masked by local GABAergic inhibition.

The existence of overlapping thalamocortical afferents from neighboring receptive fields has been verified in cats using intra-axonal injections of horseradish peroxidase (Landry & Deschenes, 1981; Schwark & Jones, 1989) and antidromic stimulation of thalamocortical fibers (Snow et al., 1988). Overlapping thalamocortical projections within the somatosensory cortex have also been observed in rats (Armstrong-James et al., 1991) and in monkeys (Rausell & Jones, 1995). In addition to thalamocortical overlapping afferents, there is evidence of intracortical horizontal afferents extending beyond their typical receptive field representations (Manger et al., 1997).

Although these studies improve our understanding of the neural substrates that are responsible for short-term plasticity in the somatosensory cortex, they do not address the functionality of newly reorganized representational areas. One hypothesis derived from studies described above is that newly expanded representational territories in the sensory cortex are capable of enhancing their corresponding stimulus representations (Weinberger, 1995). Evidence supporting this hypothesis reflects the long-term reorganizational processes that occur in response to persistent changes in sensory input. Only a few studies have addressed this issue during short-term reorganizational plasticity.

Two of these studies quantified the minimum stimulus intensities necessary to evoke a sensory response (stimulus intensity thresholds) within appropriate receptive field representations in sensory cortex. These stimulus intensity thresholds were compared to those obtained within a reorganized representational territory immediately after sensory denervation. One study measured multiunit responses to increasing decibels within reorganized frequency bands of the primary auditory cortex (Robertson & Irvine, 1989). The other study measured single-unit responses to increasing stimulus contrast within reorganized primary visual cortex (Chino et al., 1995). These two studies found that newly emerged responses within denervated areas of the auditory and visual cortices are not immediately sensitive to low-threshold stimulation. This suggests that the newly reorganized sensory cortex may not immediately enhance stimulus representations effectively. Direct evidence of this phenomenon in the somatosensory cortex is lacking. However, studies of this issue in the somatosensory cortex have demonstrated that the response characteristics within a newly reorganized territory (e.g., spikes/stimulus and response latency) are similar to normal responses (Doetsch et al., 1996; Schroeder et al.,

1997). This discrepancy may suggest that receptive fields are maintained differently within these cortices. It is also possible that this discrepancy may be due to methodologic differences.

To address this issue, we quantified and compared minimal force thresholds for evoking cortical responses in the somatosensory cortex before and immediately after a peripheral nerve injury (Barbay et al., 1999). This procedure was performed in adult rats using a crush injury of the sciatic nerve. Similar procedures have been well documented in the literature as a model for cortical plasticity in the somatosensory cortex (Cusick et al., 1990; Wall & Cusick, 1984).

In general, a sciatic nerve crush limits the cutaneous hindlimb representation in the cortex to input from the saphenous nerve. Because these nerves are isolated in the hindlimb, it is easy to crush the sciatic nerve while leaving the saphenous nerve completely intact. Immediately after sciatic input to the cortex is eliminated, stimulation of saphenous innervated skin evokes novel cutaneous responses within the former sciatic territory in the somatosensory cortex. The sciatic territory is determined (i.e., mapped) by multiunit physiologic recording techniques prior to sciatic nerve denervation. The border between sciatic and saphenous responses in the cortex is used to determine novel saphenous responses with the same physiologic mapping techniques.

In our study, natural stimulation was applied to the sciatic and saphenous innervated skin of the hindlimb (Wall & Cusick, 1984) by force-calibrated monofilaments (Semmes-Weinstein monofilaments). These monofilaments are nylon fibers of varying diameters, which are used to apply increasing force systematically to the skin. Since it is difficult to distinguish cutaneous responses from proprioceptive responses at high stimulus intensities, a criterion for the maximum force used to elicit a reliable cutaneous response was determined. This criterion was based on similar forces used in humans (see Schmidt, 1986) and corresponds to the force used to record evoked responses in somatosensory area 3b in primates (Nudo et al., 1997).

The results of this experiment show that low-threshold stimulation of saphenous innervated skin, applied immediately after a sciatic crush, is easily detected within the former sciatic territory (Fig. 9-5). Furthermore, the force used to evoke multiunit responses within the former sciatic territory is not significantly different from that observed before a sciatic nerve crush within the typical saphenous territory. These findings support the hypothesis that short-term plasticity in the somatosensory cortex results in functional changes that are immediately realized and therefore capable of enhancing stimulus representations effectively. However, these findings do not rule out the possibility that high-threshold afferents also overlap into neighboring representational areas. In fact, several high-threshold sites were observed, but it could not be determined if these sites were high-threshold cutaneous sites or typical noncutaneous sites from deep tissue stimulation (Chapin & Lin, 1984).

In a subsequent study in the rat, we tracked the reorganization of former sciatic territory at 2 months ($n = 6$) and 4 months ($n = 5$) after a sciatic nerve crush (Barbay et al., 1998). Our findings were consistent with the hypothesis that long-

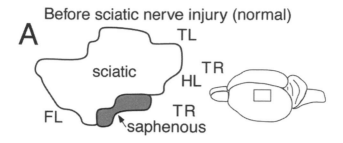

Before sciatic nerve injury (normal)

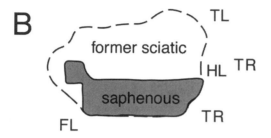

Immediately after sciatic nerve injury

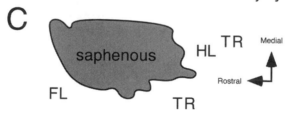

7-9 months after sciatic nerve injury

Figure 9-5. Short-term and long-term changes in the somatosensory cortex of the rat after a sciatic nerve injury. Immediately after the injury, much of the former sciatic territory responds to input from the saphenous nerve. These responses are indistinguishable from normal saphenous responses with respect to stimulus sensitivity. Several months after sciatic nerve section and ligation, the saphenous nerve representation occupies almost the entire area that formerly responded to sciatic nerve input. (A and B) Adapted from Barbay et al. (1999). (C) Adapted from Cusick et al. (1990). The inset shows the location of the hindpaw representation in the rat somatosensory cortex.

term plasticity is characterized by a slowly progressive increase in synaptic efficacy. First, saphenous representations within the former sciatic territory were more extensive than that observed immediately after a sciatic nerve crush. Second, the stimulus intensity thresholds for these novel saphenous responses that were observed 2 and 4 months after the sciatic nerve crush were no different from the mean thresholds used to evoke normal saphenous responses. Third, because sciatic

input into the somatosensory cortex is reinstated over time after a crush injury, there was significant recovery of sciatic representations at 2 months; by 4 months, the cortical representational topography appeared to be normal. These findings suggest that after peripheral nerve damage and regeneration, normal functional topopraphy in the somatosensory cortex can be reestablished. Fourth, the mean stimulus intensity thresholds for sciatic responses reinstated 2 and 4 months after the sciatic nerve crush were higher than the mean thresholds used to evoke normal sciatic responses, but were still within normal limits. A fifth observation was that there were more noncutaneous responses within the former sciatic territory 2 months after the sciatic crush than there were either immediately after or at 4 months after the sciatic nerve crush. Although we could not determine if these were high-threshold cutaneous responses, their emergence 2 months after the sciatic nerve crush followed by their disappearance 4 months after the crush, when sciatic responses were reinstated, suggests that these may have been high-threshold sciatic and/or saphenous responses.

This interpretation is consistent with the expansion of saphenous representation observed after chronic sciatic nerve damage (Cusick et al., 1990). In their study, Cusick et al., permanently eliminated sciatic input to the cortex surgically, by transection and ligation of the sciatic nerve, or pharmacologically by applying a neurotoxin to the sciatic nerve. Both treatments prevented regeneration of the sciatic nerve. There was an immediate expansion of saphenous representation within the former sciatic territory similar to what we found following a sciatic crush injury. In addition to this immediate expansion of the saphenous territory, a slow progression of saphenous expansion was observed. Eventually, by 7 to 9 months after chronic sciatic denervation, the entire former sciatic territory responded to stimulation of saphenous innervated skin (Fig. 9-5).

Therefore, it is reasonable to assume that the gradual emergence of saphenous representation within the former sciatic territory in Cusick et al.'s experiment, as well as ours, reflects a gradual increase in sensitivity in which the stimulus intensity needed to evoke a saphenous response is reduced over time. This process may also reflect the gradual reinstatement of sciatic sensitivity observed in our study.

Cellular Correlates of Cortical Map Plasticity: Changes in Neuron Structure

As described above, changes in the functional organization of the mammalian cortex have been demonstrated after several manipulations, including peripheral deafferentation (Barbay et al., 1999; Darian-Smith & Gilbert, 1994; Donoghue et al., 1990), intracortical stimulation (Nudo et al., 1990), cortical lesions (Carmichael et al., 1997; Nudo & Milliken, 1996), local administration of neurochemicals (Jacobs & Donoghue, 1991), and behavioral training (Kleim et al., 1998; Nudo et al., 1996a; Recanzone et al., 1992, 1993). The results of these experiments suggest that cortical reorganization can be both rapid and enduring. Within the rodent motor cortex, for example, the administration of GABAergic antagonists can induce the expansion of neighboring movement representations within minutes (Jacobs

& Donoghue, 1991), as can repeated intracortical stimulation (Nudo et al., 1990). Similarly, within the sensory cortex, peripheral denervation can lead to the immediate expansion of sensory representations (Barbay et al., 1999; Chino et al., 1992; Robertson & Irvine, 1989). Although the specific cellular processes underlying this plasticity remain to be determined, changes in synaptic strength are probably involved. The rapidly occurring changes in the functional topography of the cortex described above have been proposed to be mediated by the unmasking of latent excitatory connections via the inhibition of local inhibitory synapses (Hicks & Dykes, 1983; Jacobs & Donoghue, 1991). Changes in the relative levels of synaptic excitation and inhibition provide an attractive model of neural processes by which *rapidly* occurring changes in cortical organization could occur. However, this seems an unlikely mechanism for producing *long-term* changes in cortical function.

More lasting changes in cortical function might require modifications in the topography of synaptic connectivity involving changes in neuronal morphology. Indeed, changes in neuron structure have been observed after manipulations that also induce functional reorganization. Peripheral deafferentation (Bishop, 1982; Darian-Smith & Gilbert, 1994; Friedlander et al., 1991), repetitive electrical stimulation (Hawrylak et al., 1993; Keller et al., 1992), and cortical lesions (Carmichael et al., 1997) have all been associated with altered neuron structure. For example, small scotomas placed in the cat retina led to functional expansion of nondeprived areas of the visual cortex into deprived areas (Gilbert & Weisel, 1992; Kaas et al., 1990). This expansion was accompanied by the sprouting of intracortical axons from nondeprived to deprived areas (Darian-Smith & Gilbert, 1994). Axonal sprouting was also observed within monocularly deprived regions of kitten visual cortex, where there was an increase in the number of axonal varicosities making contact with multiple postsynaptic partners (Friedlander et al., 1991). Similar results were found in the rat somatosensory cortex, where small infarcts in the barrel subfield resulted in axonal sprouting in the surrounding cortex (Carmichael et al., 1997).

Changes in neuronal morphology might also support the functional reorganization observed within the motor cortex after skill learning. Nudo et al. (1996a) demonstrated a learning-dependent expansion of digit representation within the primary motor cortex of squirrel monkeys trained on a fine digit task that was not simply due to increased use (Nudo et al., 1997; Plautz et al., 1995). Similarly, Kleim et al. (1998) showed that rats trained on a skilled reaching task exhibited an increase in wrist and digit representations within the caudal forelimb area (CFA) of the motor cortex in comparison to rats trained on a simple bar-pressing task (Fig. 9-6). Interestingly, no differences in the topography of movement representations between these two conditions were found within the rostral forelimb area (RFA) or the hindlimb area (HLA). The notion that this functional plasticity is accompanied by structural plasticity is supported by experiments showing that training on a similarly skilled reaching task led to dendritic hypertrophy within the motor cortex. The pyramidal cells of reach-trained animals exhibited an increase in the amount of dendritic material in the hemisphere contralateral to the trained paw in comparison to nontrained controls (Greenough et al., 1985; Withers & Greenough, 1989).

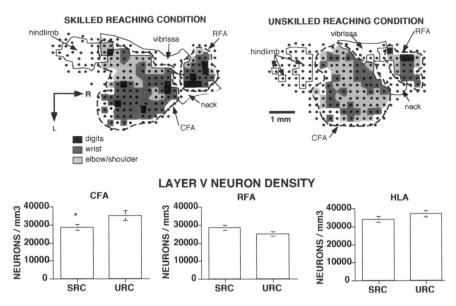

Figure 9-6. Reorganization of motor representations after skilled reach training in rats. Animals in the skilled reaching condition exhibited an increase in wrist and digit representations and a decrease in elbow/shoulder representations in the caudal forelimb area (CFA) in comparison to animals in the unskilled reaching condition (URC). No differences in movement topography were found in the rostral forelimb area (RFA). The skilled reach training animals also had a significantly reduced neuron density within layer V of the CFA in comparison to the unskilled reach training animals. No differences in neuron density were found in either the RFA or the hindlimb area (HLA). These results suggest that changes in neuronal morphology support the functional reorganization observed within the motor cortex following skill learning.

Similarly, layer V pyramidal cells of rats trained to recoil a length of string (requiring the skilled use of both paws) showed a bilateral increase in dendritic arbor in comparison to nontrained controls (Kolb, 1995). The increase in dendritic arbor probably reflects increased synapse numbers, as rats trained on a complex motor learning task had significantly more synapses per neuron within the motor cortex than did both active and inactive controls (Kleim et al., 1996).

Although the regions of cortex examined in these anatomic studies were not physiologically defined, the measurements were probably taken within the CFA, given the stereotaxic coordinates reported and the large size of this subregion (Kleim et al., in press; Neafsey et al., 1986). Because skilled reach training led to functional reorganization within the CFA, but not within the RFA or HLA (Kleim et al., 1998), it would be interesting to examine how the changes in neuronal morphology are distributed across the three physiologically defined subregions. By examining neuron density within the three subregions of the motor cortex from rats in either a Skilled Reaching Condition (SRC) or an Unskilled Reaching Condition

(URC), we correlated changes in neuropil volume with changes in the topography of movement representations within the same animals. The results of this experiment showed that the SRC animals had a significantly greater area of both digit and wrist movements than the URC within the CFA (Kleim et al., 1998). The increase in digit and wrist representations appeared to occur at the expense of elbow/shoulder representations, as SRC animals had significantly reduced areal representations of elbow/shoulder movements in comparison to URC animals. There were no between-group differences in the area of movement representations in either the RFA or the HLA. The SRC animals also had a significantly reduced neuron density within layer V of the CFA in comparison to the URC animals (Fig. 9-6). No differences in neuron density between the SRC and URC animals were found in either the RFA or the HLA (Fig. 9-6). Changes in neuron density are indicative of an increase in the volume of neuropil due to increases in dendritic arbor (Greenough et al., 1985; Volkmar & Greenough, 1972), synapse number (Black et al., 1987; Kleim et al., 1996, 1997; Turner & Greenough, 1985), glial material (Anderson et al., 1994), and cerebrovasculature (Black et al., 1987). The expanded neuropil pushes neurons apart, resulting in a decrease in the number of neurons per unit volume of cortex (Kleim et al., 1996; Turner & Greenough, 1985). Thus the functional reorganization of the CFA associated with skilled-reaching training was accompanied by an increase in neuropil within this same region. The RFA and HLA did not show any learning-dependent changes in movement topography or neuron density. Although preliminary, these results suggest that changes in neuron structure correlate with the functional reorganization of movement representations within the rodent motor cortex. Further work is being done to determine whether this decrease in neuron density also reflects an increase in the number of synapses per neuron, as it has in previous studies (Black et al., 1990; Kleim et al., 1996; Turner & Greenough, 1985).

It is tempting to speculate that the behavioral recovery and cortical reorganization observed in the motor cortex after focal infarct and subsequent rehabilitative training (Nudo et al., 1996b) may also involve changes in neuronal morphology. In support of this idea, use-dependent dendritic (Jones & Schallert, 1994) and synaptic growth (Jones et al., 1996) has been observed in the rat motor cortex after electrolytic lesions in the contralateral hemisphere (see Chapter 8).

Concluding Remarks

While the plasticity studies of the past decade have suggested provocative hypotheses regarding the neural bases for recovery of function, several important issues still need to be addressed. First, while the current data are compelling, the functional meaning of plastic change after injury is not yet clear. Recent neuroimaging data from human stroke patients confirm many of the neurophysiologic findings in primates. That is, the size of specific motor representations is altered during motor recovery (Chollet et al., 1991; Cohen et al., 1993; Cramer et al., 1997; Freund, 1996; Rossini et al., 1998; Weiller et al., 1992). However, the changes over long time courses after cortical injury may be adaptive, maladaptive, or epiphenomenal, and distinctions among the three alternatives may not always be obvious. There is an immediate need for more and better correlational studies in animals and humans that relate neurophysiologic and neuroimaging data to functional outcomes. Second, while the primary motor cortex provides a handy window into the spatial distribution of movement representations in the motor system, a more integrative picture of reorganization in other cortical and subcortical motor regions is needed. Third, the interactive effects of various other modulators of plasticity (behavioral, pharmacologic, etc.) need to be addressed in more detail. It is now clear that specific behavioral experiences modulate cortical function after injury and may be as potent as pharmacologic agents in improving motor function after stroke (Feeney & Sutton, 1987). Fourth, dynamic processes triggered by neuronal injury occur for long periods of time after the injury. It is important to address the issue of critical, or sensitive, periods for each of these modulators. While these challenges are significant, the tools are now available to address the complex questions of neural recovery in detail from the molecular to the behavioral level.

These studies will have important implications for rehabilitation of brain-injured humans. While the basic neurochemical principles underlying neuronal death after injury have led to exciting advances in the treatment of acute stroke and traumatic brain injury, the neural principles governing recovery over the ensuing weeks, months, and years remain puzzling. Further knowledge of the effects of use and disuse on neurophysiologic and neuroanatomic organization may lead to new therapeutic strategies based on underlying principles of neuronal plasticity.

ACKNOWLEDGMENTS

This work was supported by the National institute of Neurological Diseases and Stroke (NS30853), the Kansas Claude D. Pepper Center for Independence in Older Americans (National Institute on Aging Grant AG14635), the Natural Sciences and Engineering Research Council of Canada, a center grant from the National Institute of Child Health and Human Development (HD02528), and the American Heart Association.

References

Alloway, K.D., Rosenthal, P., and Burton, H. (1989) Quantitative measurements of receptive field changes during antagonism of GABAergic transmission in primary somatosensory cortex of cats. *Experimental Brain Research,* 78:514–532.

Anderson, B.J., Li, X., Alcantara, A.A., Isaacs, K.R., Black, J.E., and Greenough, W.T. (1994) Glial hypertrophy is associated with synaptogenesis following motor skill learning, but not with angiogenesis following exercise. *Glia,* 11:73–80.

Armstrong-James, M., Callahan, C.A., and Friedman, M.A. (1991) Thalamo-cortical processing of vibrissal information in the rat. I. Intracortical orgins of surround but not centre-receptive fields of layer IV neurons in the rat S1 barrel field cortex. *Journal of Comparative Neurology,* 303:193–210.

Asanuma, H., and Rosén I. (1972) Topographical organization of cortical efferent zones projecting to distal forelimb muscles in the monkey. *Experimental Brain Research,* 14: 243–256.

Barbay, S., Peden, E.K., and Falchook, G., Nudo, R.J. (1999) Sensitivity of neurons in somatosensory cortex (S1) to cutaneous stimulation of the hindlimb immediately following a sciatic nerve crush. *Somatosensory and Motor Research*, 16:103–114.

Barbay, S., Peden, E.K., Falchook, G., and Nudo, R.J. (1998) Sensitivity of cutaneous hindlimb responses in somatosensory cortex (S1) of the rat two and four months after a sciatic nerve crush. *Society for Neuroscience Abstracts*, 24:635.

Bishop, B. (1982) Neural plasticity: Part 3: Responses to lesions in the peripheral nervous system. *Physical Therapy*, 62:1275–1282.

Black, J.E., Isaacs, K.R., Anderson, B.J., Alcantara, A.A., and Greenough, W.T. (1990) Learning causes synaptogenesis whereas motor activity causes angiogenesis in crebellar cortex of adult rats. *Proceedings of the National Academy of Sciences of the USA*, 87:5568–5572.

Black, J.E., Sirevaag, A.M., and Greenough, W.T. (1987) Complex experience promotes capillary formation in young rat visual cortex. *Neuroscience Letters*, 83:351–355.

Buonomano, D.V., and Merzenich, M.M. (1998) Cortical plasticity: From synapses to maps. *Annual Review of Neuroscience*, 21:149–186.

Carmichael, S.T., Wei, L., Rovainen, C.M., and Woolsey, T.A. (1997) Anatomical and metabolic changes in peri-infarct cortex after focal stroke in the rat. *Society for Neuroscience Abstracts*, 23:1378.

Chapin, J.K., and Lin, C.S. (1984) Mapping the body representation in the S1 cortex of anesthetized and awake rats. *Journal of Comparative Neurology*, 229:199–213.

Cheney, P.D., and Fetz, E.E. (1985) Comparable patterns of muscle facilitation evoked by individual corticomotoneuronal (CM) cells and by single intracortical microstimuli in primates: Evidence for functional groups of CM cells. *Journal of Neurophysiology*, 53:786–804.

Chino, Y.M., Kaas, J.H., Smith, E.L., Langston, A.L., and Cheng, H. (1992) Rapid reorganization of cortical maps in adult cats following restricted deafferentation in retina. *Vision Research*, 32:789–796.

Chino, Y.M., Smith, E.L., Kaas, J.H., Sasaki, Y., and Cheng, H. (1995) Receptive-field properties of deafferentated visual cortical neurons after topographic map reorganization in adult cats. *Journal of Neuroscience*, 15:2417–2433.

Chollet, F., DiPiero, V., Wise, R.J., Brooks, D.J., Dolan, R.J., and Frackowiak, R.S. (1991) The functional anatomy of motor recovery after stroke in humans: A study with positron emission tomography. *Annals of Neurology*, 29:63–71.

Clark, S.A., Allard, T., Jenkins, W.M., and Merzenich, M.M. (1988) Receptive fields in the body-surface map in adult cortex defined by temporally correlated inputs. *Nature*, 332:444–445.

Classen, J., Liepert, J., Wise, S.P., Hallett, M., and Cohen L.G. (1998) Rapid plasticity of human cortical movement representation induced by practice. *Journal of Neurophysiology*, 79:1117–1123.

Cohen, L.G., Brasil-Neto, J.P., Pascual-Leone, A., and Hallett M. (1993) Plasticity of cortical motor output organization following deafferentation, cerebral lesions, and skill acquisition. *Advances in Neurology*, 63:187–200.

Cramer, S.C., Nelles, G., Benson, R.R., Kaplan, J.D., Parker, R.A., Kwong, K.K. Kennedy, D.N., Finklestein, S.P., and Rosen, B.R. (1997) A functional MRI study of subjects recovered from hemiparetic stroke. *Stroke*, 28:2518–2527.

Cusick, C.G., Wall, J.T., Whiting, J.H., and Wiley R.G. (1990) Temporal progression of cortical reorganization following nerve injury. *Brain Research*, 537:355–358.

Darian-Smith, C., and Gilbert, C.D. (1994) Axonal sprouting accompanies functional reorganization in adult striate cortex. *Nature*, 368:737–740.

Doetsch, G.S., Harrison, T.A., MacDonald, A.C., and Litaker, M.S. (1996) Short-term plasticity in primary somatosensory cortex of the rat: Rapid changes in magnitudes and latencies of neuronal responses following digit denervation. *Experimental Brain Research,* 112:505–512.

Donoghue, J.P., and Sanes, J.N. (1988) Organization of adult motor cortex representation patterns following neonatal forelimb nerve injury in rats. *Journal of Neuroscience,* 8: 3221–3232.

Donoghue, J.P., Suner, and S., Sanes, J.N. (1990) Dynamic organization of primary motor cortex output to target muscles in adult rats. II. Rapid reorganization following motor nerve lesions. *Experimental Brain Research,* 79:492–503.

Duncan, P.W., and Lai S.M. (1997) Stroke recovery. *Topics in Stroke Rehabilitation,* 4:51–58.

Dykes, R.W., Landry, P., Metherate, R., and Hicks, T.P. (1984) Functional role of GABA in cat primary somatosensory cortex: Shaping receptive fields of cortical neurons. *Journal of Neurophysiology,* 52:1066–1093.

Edelman, G.M. (1993) Neural Darwinism: Selection and reentrant signaling in higher brain function. *Neuron,* 10:115–125.

Elbert, T., Pantev, C., Wienbruch, C., Rockstroh, B., and Taub E. (1995) Increased cortical representation of the fingers of the left hand in string players. *Science,* 270:305–307.

Feeney, D.M., and Sutton R.L. (1987) Pharmacotherapy for recovery of function after brain injury. *CRC Critical Review of Neurobiology,* 3:135–197.

Florence, S.L., Garraghty, P.E., Wall, J.T., and Kaas, J.H. (1994) Sensory afferent projections and area 3b somatotopy following median nerve cut and repair in macaque monkeys. *Cerebral Cortex,* 4:391–407.

Franz, S.I. (1915) Variations in distribution of the motor centers. *Psychological Monographs,* 19:80–162.

Franz, S.I., Scheetz, M.E., and Wilson, A.A. (1915) The possibility of recovery of motor function in long-standing hemiplegia. *Journal of the American Medical Association,* 65: 2150–2154.

Freund, H.J. (1996) Remapping the brain. *Science,* 272:1754.

Friedlander, M.J., Martin, K.A., and Wassenhove-McCarthy, D. (1991) Effects of monocular visual deprivation on geniculo-cortical innervation of area 18 in the cat. *Journal of Neuroscience,* 11:3268–3288.

Friel, K.M., and Nudo, R.J. (1998a) Recovery of motor function after focal cortical injury in primates: Compensatory movement patterns used during rehabilitative training. *Somatosensory and Motor Research,* 15:173–189.

Friel, K.M., and Nudo, R.J. (1998b) Restraint of the unimpaired hand is not sufficient to retain spared hand representation after focal cortical injury. *Society for Neuroscience Abstracts,* 24:405.

Fritsch, G., and Hitzig, E. (1870) Über die elektrische Erregbarkeit des Grosshirns. *Archiv für Anatomie und Physiologie,* 37:300–332.

Garraghty, P.E., and Kaas, J.H. (1991) Large-scale functional reorganization in adult monkey cortex after peripheral nerve injury. *Proceedings of the National Academy of Sciences of the USA,* 88:6976–6980.

Gilbert, C.D., and Weisel, T.N. (1992) Receptive field dynamics in adult primary visual cortex. *Nature,* 356:150–152.

Glees, P., and Cole, J. (1950) Recovery of skilled motor functions after small repeated lesions in motor cortex in macaque. *Journal of Neurophysiology,* 13:137–148.

Gould, H.J.I., Cusick, C.G., Pons, T.P., and Kaas, J.H. (1986) The relationship of corpus callosum connections to electrical stimulation maps of motor, supplementary motor, and the frontal eye fields in owl monkeys. *Journal of Comparative Neurology,* 247: 297–325.

Grafton, S.T., Mazziotta, J.C., Presty, S., Friston, K.J., Frackowiak, R.S.J., and Phelps, M.E. (1992) Functional anatomy of human procedural learning determined with regional cerebral blood flow and PET. *Journal of Neuroscience,* 12:2542–2548.

Graham Brown, T., and Steward, R.M. (1916) On disturbances of the localization and discriminations of sensations in cases of cerebral lesions, and on the possibility of the recovery of these functions after a process of training. *Brain,* 39:348–454.

Greenough, W.T., Larson, J.R., and Withers, G.S. (1985) Effects of unilateral and bilateral training in a reaching task on dendritic branching of neurons in the rat motor-sensory forelimb cortex. *Behavioral and Neural Biology,* 44:301–314.

Gresham, G.E., Duncan, P.W., Stason, W.B., et al. (1995) *Post-stroke Rehabilitation. Clinical Practice Guideline, No. 16.* AHCPR Publication No. 95-0662. Rockville, MD: U.S. Department of Health and Human Services. Public Health Service, Agency for Health Care Policy and Research.

Hawrylak, N., Chang, F.L., and Greenough W.T. (1993) Astrocytic and synaptic response to kindling in hippocampal subfield CA1. II. Synaptogenesis and astrocytic process increases to in vivo kindling. *Brain Research,* 603:309–316.

Hicks, T.P., and Dykes, R.W. (1983) Receptive field size for cetain neurons in primary somatosensory cortex is determined by GABA-mediated intracortical inhibition. *Brain Research,* 274:160–164.

Huntley, G.W., and Jones, E.G. (1991) Relationship of intrinsic connections to forelimb movement representations in monkey motor cortex: A correlative anatomical and physiological study. *Journal of Neurophysiology,* 66:390–413.

Jacobs, K.M., and Donoghue, J.P. (1991) Reshaping the cortical motor map by unmasking latent intracortical connections. *Science,* 251:944–947.

Jenkins, I.H., Brooks, D.J., Nixon, P.D., Frackowiak, S.J., and Passingham, R.E. (1994) Motor sequence learning: A study with positron emission tomography. *Journal of Neuroscience,* 14:3775–3790.

Jenkins, W.M., Merzenich, M.M., Ochs, M.T., Allard, T., and Guic-Robles, E. (1990) Functional reorganization of primary somatosensory cortex in adult owl monkeys after behaviorally controlled tactile stimulation. *Journal of Neurophysiology,* 63:82–104.

Jones, T.A., Kleim, J.A., and Greenough, W.T. (1996) Synaptogenesis and dendritic growth in the cortex opposite unilateral sensorimotor cortex damage in adult rats: A quantitative electron microscopic examination. *Brain Research,* 733:142–148.

Jones, T.A., and Schallert, T. (1994) Use-dependent growth of pyramidal neurons after neocortical damage. *Journal of Neuroscience,* 14:2140–2152.

Kaas, J.H. (1991) Plasticity of sensory and motor maps in adult mammals. *Annual Review of Neuroscience,* 14:137–167.

Kaas, J.H., Krubitzer, L.A., Chino, Y.M., Langston, A.L., Polley, E.H., and Blair, N. (1990) Reorganization of retinotopic cortical maps in adult mammals after lesions of the retina. *Science,* 248:229–231.

Karni, A., Meyer, G., Jezzard, P., Adams, M.M., Turner, R., and Ungerleider, L.G. (1995) Functional MRI evidence for adult motor cortex plasticity during motor skill learning. *Nature,* 377:155–158.

Karni, A., Meyer, G., Rey-Hipolito, C., Jezzard, P., Adams, M.M., Turner, R., and Ungerleider, L.G. (1998) The acquisition of skilled motor performance: Fast and slow experience-driven changes in primary motor cortex. *Proceedings of the National Academy of Sciences of the USA,* 95:861–868.

Keller, A. (1993) Intrinsic synaptic organization of the motor cortex. *Cerebral Cortex,* 3: 430–441.

Keller, A., Arissian, K., and Asanuma, H. (1992) Synaptic proliferation in the motor cortex of adult cats after long-term thalamic stimulation. *Journal of Neurophysiology,* 68:295–308.

Kleim, J.A., Ballard, D., Vij, K., and Greenough, W.T. (1997) Learning dependent synaptic modifications in the cerebellar cortex of the adult rat persist for at least four weeks. *Journal of Neuroscience,* 17:717–721.

Kleim, J.A., Barbay, S., and Nudo, R.J. (1998) Functional reorganization of the rat motor cortex following motor skill learning. *Journal of Neurophysiology,* 80:3321–3325.

Kleim, J.A., Lussnig, E., Schwarz, E.R., Comery, T.A., and Greenough, W.T. (1996) Synaptogenesis and Fos expression in the motor cortex of the adult rat after motor skill learning. *Journal of Neuroscience,* 16:4529–4535.

Kolb, B. (1995) *Brain Plasticity and Behavior.* Mahwah, NJ: Erlbaum.

Landry, P., and Deschenes, M. (1981) Intracortical arborizations and receptive fields of identified ventrobasal thalamocortical afferents to the primary somatic sensory cortex in the cat. *Journal of Comparative Neurology,* 199:345–371.

Lashley, K.S. (1924) Studies of cerebral function in learning: V. The retention of motor habits after destruction of the so-called motor areas in primates. *Archives of Neurology and Psychiatry,* 12:249–276.

Lashley, K.S. (1938) Factors limiting recovery after central nervous system lesions. *Journal of Nervous and Mental Disease,* 88:733–755.

LeVere, T.E. (1980) Recovery of function after brain damage: A theory of the behavioral deficit. *Physiological Psychology,* 8:297–308.

Leyton, A.S.F., and Sherrington, C.S. (1917) Observations on the excitable cortex of the chimpanzee, orang-utan and gorilla. *Quarterly Journal of Experimental Physiology,* 11: 135–222.

Liepert, J., Miltner, W.H.R., Bauder, H., Sommer, M., Dettmers, C., Taub, E., and Weiller, C. (1998) Motor cortex plasticity during constraint-induced movement therapy in stroke patients. *Neuroscience Letters,* 250:5–8.

Manger, P.R., Woods, T.M., Munoz, A., and Jones, E.G. (1997) Hand/face border as a limiting boundary in the body representation in monkey somatosensory cortex. *Journal of Neuroscience,* 17:6338–6351.

Merzenich, M.M. (1985) Sources of intraspecies and interspecies cortical map variability in mammals. In M.J. Cohen and F. Strumwasser (eds.), *Comparative Neurobiology: Modes of Communication in the Nervous System.* New York: Wiley, pp. 105–116.

Merzenich, M.M., Kaas, J.H., Wall, J.T., Sur, M., Nelson, R.J., and Felleman, D.J. (1983) Progression of change following median nerve section in the cortical representation of the hand in areas 3b and 1 in adult owl and squirrel monkeys. *Neuroscience,* 10:639–665.

Merzenich, M.M., Nelson, R.J., Stryker, M.P., Cynader, M.S., Schoppmann, A., and Zook, J.M. (1984) Somatosensory cortical map changes following digit amputation in adult monkeys. *Journal of Comparative Neurology,* 224:591–605.

Neafsey, E.J., Bold, E.L., Haas, G., Hurley-Gius, K.M., Quirk, G., and Sievert, C.F. (1986) The organization of rat motor cortex: A microstimulation mapping study. *Brain Research Reviews,* 11:77–96.

Nudo, R.J., Jenkins, W.M., and Merzenich, M.M. (1990) Repetitive microstimulation alters the cortical representation of movements in adult rats. *Somatosensory and Motor Research,* 7:463–483.

Nudo, R.J., Jenkins, W.M., Merzenich, M.M., Prejean, T., and Grenda, R. (1992) Neurophysiological correlates of hand preference in primary motor cortex of squirrel monkeys. *Journal of Neuroscience,* 12:2918–2947.

Nudo, R.J., and Milliken, G.W. (1996) Reorganization of movement representations in primary motor cortex following focal ischemic infarcts in adult squirrel monkeys. *Journal
of Neurophysiology,* 75:2144–2149.

Nudo, R.J., Milliken, G.W., Jenkins, W.M., and Merzenich, M.M. (1996a) Use-dependent
alterations of movement representations in primary motor cortex of adult squirrel monkeys. *Journal of Neuroscience,* 16:785–807.

Nudo, R.J., Plautz, E.J., and Milliken, G.W. (1997) Adaptive plasticity in primate motor
cortex as a consequence of behavioral experience and neuronal injury. *Seminars in Neuroscience,* 9:13–23.

Nudo, R.J., Wise, B.M., SiFuentes, F., and Milliken, G.W. (1996b) Neural substrates for the
effects of rehabilitative training on motor recovery after ischemic infarct. *Science,* 272:
1791–1794.

Ogden, R., and Franz, S.I. (1917) On cerebral motor control: The recovery from experimentally produced hemiplegia. *Psychobiology,* 1:33–50.

Ostendorf, C.G., and Wolf, S.L. (1981) Effect of forced use of the upper extremity of a hemiplegic patient on changes in function. A single case design. *Physical Therapy,*
61:1022–1028.

Pascual-Leone, A., Grafman, J., and Hallett, M. (1994) Modulation of cortical motor output
maps during development of implicit and explicit knowledge. *Science,* 263:1287–1289.

Pascual-Leone, A., Nguyet, D., Cohen, L.G., Brasil-Neto, J.P., Cammarota, A., and Hallett, M.
(1995) Modulation of muscle responses evoked by transcranial magnetic stimulation
during the acquisition of new fine motor skills. *Journal of Neurophysiology,* 74:1037–
1045.

Penfield, W., and Boldrey, E. (1937) Somatic motor and sensory representation in the cerebral cortex of man as studied by electrical stimulation. *Brain,* 60:389–443.

Plautz, E.J., Milliken, G.W., and Nudo, R.J. (1995) Differential effects of skill acquisition
and motor use on the reorganization of motor representations in area 4 of adult squirrel
monkeys. *Society for Neuroscience Abstracts,* 21:1902.

Pons, T.P., Garraghty, P.E., Ommaya, A.K., Taub, E., and Mishkin, M. (1991) Massive cortical reorganization after sensory deafferenation in adult macaques. *Science,* 252:1857–
1860.

Rausell, E., and Jones, E.G. (1995) Extent of intracortical arborization of thalamocortical
axons as a determinant of representational plasticity in monkey somatic sensory cortex.
Journal of Neuroscience, 15:4270–4288.

Recanzone, G.H., Merzenich, M.M., Jenkins, W.M., Grajski, K.A., and Dinse, H.R. (1992)
Topographic reorganization of the hand representation in cortical area 3b of owl monkeys trained in a frequency discrimination task. *Journal of Neurophysiology,* 67:1031–
1056.

Recanzone, G.H., Schreiner, G.E., and Merzenich, M.M. (1993) Plasticity in the frequency
representation of primary auditory cortex following discrimination training in adult owl
monkeys. *Journal of Neurophysiology,* 13:87–103.

Robertson, D., and Irvine, D.R.F. (1989) Plasticity of frequency organization in auditory
cortex of guinea pigs with partial unilateral deafness. *Journal of Comparative Neurology,*
282:456–471.

Rossini, P.M., Caltagirone, C., Castriota-Scanderbeg, A., Cicinelli, P., Del Gratta, C., De-
martin, M., Pizzella, V., Traversa, R., and Romani, G.L. (1998) Hand Motor cortical area

reorganization in stroke: A study with fMRI, MEG and TCS maps. *NeuroReport,* 9: 2141–2146.

Sanes, J.N., Donoghue, J.P., Thangaraj, V., Edelman, R.R., and Warach, S. (1995) Shared neural substrates controlling hand movements in human motor cortex. *Science,* 268: 1775–1777.

Schieber, M.H., and Deuel, R.K. (1997) Primary motor cortex reorganization in a long-term monkey amputee. *Somatosensory and Motor Research,* 14:157–167.

Schlaug, G., Knorr, U., and Seitz, R.J. (1994) Inter-subject variability of cerebral activations in acquiring a motor skill: a study with positron emission tomography. *Experimental Brain Research,* 98:523–534.

Schmidt, R.F. (1986) Somatovisceral sensibility. In *Fundamentals of Sensory Physiology.* R.F. Schmidt (ed.), New York: Springer, pp. 30–67.

Schroeder, C.E., Seto, S., and Garraghty, P.E. (1997) Emergence of radial nerve dominance in median nerve cortex after median nerve transection in an adult squirrel monkey. *Journal of Neurophysiology,* 77:522–526.

Schwark, H.D., and Jones, E.G. (1989) The distribution of intrinsic cortical axons in area 3b of cat primary somatosensory cortex. *Experimental Brain Research,* 78:501–513.

Seitz, R.J., Roland, R.E., Bohm, C., Greitz, T., and Stone-Elander, S. (1990) Motor learning in man: A positron emission tomographic study. *NeuroReport,* 1:57–60.

Snow, P.J., Nudo, R.J., Rivers, W., Jenkins, W.M., and Merzenich, M.M. (1988) Somatotopically inappropriate projections from thalamocortical neurons to the SI cortex of the cat demonstrated by the use of intracortical microstimulation. *Somatosensory Research,* 5:349–372.

Stein, D.G. (1998) Brain injury and theories of recovery. In L. Goldstein (ed.), *Restorative Neurology: Advances in Pharmacotherapy for Recovery After Stroke.* Armonk, NY: Futura, pp. 1–34.

Taub, E. (1980) Somatosensory deafferentation research with monkeys: Implications for rehabilitation medicine. In L. P. Ince (ed.), *Behavioral Psychology in Rehabilitation Medicine: Clinical Applications.* New York: Williams & Wilkins, pp. 371–401.

Taub, E. (1994) Overcoming learned nonuse: A new approach to treatment in physical medicine. In J. G. Carlson, A. R. Seifert, and N. Birbaumer (eds.), *Clinical Applied Psychophysiology.* New York: Plenum Press, pp. 185–220.

Taub, E., and Wolf, S.L. (1997) Constraint induced movement techniques to facilitate upper extremity use in stroke patients. *Topics in Stroke Rehabilitation,* 3:38–61.

Tower, S.S. (1940) Pyramidal lesions in the monkey. *Brain,* 63:36–90.

Triggs, W.J., Calvanio, R., Macdonnel, R.A.L., Cros, D., and Chiappa, K.H. (1994) Physiological motor asymmetry in human handedness: evidence from transcranial magnetic stimulation. *Brain Research,* 636:270–276.

Turner, A.M., and Greenough, W.T. (1985) Differential rearing effects on rat visual cortex synapses. I. Synaptic and neuronal density and synapses/neuron. *Brain Research,* 329: 195–203.

Volkmann, J., Schnitzler, A., Witte, O.W., and Freund, H.-J. (1998) Handedness and asymmetry of hand representation in human motor cortex. *Journal of Neurophysiology,* 79:2149–2154.

Volkmar, F.R., and Greenough, W.T. (1972) Rearing complexity affects branching of dendrites in the visual cortex of the rat. *Science,* 176:1445–1447.

Wade, D.T., Wood, V.A., and Langston-Hewer, R.L. (1985) Recovery after stroke: the first three months. *Journal of Neurology, Neurosurgery and Psychiatry,* 48:7–13.

Wall, J.T., and Cusick, C.G. (1984) Cutaneous responsiveness in primary somatosensory (S-I) hindpaw cortex before and after partial hindpaw deafferentation in adult rats. *Journal of Neuroscience,* 4:1499–1515.

Wall, J.T., Huerta, M.F., and Kaas, J.H. (1992) Changes in the cortical map of the hand following postnatal median nerve injury in monkeys: Modification of somatotopic aggregates. *Journal of Neuroscience,* 12:3445–3455.

Wassermann, E.M., McShane, L.M., Hallett, M., and Cohen, L.G. (1992) Noninvasive mapping of muscle representations in human motor cortex. *Electroencephalography and Clinical Neurophysiology,* 85:1–8.

Weiller, C., Chollet, F., Friston, K.J., Wise, R.J.S., and Frackowiak, R.S.J. (1992) Functional reorganization of the brain in recovery from striatocapsular infarction in man. *Annals of Neurology,* 31:463–472.

Weinberger, N.M. (1995) Dynamic regulation of receptive fields and maps in the adult sensory cortex. *Annual Review of Neuroscience,* 18:129–158.

Withers, G.S., and Greenough, W.T. (1989) Reach training selectively alters dendritic branching in subpopulations of Layer II/III pyramids in rat motor-somatosensory forelimb cortex. *Neuropsychologia,* 27:61–69.

Wolf, S.L., Lecraw, D.E., Barton, L.A., and Jann, B.B. (1989) Forced use of hemiplegic upper extremities to reverse the effects of learned nonuse among chronic stroke and head-injured patients. *Experimental Neurology,* 104:125–132.

Xerri, C., Merzenich, M.M., Peterson, B.E., and Jenkins, W. (1998) Plasticity of primary somatosensory cortex paralleling sensorimotor skill recovery from stroke in adult monkeys. *Journal of Neurophysiology,* 79:2119–2148.

II

Developmental Studies
of Neuroplasticity

10

Spatial Cognitive Development Following Prenatal or Perinatal Focal Brain Injury

JOAN STILES

A long-standing question in the study of development following early focal brain injury is whether it is possible to document specific disorders associated with early localized brain injury. Early studies indicated that the consequences of early focal brain injury are minimal. From these data it appeared that children are quite resilient, in comparison with adults, in that they recover, or more precisely acquire, cognitive functioning following injury to the brain that would leave adults permanently impaired (Alajouanine & Lhermitte, 1965; Brown & Jaffe, 1975; Carlson et al., 1968; Gott, 1973; Hammill & Irwin, 1966; Krashen, 1973; Lenneberg, 1967; McFie, 1961; Reed & Reitan, 1971). However, more recent retrospective studies of adults and older children whose injuries occurred early in life have provided evidence of subtle, persistent cognitive deficits within the general pattern of recovery (Day & Ulatowska, 1979; Dennis, 1980; Dennis & Kohn, 1975; Dennis & Whitaker, 1976; Kohn, 1980; Kohn & Dennis, 1974; Rudel & Teuber, 1971; Rudel et al., 1974; Vargha-Khadem et al., 1983, 1985; Woods, 1980; Woods & Carey, 1979). A limiting factor in all of this early work was its reliance on retrospective accounts of development in which the outcome of development following early injury is used to infer developmental process.

In order to define the effects of early neurological injury, it is necessary to take a prospective approach in which children are identified early in life and followed longitudinally. Such an approach makes it possible to address a critical set of questions: Is impairment evident early in life? Does the profile of deficit in children appear to be similar to that in adults with injury to comparable brain areas? Is there evidence of change in the profile of deficit across the course of development? To date, the few prospective studies of development following early brain injury have focused on either language or general cognitive ability as assessed by standardized

201

tests. Studies by Aram and colleagues (Aram, 1988; Aram et al., 1983, 1986; Rankin et al., 1981) have shown that preschool children with early-occurring focal brain injury have subtle linguistic and cognitive deficits. Further, longitudinal follow-up studies suggest that these early deficits persist throughout the school-age period (Aram, 1988). Bates (et al., 1991; Bates et al., 1997) and colleagues have provided detailed longitudinal accounts of early language impairment in the focal lesion (FL) population. Beginning in the first year of life, they have documented deficits in phonological, lexical, and morphosyntactic processing. By the late preschool period, most of these children appear to catch up in that their use of lexical and morphosyntactic structures falls within the normal range. However, analysis of discourse in the school-age period suggests continuing subtle linguistic impairment (Reilly et al., 1998). These studies are important because they provide strong evidence of functional deficits following early injury. However, additional work is needed, particularly for nonlinguistic functions.

Spatial cognitive processing is an important domain that has received little attention in the study of the child FL population. The ongoing longitudinal study of spatial cognitive development in children with early focal brain injury described here is the only major prospective study focused specifically on the development of spatial cognition in this population. When we began, virtually nothing was known about visuospatial processing in children with focal brain injury. Over the past decade, we have made considerable progress in identifying and defining profiles of specific deficits and development in this domain.

Spatial cognition refers to a wide array of abilities, from simple object localization, to the ability to mentally transpose or rotate an imagined object, to the complex computations required for cartography or navigation. The studies described here provide detailed assessments of one basic aspect of spatial cognition: spatial pattern analysis. *Spatial analysis* is defined as the ability to specify the parts and the overall configuration of a visually presented pattern and to understand how the parts are related to form a whole. It thus involves the ability both to segment a pattern into a set of constituent parts and to integrate those parts into a coherent whole. This definition is consistent with other descriptions of pattern analysis found in both adult and child literatures (e.g., Delis et al., 1986, 1988; Garner, 1974; Kemler, 1983; Palmer, 1977, 1980; Palmer & Bucher, 1981; Robertson & Delis, 1986; Smith & Kemler, 1977; Vurpillot, 1976). A variety of factors have been reported to affect spatial analysis. Among these are neurological and developmental status. Both of these factors have a direct bearing on our assessment of spatial analytic ability in children with focal brain injury.

Adults with Focal Brain Injury

Studies of adults have shown that focal brain injury results in disorders of spatial analytic functioning. These studies suggest that different patterns of spatial deficit are associated with left hemisphere (LH) and right hemisphere (RH) lesions (e.g., Arena & Gainotti, 1978; Delis et al., 1988; Delis et al., 1986; Gainotti & Tiacci,

1970; Lamb & Robertson, 1988, 1989, 1990; McFie & Zangwill, 1960; Piercy et al., 1960; Ratcliff, 1982; Robertson & Delis, 1986; Robertson & Lamb, 1988; Swindell et al., 1988; Wasserstein et al., 1987). Injury to LH brain regions results in disorders involving difficulty defining the parts of a spatial array. For example, in drawing, patients with LH injury tend to oversimplify spatial patterns and omit details. On perceptual judgment tasks, they rely on overall configural cues and ignore specific elements. By contrast, patients with RH lesions have difficulty with the configural aspects of spatial analysis. In drawing, they include details but fail to maintain a coherent organization among the elements. On perceptual judgment tasks, they focus on the parts of the pattern without attending to the overall form.

Normal Development of Spatial Analytic Processing

Over the past 10 years, a major line of work in our laboratory has been the study of spatial analysis in normally developing children. That work has yielded two major findings. First, children as young as 3 years of age are capable of analyzing visually presented arrays by segmenting out relevant elements and integrating them to form coherent wholes. Second, there is evidence of systematic change in the character of that analysis (Akshoomoff & Stiles, 1995a, 1995b; Feeney & Stiles, 1996; Stiles, 1995a; Stiles & Stern, submitted; Stiles et al., 1991; Stiles-Davis, 1988; Tada & Stiles, 1996). Data from a large series of studies using different measures and testing children ranging in age from 3 to 12 years show that initially children segment out well-formed, independent units and use simple combinatorial rules to integrate the parts into the overall configuration. With development, change is observed in both the nature of the parts and the relations children use to organize the parts. Further, pattern complexity affects how children approach the problem of analysis. In studies of both preschool (Feeney & Stiles, 1996; Stiles & Stern, submitted; Tada & Stiles, 1996) and school-age children (Akshoomoff & Stiles, 1995a, 1995b), we have found that the ways in which children approach the task of analyzing a spatial pattern depend on a wide array of factors that are related to both the information presented in the pattern itself and the strategies the child uses to process the array. How the child interprets the structure of the array depends on the interaction between the amount of information in the array and the strategy employed.

Spatial Analytic Processing in Children with Focal Brain Injury

The studies we have conducted over the past 10 years have begun to provide detailed profiles of deficit and recovery for spatial functioning associated with early lateralized brain injury. Different profiles have been observed, depending on the side of the injury, and these differences are consistent with patterns of deficit observed among adults with either right or left posterior brain injury. On construction and perception tasks, children with RH injury have difficulty with spatial integration.

While they are able to segment a spatial form into its elements, they have difficulty organizing those elements to form a coherent whole. The profile of spatial deficit for children with LH injury is quite different from that of children with RH injury. Children with LH injury oversimplify complex spatial forms and fail to encode the details or elements of these forms.

In addition to documenting patterns of specific deficits, we have provided some evidence of functional recovery. Longitudinal data indicate that with development children with both LH and RH injury show considerable behavioral improvement, eventually achieving ceiling-level performance on most spatial construction tasks. However, the time course over which this improvement occurs is protracted, and in cases where we have examined the underlying processes associated with recovery, anomalous processing profiles have emerged. Thus, although this work provides evidence of both initial deficit and subsequent recovery, the particular patterns of developmental delay raise important questions about the nature of development and functional recovery in this population. There are clearly specific and distinguishable patterns of deficit following early focal brain injury and there is development, but how persistent are those deficits? Does the pattern of behavioral improvement observed in the longitudinal data index generalized recovery of function with development, or do the data reflect a more limited pattern of compensation?

Children with Focal Brain Injury

Children in the FL population all suffered a single unilateral focal brain lesion within the first 6 months of life. The specific inclusionary criteria were:

1. Presence of a single unilateral brain lesion documented by a computed tomography (CT) or magnetic resonance imaging (MRI) scan
2. Onset of the lesion prior to 6 months of age
3. Normal or corrected to normal vision
4. Normal or corrected to normal hearing

Children were excluded from the study if any of the following were found:

1. Evidence of multiple lesions
2. Age of lesion onset later than 6 months of age
3. Medical history of a condition that might cause more global damage (e.g., severe closed head trauma, bacterial meningitis, encephalitis, or severe asphyxia)
4. Evidence of an evolving lesion such as a brain tumor or arteriovenous malformation
5. History of a neurosurgical procedure (e.g., ventriculoperitoneal shunt)

The most common cause of injury in this population was stroke. The presence of brain insult was typically identified in one of three ways: (*1*) neonatal seizures, (*2*) hemiplegia, or (*3*) routine ultrasound examination for other medical reasons (meconium staining, premature birth, etc.). In general, children in the FL population do well behaviorally, both individually and as a group. They typically score within the normal range on standardized IQ measures and attend public schools.

Studies of Spatial Processing in Children with Focal Brain Injury

The main goal of the studies described here was to provide detailed assessments of spatial analytic processing in children with pre- or perinatal focal brain injury. Many of the studies used construction-based tasks to assess processing abilities. Construction tasks are a rich source of information on both the products of construction efforts and the processes by which those products are achieved. A recurrent theme throughout these studies is the understanding of the process. As demonstrated by the studies described below, looking not just at *what* a child does but also *how* she or he does it can provide important data about deficits and development in this population.

Spatial Classification. Our study of spatial classification (Stiles-Davis et al., 1985) was the first to explicitly establish a specific disorder of spatial integrative ability in 2- to 3-year-olds with RH injury. In this study, children were presented with stimulus sets containing two classes of objects and simply encouraged to play with them. This procedure elicits systematic class-grouping activity in both normal children and those with focal brain injury. The results showed that children with RH injury were selectively impaired in their ability to form spatial groupings. Specifically, while RH-injured children stacked objects or placed one object within another, they did not place objects next to one another to extend their constructions out in space. Normal and LH-damaged children regularly placed objects next to each other as early as 24 months of age. A second task using a temporal measure of classification showed that the RH children were not impaired in their ability to form simple class relations. Thus the impairment on the spatial classification task reflected a primary disorder of spatial grouping rather than a disorder of classification per se. These findings suggested very limited development of spatial integrative ability for children with RH damage.

Spontaneous Block Construction in the Preschool Children. To elaborate the spatial classification findings, we conducted a large study focused on the ways in which 3- and 4-year-old children with focal brain injury spontaneously organize blocks into spatial groupings (Stiles & Nass, 1991; also see Stiles-Davis, 1988, for data on normal children). The study included two experiments. The first was a cross-sectional examination of 20 children tested at ages 3 and 4 (5 children with RH injury and 5 with LH injury at each age were included). The second experiment was a longitudinal case study of six children (three RH and three LH) tested at ages 3 and 4. The longitudinal data were intended to provide converging evidence of developmental patterns observed in the cross-sectional experiment. The data from both experiments were evaluated using eight measures of spatial grouping activity.

The results of this study of spontaneous block play showed that focal brain injury affected grouping activity for children with both RH and LH injury. Overall, performance of both groups was below that of normal children at 3 and 4 years of age. The profiles of deficit differed, however, for the two lesion groups. Children with RH injury were impaired on all measures of spatial construction at age 3. By age 4, development was observed on low-level measures assessing children's ability to combine pairs of objects. However, impairment was still observed on more global measures of organization. The behavior typical of this pattern of results was one in which children systematically placed blocks one by one in disordered heaps. In contrast, while children with LH injury at age 4 continued to produce fewer local-level relations, they showed a more normal pattern of development in the kinds of global structures they produced. Like normal 4-year-old children they generated arches, enclosures, and symmetries. The findings for both the RH and LH groups were consistent for the cross-sectional and longitudinal experiments. The pattern for the RH group extends our findings of spatial integrative deficit early in the preschool period. The finding of impaired development for the children with LH injury is the first report of a spatial deficit in this group.

Copying Model Block Constructions. To pursue the findings of the original study of spontaneous block construction in a more systematic fashion, we designed a second study in which children were asked to copy a specific set of model block constructions. In this study of 3- to 6-year-olds (Stiles et al., 1996), measures of both construction accuracy (the "product" measure) and construction strategy (the "process" measure) were employed to provide a more detailed description of spatial impairment in children with both RH and LH injury. In this task, children were presented with simple block models (e.g., a line of blocks or a double arch) and asked to reproduce them with the model present. Children with LH injury initially showed a delay, producing simplified constructions. By the time they were 4 years old, they showed an interesting dissociation in performance. Most of the children were able to produce accurate copies of the target constructions; however, the procedures they used in copying the forms were greatly simplified. This dissociation between product and process, which is not observed among normally developing children, persisted at least through age 6.

Children with RH injury were also initially delayed on the block-copying task. At age 3, these children produced only very simple constructions (such as stacks or lines), regardless of the model presented. At about 4 years of age, they produced more complex but disordered, poorly configured constructions. At this time, the procedures used to generate these ill-formed constructions were comparable to those of age-matched controls. Thus, at age 4, the children with RH injury showed evidence of a dissociation between product and process; they were able to use complex construction procedures, but the products of their efforts were poor. By age 6, the performance profile for this group of children had changed. They were able to copy the target construction accurately, but like their LH-injured peers, they now used simple construction procedures. It appeared that although the children with RH injury were capable of using complex construction procedures, they were unable to use these procedures to generate accurate spatial products. Limits on their ability to analyze the spatial pattern forced them to simplify their approach to construction, and this allowed them, by age 6, to produce accurate copies of the model block constructions.

This study suggests that there is impairment in spatial processing following early injury and that there is compensation with development. However, close examination of how spatial constructions are generated suggests a persistent deficit. These findings have been replicated in a study of Italian and American children with localized brain injury (Vicari et al., 1998). In addition, this study showed that the profiles of deficit were evident in children with isolated RH or LH subcortical injury, as well as in children with injury involving both cortical and subcortical areas.

Free Drawing. Data from another type of spatial construction task provide additional evidence of a spatial integration deficit in children with RH injury. In an early paper (Stiles-Davis et al., 1988), we reported drawing disorders in two 5-year-old children with RH injury similar to those reported for RH-injured adults. Figure 10-1 shows examples of the drawings produced by children in this study. In drawing houses, RH-injured children included appropriate parts, but failed to arrange them in spatially organized ways. This is consistent with reports of adults with similar injury. They depict people with hair coming from all sides of the head and with body parts not clearly distinguished. This is consistent with Swindell and colleagues' (1988) characterization of the human figure drawings of adult patients with RH injury as "scattered, fragmented, and disorganized . . . subjects often overscored lines and added extraneous scribblings" (p. 19). These deficits were not observed in age- and IQ-matched children with LH injury, nor were they observed in age-matched, normally developing control children.

Although the children with RH injury showed marked deficits of spatial integration at age 5, our longitudinal data provide evidence that there is considerable improvement on this task with age. Figure 10-2 provides examples of a longitudinal series of house drawings produced by children with RH injury. It is clear that with age, the quality of the children's drawings improves. However, another notable feature of these series, is the similarity of drawings from one testing session to the next. Drawings produced even years apart are very similar. These longitudinal series suggest that one possible avenue for the improvement observed in this task may be the development of compensatory drawing strategies, specifically the development of graphic formulas (Stiles et al., 1997). It is possible that the children are able to develop formulaic strategies over time for generating specific graphic objects such as houses. However, such a strategy should be quite limited, suggesting that while performance on a specific, practiced set of drawings might improve, that improvement should not extend to a wider range of drawings. Children's reliance on graphic formulas was tested using a task developed by Karmiloff-Smith (1990) in which children are asked first to draw a house and then an "impossible house, a house that couldn't possibly be." Our own data from more than 100 normally developing 6- to 12-year old children showed that by far the most typical solution to this task is to distort the spatial configuration of the house. Data from children with LH injury are indistinguishable from those of normal children. However, in both our cross-sectional samples ($n = 9$ children between 8 and 13 years of age)

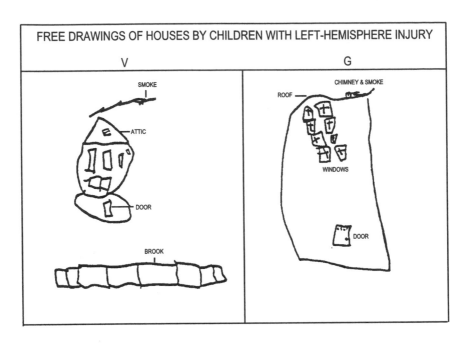

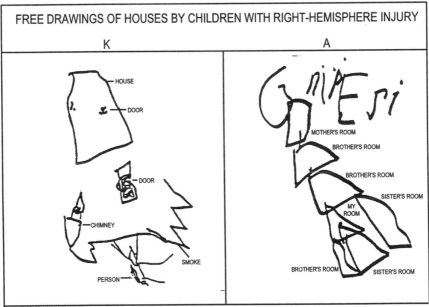

Figure 10-1. Free drawings of a house produced by LH- and RH-injured children. Labels indicate elements named spontaneously by each child. From "Drawing ability in four young children with congenital unilateral brain lesions" by J. Stiles-Davis, J. Janowsky, M. Engel, and R. Nass, 1988, *Neuropsychologia,* 26(3), p. 365. Copyright 1988 by Pergamon Press. Reprinted with permission.

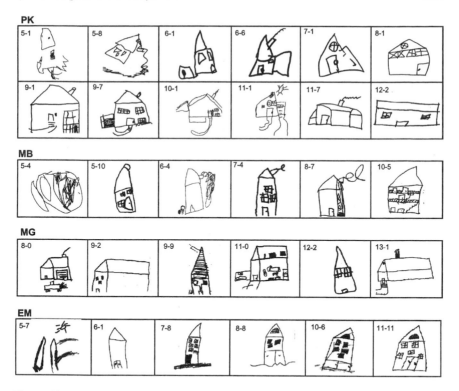

Figure 10-2. A longitudinal series of house drawings by four children with RH injury. For those children tested in the late preschool period (PK and MB), the initial disorganization of the drawing is evident. In each case, the drawings improve with development. Note the consistency of the drawing across testing sessions. From "The development of drawing in children with congenital focal brain injury" by J. Stiles, D. Trauner, M. Engel, and R. Nass, 1997, *Neuropsychologia,* 35(3), p. 303. Copyright 1997 by Elsevier Science Ltd. Adapted with permission.

and our longitudinal samples ($n = 6$ children tested annually from 6 to 12 years of age) of children with RH injury, configural distortion was not used. Instead, as illustrated in Figure 10-3, these children derived a number of nonconfigurational solutions for solving the problem, including verbal description (drawing an identical house and then describing something impossible inside), formula substitution (drawing another formulaic object and asserting that it was a house), reduction (putting a dot on the page and saying that the house was very small), and invisibility. These are all good strategies that indicate an understanding of the task. The notable absence of configural distortion strategies among the RH sample suggests that the children are limited in their ability to analyze or reanalyze the spatial array.

Copying Geometric Forms. Data from two simple copying tasks are consistent with the findings reported for the free drawing tasks. Children showed initial impairment

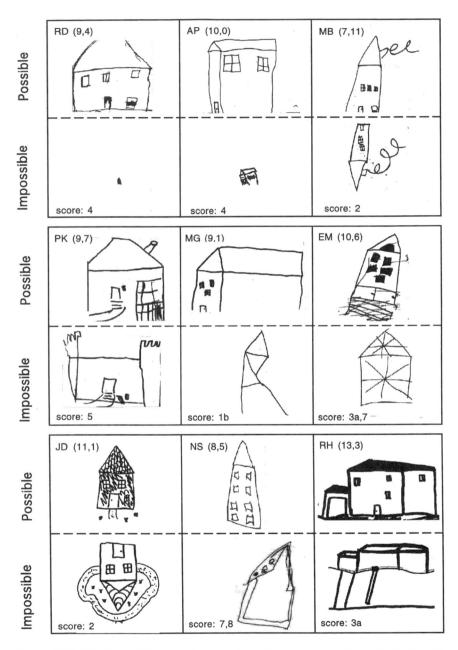

Figure 10-3. The impossible house drawings from the cross-sectional sample of nine children with RH injury. The age on testing is given in the upper left corner. The assigned category score(s) is indicated at the lower left. From "The development of drawing in children with congenital focal brain injury" by J. Stiles, D. Trauner, M. Engel, and R. Nass, 1997, *Neuropsychologia,* 35(3), p. 308. Copyright 1997 by Elsevier Science Ltd. Reprinted with permission.

on a memory reproduction task using hierarchically organized forms and on a task requiring them to copy simple geometric forms (Stiles et al., submitted). A typical hierarchical stimulus consists of a large letter (the global level) composed of appropriately arranged smaller letters (the local level)—for example, a large H made of small Ss. Hierarchical forms are particularly good experimental stimuli because they contain comparable information at both the global (overall configuration) and local (pattern detail) levels and thus provide a powerful means for examining possible dissociations in spatial analytic processing. On the hierarchical forms task, 5- to 6-year-old children were first shown a hierarchical letter or form pattern and told that they would be asked to reproduce it from memory. On testing, the children with LH injury had difficulty remembering the local-level elements, while the children with RH injury appear to remember the global structure but had difficulty reproducing it accurately. The findings from this task are similar to those for adult patients with unilateral focal brain injury.

The copying task required 3- to 5-year-old children to copy simple forms such as a plus, an X, and an asterisk. In the preschool period, the performance of normally developing children changes systematically on this task (Feeney & Stiles, 1996; Tada & Stiles, 1996), with adult-like performance achieved by 5 years of age. Comparison of the FL groups with normally developing children on this task revealed that children with RH injury were initially delayed on this task and continued to show evidence of impairment across the preschool period. By contrast, the performance of children with LH injury was indistinguishable from that of normally developing children by age 4 and showed the normal profile of improvement.

Copying the Rey Osterreith Complex Figure. A parallel set of findings was observed in older children using a more difficult construction task, the Rey Osterreith Complex Figure Copying task. Even cursory examination of the data suggested that children with either RH or LH injury had difficulty with the task. However, we could not evaluate their performance effectively because the existing child scoring systems did not adequately capture normal developmental change in performance on this task. To solve this problem, we completed a series of studies with a large sample of normally developing 6- to 12-year-olds (Akshoomoff & Stiles, 1995a, 1995b). In those studies, we adapted a new scoring system recently developed for use with adult data (Stern et al., 1994), and we developed an additional set of process measures. This composite scoring system provided a systematic account of normal developmental change on this task. The results of those studies allowed us to assess the data from the FL population (Akshoomoff & Stiles, in press). Preliminary examination of longitudinal data from 7 children and cross-sectional data from 21 children showed that the drawings by the younger (ages 6–7) FL children were sparser and less accurate than those of normal children of the same age. However, there were no striking differences between the young children with early LH and RH injury. With development, the limited available data suggest that performance improves considerably. By the time the children were 9 to 10 years old, they were able to produce reasonably accurate copies of the Rey figure. However, analysis of *how* they generated the form indicated that they used very simple construction procedures. The failure to find differences between the RH and LH groups on the Rey copying task could reflect underlying task demands that place equal emphasis on the segmentation and integrative processes and thus equally disrupt performance on the task. More likely, we simply do not yet have enough data from children in the 7- to 10-year age range to detect systematic differences in the performance of the two groups. None the less, the two main findings from the Rey copying data (i.e., early initial delay and later dissociation of product and process) mirror those found in our study of block construction in preschool children. In both studies, initial delay was observed for children with both RH and LH injury, suggesting that the ability both to identify the elements of a pattern and to integrate those elements is necessary for this task, and that a deficit in either aspect of spatial analysis affects performance. Later, the children are able to compensate for their deficits, producing accurate copies of the model forms. However, for both the block construction task and the Rey copying task, the procedures used are simplified. This similarity of performance profiles across measures and at different developmental time periods may provide the basis for developing a model of compensatory change in this population.

Defining the Nature of Developmental Change in the Focal Lesion Population

These studies of the development of spatial analytic processing in children with early focal brain injury provide important clues to the problem of defining the processes that underlie development following early localized brain injury. The contributions of this work come in part from the studies themselves and in part from the profiles of deficit and change within the domain of visuospatial processing they have generated. However, another important factor is the context in which this work has been done. All of the work on visuospatial processing reported here has been done in association with investigators studying development in other cognitive domains. Thus we have collaboratively developed profiles of linguistic, affective, and spatial development on the same population of children. One of the most notable features of this extended body of data is that the cross-domain profiles do not always provide the same answers to the three critical questions raised earlier. Language and visuospatial processing, for example, provide different answers to the questions of initial deficit, mapping to adult profiles of deficit, and change over time. The contrast between the developmental profiles of language and visuospatial processing has provided interesting and important insights into the process of developmental change following early insult.

When we began our work, our goal was to use the prospective approach to investigate processes of recovery and/or compensation as they occur in real developmental time. For spatial analytic processes, deficits in visuospatial processing are evident as early as we have been able to test for them; the specific features of deficit map well onto those regions of the brain associated with particular deficits in adults; and the deficits, although subtle, persist over time. Data from our longitudinal studies of language provide a very different picture of development following early brain injury. Language deficits are evident from the earliest stages of language acquisition, but the specific features of deficit do not map well to the adult profile. Further, children show considerable improvement over time, achieving normal levels of performance in both the semantic and grammatical aspects of language by age 5 (Bates et al., 1997; Reilly et al., 1998). Subtle deficits in discourse and narrative production are evident in the school-age period, but the pattern of deficit is uniform across the lesion population. The site of the lesion does not appear to affect the pattern of later deficit.

The specific features of developmental profiles obtained for different behavioral domains suggest that data from any single domain may present only one part of a complex puzzle, which if considered in isolation may lead to very limited, and possibly inaccurate, conclusions about the nature of development following early injury. One of our most important insights to date has been that the processes underlying functional recovery do not require us to posit special mechanisms such as selective preservation or crowding (see Stiles, 1995b, 1998, in press). The profiles of development observed in our longitudinal data can be accounted for by the same mechanisms that underlie normal brain development.

The normally developing brain is dynamic and plastic. Initially, there is a profusion of connections throughout the brain. With development, many of these early connections are withdrawn and others are stabilized. This selective stabilization process is presumed to be the product of competitive processes that are driven to a large extent by input. The structure and organization of the mature normal brain are the products of these plastic, competitive processes. It should also be noted that the capacity for plastic change is never completely lost. Indeed, recent animal studies have shown that, across a range of mammalian species, patterns of neural connectivity in the adult organism are altered by changes in input to the system (Kaas, 1991; Merzenich & Jenkins, 1995; Pons, 1995). In short, plasticity is a central feature of brain development; it is not a systemic response to pathological insult.

When plasticity is viewed as a necessary part of brain development rather than as a possible alternative in the case of early insult, a very different perspective on the effects of early brain injury on development emerges. The developing brain is a dynamic, responsive, and, to some extent, self-organizing system. Early injury constitutes a perturbation of normal development. Specific neural resources are lost, and there should be consequent impairment of the system. That is precisely what we observe in both language and visuospatial processing. However, it is also a developing system and therefore a system with an exuberance of resources, the fate of which are determined in large measure by input. Thus, the magnitude and duration of the initial impairment may well depend on a range of factors such as the timing of the insult, the extent and location of the injury, and the specificity of the neural substrate for the function under consideration. Spatial information processing is a phylogenetically older function than language processing, and its neural substrate may be much more highly specified and constrained during development than the neural substrate required for language acquisition. However, it is also clear that the effects of early injury on spatial processing are markedly attenuated relative to those of later injury. This suggests that the capacity for reorganization and functional compensation is retained *within* this more constrained system.

ACKNOWLEDGMENT

This work was supported by NICHHD Grant R01-HD25077, NINDS Grant P50-NS22343, and NIDCD Grant P50-DC01289. The author wishes to thank the parents and children for their participation in the studies presented in this chapter.

References

Akshoomoff, N.A., and Stiles, J. (1995a) Developmental trends in visuospatial analysis and planning: I. Copying a complex figure. *Neuropsychology,* 9(3):364–377.

Akshoomoff, N.A., and Stiles, J. (1995b) Developmental trends in visuospatial analysis and planning: II. Memory for a complex figure. *Neuropsychology,* 9(3):378–389.

Akshoomoff, N.A., and Stiles, J. (in press) Children's Performance on the Rey-Osterrieth Complex Figure and the development of spatial analysis. In J. Knight and E. Kaplan (eds.), *The Handbook of Rey-Osterrieth Complex Figure Usage: Clinical and Research Applications.*

Alajouanine, T., and Lhermitte, F. (1965) Acquired aphasia in children. *Brain,* 88(4): 653–662.

Aram, D.M. (1988) Language sequelae of unilateral brain lesions in children. In F. Plum, (ed.), *Language Communication and the Brain.* New York: Raven Press, pp. 171–197.

Aram, D.M., Ekelman, B.L., and Whitaker, H.A. (1986) Spoken syntax in children with acquired unilateral hemisphere lesions. *Brain and Language,* 27(1):75–100.

Aram, D.M., Rose, D.F., Rekate, H.L., and Whitaker, H.A. (1983) Acquired capsular/ striatal aphasia in childhood. *Archives of Neurology,* 40:614–617.

Arena, R., and Gainotti, G. (1978) Constructional apraxia and visuoperceptive disabilities in relation to laterality of cerebral lesions. *Cortex,* 14(4):463–473.

Bates, E., and Thal, D. (1991) Associations and dissociations in language development. In J. Miller (ed.), *Research on Child Language Disorders: A Decade of Progress.* Austin, TX: Pro-Ed, pp. 145–168.

Bates, E., Thal, D., Trauner, D., Fenson, J., Aram, D., Eisele, J., and Nass, R. (1997) From first words to grammar in children with focal brain injury. In D. Thal and J. Reilly (eds.), Special Issue on Origins of Communication Disorders, *Developmental Neuropsychology,* 13(3):275–343.

Brown, J.W., and Jaffe, J. (1975) Hypothesis on cerebral dominance. *Neuropsychologia,* 13(1):107–110.

Carlson, J., Netley, C., Hendrick, E., and Pritchard, J. (1968) A reexamination of intellectual abilities in hemidecorticated patients. *Transactions of the American Neurological Association,* 93:198–201.

Day, P.S., and Ulatowska, H.K. (1979) Perceptual, cognitive, and linguistic development after early hemispherectomy: Two case studies. *Brain and Language,* 7(1):17–33.

Delis, D.C., Kiefner, M.G., and Fridlund, A.J. (1988) Visuospatial dysfunction following unilateral brain damage: Dissociations in hierarchical hemispatial analysis. *Journal of Clinical and Experimental Neuropsychology,* 10(4):421–431.

Delis, D.C., Robertson, L.C., and Efron, R. (1986) Hemispheric specialization of memory for visual hierarchical stimuli. *Neuropsychologia,* 24(2):205–214.

Dennis, M. (1980) Capacity and strategy for syntactic comprehension after left or right hemidecortication. *Brain and Language,* 10(2):287–317.

Dennis, M., and Kohn, B. (1975) Comprehension of syntax in infantile hemiplegics after cerebral hemidecortication. *Brain and Language,* 2(4):472–482.

Dennis, M., and Whitaker, H.A. (1976) Language acquisition following hemidecortication: Linguistic superiority of the left over the right hemisphere. *Brain and Language,* 3:404–433.

Feeney, S.M., and Stiles, J. (1996) Spatial analysis: An examination of preschoolers' perception and construction of geometric patterns. *Developmental Psychology,* 32(5):933–941.

Gainotti, G., and Tiacci, C. (1970) Patterns of drawing disability in right and left hemispheric patients. *Neuropsychologia,* 8:379–384.

Garner, W.R. (1974) *The Processing of Information and Structure.* Potomac, MD: Erlbaum.

Gott, P.S. (1973). Cognitive abilities following right and left hemispherectomy. *Cortex,* 9(3):266–274.

Hammill, D., and Irwin, O.C. (1966) I.Q. differences of right and left spastic hemiplegic children. *Perceptual and Motor Skills,* 22(1):193–194.

Kaas, J.H. (1991). Plasticity of sensory and motor maps in adult mammals. *Annual Review of Neuroscience,* 14:137–167.

Karmiloff-Smith, A. (1990) Constraints on representational change: Evidence from children's drawing. *Cognition,* 34:57–83.

Kemler, D. (1983) Exploring and reexploring issues of integrality, perceptual sensitivity, and dimensional salience. *Journal of Experimental Child Psychology,* 36(3):365–379.

Kohn, B. (1980) Right hemisphere speech representation and comprehension of syntax after left cerebral injury. *Brain and Language,* 9(2):350–361.

Kohn, B., and Dennis, M. (1974) Selective impairments of visuospatial abilities in infantile hemiplegics after right cerebral hemidecortication. *Neuropsychologia,* 12(4):505–512.

Krashen, S.D. (1973) Lateralization, language learning, and the critical period: Some new evidence. *Language Learning,* 23(1):63–74.

Lamb, M.R., and Robertson, L.C. (1988) The processing of hierarchical stimuli: Effects of retinal locus, locational uncertainty, and stimulus identity. *Perception and Psychophysics,* 44(2):172–181.

Lamb, M.R., and Robertson, L.C. (1989) Do response time advantage and interference reflect the order of processing of global- and local-level information? *Perception and Psychophysics,* 46(3):254–258.

Lamb, M.R., and Robertson, L.C. (1990) The effects of visual angle on global and local reaction times depends on the set of visual angles presented. *Perception and Psychophysics,* 47(5):489–496.

Lenneberg, E.H. (1967) *Biological Foundations of Language.* New York: Wiley.

McFie, J. (1961) The effects of hemispherectomy on intellectual functioning in cases of infantile hemiplegia. *Journal of Neurology, Neurosurgery, and Psychiatry,* 24:240–249.

McFie, J., and Zangwill, O.L. (1960) Visual-constructive disabilities associated with lesions of the left cerebral hemisphere. *Brain,* 83:243–259.

Merzenich, M.M., and Jenkins, W.M. (1995) Cortical plasticity, learning, and learning dysfunction. In B. Julez and I. Kovacs (eds.), *Maturational Windows and Adult Cortical Plasticity.* Reading, MA: Addison-Wesley, pp. 247–264.

Palmer, S.E. (1977) Hierarchical structure in perceptual representation. *Cognitive Psychology,* 9:441–474.

Palmer, S.E. (1980) What makes triangles point: Local and global effects in configurations of ambiguous triangles. *Cognitive Psychology,* 12(3):285–305.

Palmer, S.E., and Bucher, N.M. (1981) Configural effects in perceived pointing of ambiguous triangles. *Journal of Experimental Psychology: Human Perception and Performance,* 7(1):88–114.

Piercy, M., Hecaen, H., and Ajuriaguerra, J. (1960) Constructional apraxia associated with unilateral cerebral lesions: Left and right sided cases compared. *Brain,* 83:225–242.

Pons, T.P. (1995) Abstract: Lesion-induced cortical placticity. In B. Julesz and I. Kovacs (eds.), *Maturational Windows and Adult Cortical Placticity.* Reading, MA: Addison-Wesley, pp. 175–178.

Rankin, J.M., Aram, D.M., and Horowitz, S.J. (1981) Language ability in right and left hemisplegic children. *Brain and Language,* 14:292–306.

Ratcliff, G. (1982) Disturbances of spatial orientation associated with cerebral lesions. In M. Potegal (ed.), *Spatial Abilities: Develpment and Physiological Foundations.* New York: Academic Press, pp. 301–331.

Reed, J.C., and Reitan, R.M. (1971) Verbal and performance differences among brain-injured children with lateralized motor deficits. *Neuropsychologia,* 9:401–407.

Reilly, J.S., Bates, E., and Marchman, V. (1998) Narrative discourse in children with early focal brain injury. In M. Dennis (ed.), Special Issue on Discourse in Children with Anomalous Brain Development or Acquired Brain Injury. *Brain and Language,* 61(3): 335–375.

Robertson, L.C., and Delis, D.C. (1986) Part-whole processing in unilateral brain damaged patients: Dysfunction of hierarchical organization. *Neuropsychologia,* 24(3):363–370.

Robertson, L.C., and Lamb, M.R. (1988) The role of perceptual reference frames in visual field asymmetries. *Neuropsychologia,* 26(1):145–152.

Rudel, R.G., and Teuber, H.L. (1971) Spatial orientation in normal children and in children with early brain damage. *Neuropsychologia,* 9:401–407.

Rudel, R.G., Teuber, H.L., and Twitchell, T. (1974) Levels of impairment of sensorimotor function in children with early brain damage. *Neuropsychologia,* 12:95–108.

Smith, L.B., and Kemler, D.G. (1977) Developmental trends in free classification: Evidence for a new conceptualization of perceptual development. *Journal of Experimental Child Psychology,* 24(2):279–298.

Stern, R.A., Singer, E.A., Duke, L.M., Singer, N.G., Morey, C.E., Daughtrey, E.W., and Kaplan, E. (1994) The Boston Qualitative Scoring System for the Rey-Osterrieth Complex Figure: Description and interrater reliability. *The Clinical Neuropsychologist,* 8:309–322.

Stiles, J. (1995a) The early use and development of graphic formulas: Two case study reports of graphic formula production by 2- to 3-year old children. *International Journal of Behavior and Development,* 18(1):127–149.

Stiles, J. (1995b) Plasticity and development: Evidence from children with early occurring focal brain injury. In B. Julesz and I. Kovacs (eds.), *Maturational Windows and Adult Cortical Plasticity.* Reading, MA: Addison-Wesley, pp. 217–237.

Stiles, J. (1998) The effects of early focal brain injury on lateralization of cognitive function. *Current Directions in Psychological Science,* 7(1):21–26.

Stiles, J. (in press) Neural plasticity and cognitive development. *Developmental Neuropsychology.*

Stiles, J., Delis, D.C., and Tada, W.L. (1991) Global-local processing in preschool children. *Child Development,* 62(6):1258–1275.

Stiles, J., Feeney, S., and Chang, R. (submitted) The early development of visuo-spatial processing in children with focal brain injury: Evidence from a copying task.

Stiles, J., and Nass, R. (1991) Spatial grouping activity in young children with congenital right or left hemisphere brain injury. *Brain and Cognition,* 15(2):201–222.

Stiles, J., and Stern. C. (submitted) Developmental change in spatial cognitive processing: Complexity effects and block construction performance in preschool children.

Stiles, J., Stern, C., Trauner, D., and Nass, R. (1996) Developmental change in spatial grouping activity among children with early focal brain injury: Evidence from a modeling task. *Brain and Cognition,* 31:46–62.

Stiles, J., Trauner, D., Engel, M., and Nass., R. (1997) The development of drawing in children with congenital focal brain injury: Evidence for limited functional recovery. *Neuropsychologia,* 35(3):299–312.

Stiles-Davis, J. (1988) Developmental change in young children's spatial grouping activity. *Developmental Psychology,* 24(4):522–531.

Stiles-Davis, J., Janowsky, J., Engel, M., and Nass, R. (1988) Drawing ability in four young children with congenital unilateral brain lesions. *Neuropsychologia,* 26(3):359–371.

Stiles-Davis, J., Sugarman, S., and Nass, R. (1985) The development of spatial and class relations in four young children with right cerebral hemisphere damage: Evidence for early and spatial-constructive deficit. *Brain and Cognition,* 4(4):388–412.

Swindell, C.S., Holland, A.L., Fromm, D., and Greenhouse, J.B. (1988) Characteristics of recovery of drawing ability in left and right brain-damaged patients. *Brain and Cognition,* 7(1):16–30.

Tada, W.L., and Stiles, J. (1996) Developmental change in children's analysis of spatial patterns. *Developmental Psychology,* 32(5):951–970.

Vargha-Khadem, F., O'Gorman, A.M., and Watters, G.V. (1983) Aphasia in children with "prenatal" versus postnatal left hemisphere lesions: A clinical and CT scan study. Presented at the 11th meeting of the International Neuropsychological Society, Mexico City.

Vargha-Khadem, F., O'Gorman, A.M., and Watters, G.V. (1985) Aphasia and handedness in relation to hemispheric side, age at injury and severity of cerebral lesion during childhood. *Brain,* 108:677–696).

Vicari, S., Stiles, J., Stern, C., and Resca, A. (1998) The role of cortical and subcortical lesions in visuospatial processing: Evidence from children with early focal brain injury. *Developmental Medicine and Child Neurology,* 40:90–94.

Vurpillot, E. (1976) *The Visual World of the Child.* London: Allen and Unwin.

Wasserstein, J., Zappulla, R., Rosen, J., and Gerstman, L. (1987) In search of closure: Subjective contour illusions, Gestalt completion test, and implications. *Brain and Cognition,* 6(1):1–14.

Woods, B.T., and Carey, S. (1979) Language deficits after apparent clinical recovery from childhood aphasia. *Annals of Neurology,* 6:405–409.

Woods, B.T. (1980) The restricted effects of right-hemisphere lesions after age one: Wechsler test data. *Neuropsychologia,* 18(1):65–70.

11

Neuroplasticity Following Traumatic Diffuse versus Focal Brain Injury in Children: Studies of Verbal Fluency

HARVEY S. LEVIN, JAMES SONG,
SANDRA B. CHAPMAN, AND HARRIET HARWARD

Development and reorganization of word production following early brain injury are reviewed in this chapter, including studies of children who sustained focal vascular lesions during the first 6 months of life and studies of recovery from traumatic brain injury. Cross-sectional and longitudinal word fluency data from an ongoing project on brain injury in children are presented, and putative mechanisms for reorganization of function are discussed.

Word Production after Focal Vascular Lesions

Neuropsychological studies of children who suffered unilateral focal vascular lesions during the first 6 months of life have often addressed language development. Productivity of speech, as measured during conversation or with structured lexical tests involving word generation, has been shown to be initially impaired in young children following unilateral focal lesions of either hemisphere (Aram et al., 1990; Bates et al., 1997; Feldman et al., 1992). Cross-sectional studies (Woods & Carey, 1979) suggest that a focal lesion of either hemisphere before 1 year of age is compatible with normal language development, whereas after that age left hemisphere lesions tend to have more adverse effects on language than right hemisphere lesions. Yet prospective, longitudinal studies have documented that many children with nontraumatic focal hemispheric lesions exhibit relatively normal rates of lexical development after an initial delay (Bates et al., 1997; Feldman et al., 1992). Feldman et al. (1992) studied nine children (five with left hemisphere lesions and four with right hemisphere lesions), aged 14–48 months, who had sustained unilateral antepartum or perinatal lesions. Serial testing on three occasions separated by about 3 months revealed that the number of different words used in conversation was initially below normal for both left and right hemisphere lesion groups. The rate of age-related improvement in verbal fluency was relatively normal for both groups, suggesting that the neural substrate for language could be established after a lesion of either hemisphere. Consistent with this interpretation of Feldman et al. (1992), the San Diego group (Bates et al., 1997) has also shown that, depending on the language measure, early right hemisphere lesions can produce greater receptive language impairment before age 5 years than early left hemisphere lesions. Although long-term follow-up data for children sustaining focal lesions during the first 6 months of life are sparse beyond age 4 or 5 years, the available evidence indicates that language development is within the normal range in most children sustaining focal vascular lesions of either hemisphere before 1 year of age. However, Bates et al. (1997) have cautioned that despite apparently normal development of language, subtle deficits might reduce the level of competence that would have emerged without the vascular insult. These observations, taken together with the findings of studies of children sustaining early epileptogenic lesions (Strauss et al., 1990), lend support to Teuber's postulation that transfer of function produces a crowding effect due to competition for computational space in the intact cerebral hemisphere.

Intrahemispheric Site of Focal Vascular Lesions

An intrahemispheric site of the lesion has been reported inconsistently due to variability in the use and quality of brain imaging, particularly in multicenter studies that have used nonuniform protocols. Bates et al. (1997) found that left temporal lesions produced more severe impairment of language development on tests of vocabulary and length of utterance than lesions without left temporal involvement. In comparison with the adult aphasia literature, the San Diego group Bates et al., 1997 has found patchy evidence of "classical language areas" that correspond to the left posterior inferior frontal region (*Broca effect*) and the posterior superior temporal region in adults. Although direct comparison of recovery from focal brain lesions in children to the outcome of left hemisphere stroke in adults is difficult, the effects of intrahemispheric localization of lesion tend to be less consistent following early brain insults in young children. Bates et al. (1997) followed up samples of children who sustained focal unilateral lesions prenatally or within 6 months after birth and assessed language functions using standardized tests and analysis of spontaneous speech samples at 10–17 months ($n = 26$), 17–31 months ($n = 29$), and 20–44 months ($n = 30$). Although there were no overall laterality of lesion effects, deficits in language production were associated with left temporal lesions and a shortened mean length of utterance was related to the presence of a frontal lesion in either hemisphere. In contrast to the temporal lobe effects on vocabulary at 17–31 months and on mean length of utterance at 20–44 months, which were confined to left hemisphere lesions, a frontal lesion of either hemisphere was associated with delays in vocabulary development in children who were 17–31 months old at the time of testing. In general, the percentage of children with focal lesions whose word production fell below the 10th percentile for age (i.e., were at risk for expressive language problems) was significant regardless of the hemisphere involved. In the children with left hemisphere lesions, concomitant left frontal and left temporal damage contributed to an adverse effect on mean length of utterance. A parallel finding was obtained for right frontal involvement in children with right hemisphere lesions.

In view of the observed variation in the effects of intrahemispheric site of lesion, depending on the age at follow-up, Bates et al. (1997) inferred that the cortical representation of language is characterized by gradual modularization due to the effects of experience; the recruitment of specific structures to support language, which varies with development; and innate features of cortical regions that predispose to specific types of computational processes that change with development. Consequently, the pattern of focal lesion effects on language in young children is more subtle, transient, and variable than to the aphasias found in adults with perisylvian lesions of the left hemisphere. Although these recent investigations of development following early vascular lesions have used well-designed measures of lexical, semantic, and syntactic aspects of language, limitations of these studies include structural brain imaging confined to clinical reports of lateralization of hemispheric lesions based on computed tomography, without detailed characterization of the intrahemispheric site of the lesion. The number of children in cells defined by intrahemispheric localization of the lesion is likely to be small due to the low incidence of this disorder.

Mechanism of Reorganization of Function

As described by Carlsson and Hugdahl in Chapter 14, their verbal dichotic listening studies have shown that about three-fourths of patients sustaining early left hemisphere lesions later exhibit a left ear advantage indicating right hemisphere specialization for language. Carlsson and Hugdahl's interpretation of their dichotic listening data is also compatible with brain imaging studies that have provided evidence of increased right hemisphere participation in language. Investigations of reorganization of function in the process of recovery from aphasia in adults have used cerebral blood flow (Papanicolaou et al., 1988), evoked potentials (Papanicolaou et al., 1988), positron emission tomography (PET; Weiller et al., 1995), and more recently, functional magnetic resonance imaging (fMRI; Buckner et al., 1996) to demonstrate that homotopic areas of the right hemisphere are recruited to subserve language in at least a subgroup of patients. However, a recent PET study of word retrieval in recovering aphasic adults revealed no evidence of laterality shift of word retrieval functions to the right temporal region (Warburton et al., 1999). Positron emission tomography studies by Chugani (1997) have shown that patients who sustained focal left hemisphere epileptogenic lesions during early childhood also exhibited increased right hemisphere activation by language processing relative to a comparison group who did not have early left hemisphere lesions. Based on cross-sectional studies of 2-deoxy-2[^{18}F]fluoro-D-glucose (FDG) PET scanning indicating that cortical glucose metabolism peaks during the 4- to 9-year age range and is followed by a decline after early adolescence, Chugani et al. (1987) interpreted these findings as evidence that the capacity for reorganization of cortical function is greatest during this period. Recent PET studies have supported the view that reorganization of language function after a focal brain lesion typically recruits the contralateral homotopic region. Using a word stem completion task as an activation condition during PET, Buckner and colleagues (1997) found right inferior frontal engagement in a patient who had sustained a left frontal ischemic stroke. The inference that word generation transferred from the left to the right inferior frontal region is consistent with PET and MRI studies showing that the left inferior frontal gyrus is frequently a site of activation in normal right-handed subjects performing word generation tasks (Phelps et al., 1997). In a PET study of six adults who were recovering from fluent aphasia secondary to a left hemisphere stroke, Weiller et al. (1995) found that repetition of pseudowords and verb generation tasks produced activation of the right middle and superior temporal gyri and the right inferior frontal area, that is, homotopic areas contralateral to the regions that were activated in healthy controls while performing these tasks.

However, there is a need for longitudinal studies of functional brain imaging with language activation to elucidate the process of reorganization of function. Unresolved issues include patient variables (e.g., size of the lesion, age at injury, age at study, time since injury, and gender) and postlesion interventions (e.g., speech and language therapy) that potentially moderate the transfer of language to homotopic regions of the right hemisphere. Variability across language domains in the potential for reorganization of function and the mechanism for transfer of function (i.e., contralateral homotopic vs. ipsilateral structures) are also poorly understood. Preliminary findings (Strauss et al., 1990) in adult patients who sustained left hemisphere epileptogenic lesions in early childhood and developed atypical (i.e., right hemisphere or bilateral) hemispheric specialization for language have revealed variability in performance across communication domains. Verbal fluency, verbal reasoning, and verbal memory did not differ in the left hemisphere versus atypical language representation groups, whereas naming and language comprehension were impaired in the patients with right hemisphere or bilateral language representation relative to the left hemisphere specialization group.

Evidence for the Crowding Hypothesis

Support for Teuber's 1979 postulation requires evidence that capacities subserved by the intact hemisphere are compromised by competing for processing resources with functions that transferred from the injured hemisphere. Preliminary observations in 27 adults with early-onset epileptogenic lesions have confirmed the compromised cognitive function, as predicted by Teuber (Strauss et al., 1990). Visuospatial skills were impaired in patients who had right hemisphere or bilateral speech representation relative to other epileptic patients who had left hemisphere specialization for speech. In a related study, Satz and colleagues (1994) qualified this finding by showing that the compromise of visuospatial and nonverbal memory skills was specific to individuals who developed atypical speech representation following development of left hemisphere epileptogenic lesion before 12 months of age. Although interhemispheric transfer of function after an early left hemisphere lesion was compatible with relatively normal language development, Satz et al. (1994) reported that the linguistic performance of these patients fell below that of a healthy comparison group. Whether this preliminary finding can be extrapolated to recovery from traumatic focal lesions in children of varying age awaits further study.

Cognitive and clinical neuroscientists have generally emphasized that interhemispheric transfer of function in humans is confined to language, and they have claimed that language develops earlier than nonverbal abilities as a substrate to support this preposition (see Chapter 14). However, this view point appears at odds with studies indicating that visual perceptual and visuospatial deficits emerge after focal lesions of either hemisphere during the perinatal period or from birth to 12 months (Stiles et al., 1996). Moreover, a recent case study suggested that visuospatial abilities might transfer to the left hemisphere following right parietal injury during the first year of life. In a case report of an adolescent who developed dyscalculia and dyslexia associated with normal visuospatial ability after sustaining a focal traumatic lesion of the right parietal region at 7 months of age, Levin et al. (1996) used fMRI to test the hypothesis that this patient's disabilities were caused by competition resulting from transfer of the right hemisphere functions to the intact left hemisphere. As shown in Plate 2, activation by performing serial subtraction was confined to the patient's left hemisphere, whereas bilateral activation was typical in normal subjects.

Epidemiology and Pathophysiology of Traumatic Brain Injury

In contrast to the low incidence of focal vascular lesions in young children, traumatic brain injury (TBI) is the most frequent cause of acquired brain injury in the pediatric population, with an incidence of about 200/100,000 (Kraus et al., 1984). The external cause of TBI varies, depending on the age of the child. Physical abuse is a common cause of head trauma in the birth to 4-year age range, and falls are frequent throughout childhood. Pedestrian motor vehicle injuries are a frequent cause of severe head injury in children, whereas the most frequent cause of severe head injury in adolescents is motor vehicle crashes. Closed-head injury (CHI) produced by sudden acceleration/deceleration of the freely moving head accounts for more than 98% of TBIs in children; by contrast, penetrating missile wounds are infrequent. Consequently, this chapter focuses on studies of children following CHI. However, there is marked heterogeneity in the pathophysiology of CHI, with varying degrees of diffuse and focal brain injury. Focal brain lesions include hematomas and contusions, which have a predilection for the prefrontal and anterior temporal regions (Adams et al., 1980; Levin et al., 1997). Diffuse brain insult primarily involves diffuse axonal injury (Adams et al., 1980) and secondary injury related to excessive release of excitotoxic amino acids (McIntosh et al., 1996). Multifocal ischemic lesions are also common after severe CHI, presumably due in part to increased intracranial pressure and secondary reduction of cerebral perfusion pressure. The concomitant focal and diffuse brain insults resulting from CHI complicate investigation of the relationship between the severity of acute injury and recovery. Later in this chapter, we suggest that the effects of focal and diffuse brain insults can be dissociated.

The Glasgow Coma Scale (GCS) of Teasdale and Jennett (1997) is the most widely accepted measure of acute impairment of consciousness, an important clinical indicator of the severity of diffuse CHI. However, the motor and verbal components of the GCS are not readily applied to infants because of the demands on expressive (e.g., "confused speech") and receptive (e.g., "obeys commands") language. As Levin et al. (1989) have shown, the verbal demands imposed by the GCS can also complicate the assessment and interpretation of impaired language in adults with left hemisphere focal brain lesions. Consequently, investigators have modified the GCS for use with infants and young children (Simpson et al., 1991).

Rationale for Studying Verbal Fluency

Measures of verbal fluency have been used extensively in studies of adults and children. Word generation is relevant to communication skills in daily living and can be quantitated in relation to established normative data based on age and gender. As shown in Figure 11-1, there is a developmental trend toward verbal fluency, with increasing disparity in performance between boys and girls as a function of age. Assessment of word finding under a time limit (typically 60 seconds for reciting as many words as possible beginning with a letter designated by the examiner and usually repeated for three letters) according to specific rules (e.g., exclusion of proper nouns) enhances the sensitivity of this test to diffuse and focal features of brain injury. Verbal fluency deficits in adults with nontraumatic left frontal lesions are more severe than those of adults with left posterior lesions or right hemisphere focal lesions (Benton, 1968). Impairment of word fluency is also related to the severity of CHI in adults (Levin et al., 1976) and children (Ewing-Cobbs et al., 1987), as measured by the GCS score and by the duration of coma. Further justification for studying word fluency follows from the finding that expressive language skills tend to be more persistently impaired than the recovered pattern of language comprehension in children after CHI (Ewing-Cobbs et al., 1987). Gaps in the literature on the effects of CHI on word fluency in children include the lack of longitudinal studies and difficulty in isolating the effects of focal versus diffuse brain injury. To address these limitations, we have analyzed cross-sectional and longitudinal word fluency data that we accrued in an ongoing project on the outcome of head injury in children.

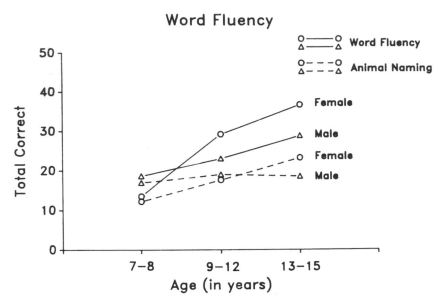

Figure 11-1. Total number of correct words plotted separately for boys and girls against age at testing for two measures of verbal fluency, including Controlled Oral Word Fluency and Animal Naming. From Levin et al. (1991). Reproduced with permission.

Cross-Sectional Study of Word Fluency after Closed Head Injury

We studied 149 head-injured children, including 111 children who sustained a severe head injury that resulted in coma and 38 children who had mild impairment of consciousness and no evidence of a brain lesion on a computed tomography (CT) scan within 24 hours after injury and on an MRI scan at least three months after injury (Table 11-1). In addition, 86 uninjured, healthy children whose distribution of demographic variables did not differ from that of the head-injured patients were recruited from the Dallas metropolitan area. As shown in Table 11-1, the children were tested at least 3 years after injury.

Administering the Word Fluency Test from the Neurosensory Center Comprehensive Examination for Aphasia (NCCEA; Spreen & Benton, 1969) involved asking the child to generate as many words as possible beginning with a specific letter in 1 minute, excluding proper nouns and the same word repeated with a different suffix. The number of words generated was summed across three letters. A Poisson distribution was used to model the distribution of verbal fluency scores. Age at the time of testing and group membership were included in the initial regression model.

Table 11-2 summarizes the verbal fluency scores of the head-injured and healthy control groups. In addition to showing an overall significant effect on the groups, pairwise comparisons revealed that the severely injured children produced fewer words than both the mildly head-injured and healthy control groups. The se-

Table 11-1. Demographic and Clinical Features of the Head Injured and Control Groups in a Cross-Sectional Study

	Controls (n = 86)		Mild CHI (n = 38)		Severe CHI (n = 111)		
	Mean	SD	Mean	SD	Mean	SD	P Value
Age at study (years)	11.3	3.1	12.1	3.3	12.3	3.5	0.11
Age at injury (years)			8.0	3.6	7.5	3.7	0.49
Months postinjury			48.8	20.8	57.3	28.2	0.09
Parental education (years)	13.8	2.5	124.4	2.5	13.5	2.3	0.16
CGS score			14.5^a	0.7	5.6^a	1.7	0.0001
Gender							
% girls	36.1		29.0		37.9		0.61
% boys	64.0		71.1		62.2		

Note: Within rows, common superscript letters denote signfiicant ($p \le .05$) pairwise contrasts.

verely injured children also committed more perseverative errors (repeating the same word) than the healthy, uninjured children. Age at the time of testing had a significant effect on the total number of correct words produced. However, there was no interaction between age at testing and injury group. These findings indicate that severe CHI can produce a persistent deficit in word fluency despite a prolonged postinjury period. To elucidate the effects of head injury on development of word fluency and the process of recovery, we also performed a longitudinal study.

Recovery and Development:Longitudinal Findings

To investigate recovery of verbal fluency, 122 head-injured children (44 with mild CHI and 78 with severe CHI) were tested serially on at least three occasions at 3, 6, 12, 21, 36, and 48 months postinjury. The study design facilitated analysis of CHI severity, age at injury, and the contribution of focal brain lesions to verbal fluency.

Table 11-2. Summary of Mean Raw Scores on Word Fluency Test by the Group in a Cross-Sectional Study

	Control (n = 86)		Mild Head Injury (n = 38)		Severe Head Injury (n = 111)	
	Mean	SD	Mean	SD	Mean	SD
Word fluency test						
Total correct	25.99^a	10.07	29.73^b	8.87	20.18^{ab}	9.90
Persev. errors	0.41^a	0.77	0.50	1.08	0.22^a	0.53
Other errors	0.93	1.30	1.03	1.24	12.73	1.89
Nonword errors	0.16	0.53	0.17	0.45	0.24	0.53

Note: Within rows, common superscript letters denote significant ($p \le .05$) pairwise contrasts.

Table 11-3. Demographic and Clinical Features of Head-Injured Groups
in Longitudinal Study

	Mild CHI (n = 44)		Severe CHI (n = 78)			
	Mean	SD	Mean	SD	Statistics	P Value
Age at injury (years)	9.8	2.8	9.6	3.2	F(1,120) = 0.09	0.76
Parental education (years)	14.5	2.5	13.9	2.4	F(1,114) = 1.65	0.20
GCS score	14.6	0.6	5.7	1.8	F(1,120) = 1035.86	0.0001
Gender						
% girls	47		42		$\chi^2(1) = 0.34$	0.56
% boys	53		58			

We conceptualized the GCS score as an index of the severity of diffuse injury, and localization of the lesion on an MRI scan (at least 3 months postinjury) characterized focal brain lesions in severely injured patients. As shown in Table 11-3, the mildly and severely head-injured groups did not differ in demographic features.

Frontal Lobe Effects

In view of the functional imaging and nontraumatic lesion studies demonstrating the contribution of the prefrontal region to verbal fluency and the preponderance of frontal lesions after CHI in children (Levin et al., 1997), we analyzed the effects of left frontal and right frontal lesions in comparison with the effects on other severely injured children who did not have left frontal or right frontal lesions (although lesions in other locations may have been present). Among 122 patients, 18 mildly, and 36 severely head-injured children who completed serial tests of fluency on all four occasions (i.e., at 3, 12, 21, and 36 months postinjury) were included in the analysis of the lesion effect. These subgroups did not differ in demographic features. As shown in Figure 11-2A, children who sustained left frontal lesions produced fewer words at 3 months postinjury than other severely injured children and those with mild CHI. However, the contribution of left frontal lesions to word fluency was diminished by 12 months. In contrast, the effect of right frontal lesions was not significant even at 3 months postinjury compared to the effect when severe head injury was not complicated by a right frontal lesion (Fig. 11-2B).

Analysis of the Process of Change Using Growth Curves

To analyze the process of change over the 3-year follow-up period, we used individual growth curves that modeled the intraindividual rate of change over serial assessments. This analysis of the process of change (Francis et al., 1991) was facilitated by the multiple time points of measurement and the sensitivity of the verbal fluency test to change. Severity of injury (GCS score) was an independent variable, and age at injury and the postinjury interval were covariates in this analysis. We postulated that severe diffuse axonal injury, as indexed by the GCS score,

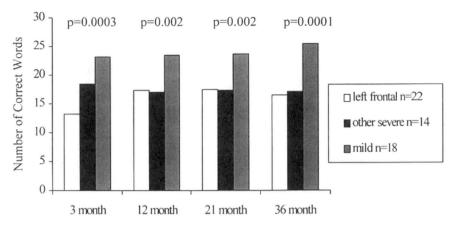

Figure 11-2A. Histogram depicting the left frontal lesion effect on word fluency plotted over serial follow-up intervals. The presence of a left frontal lesion contributed to impaired word fluency at 3 months postinjury compared to the performance of other severely injured children without left frontal lesions, but this effect resolved by 12 months. *P* values at 3 months: 0.0001 (left vs. mild), 0.03 (left vs. other severe), and 0.05 (other severe vs. mild).

occurring in early childhood would disrupt development of white matter connections to a greater extent than a similar injury sustained in late childhood or adolescence. In contrast, the effects of a mild head injury were postulated to be subtle and transient irrespective of the age at injury.

Figure 11-3 plots the growth curves of 122 CHI patients for the number of correct words according to age at injury and severity of injury. For the groups who

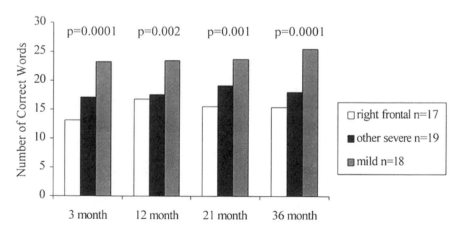

Figure 11-2B. Histogram depicting the effect of right frontal lesions in children sustaining severe CHI. There was no significant effect of right frontal lesions relative to the finding obtained in severely brain-injured children with no right frontal lesion. *P* values at 3 and 31 months: 0.08 and 0.12 (right vs. other severe).

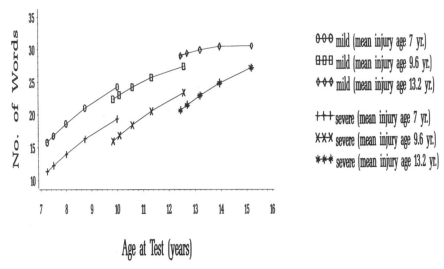

Age at Test (years)

Figure 11-3. Mean number of words recalled by 122 children with mild and severe CHI children three age-at-injury groups. The process of change analysis revealed a significant three-way interaction among CHI severity, age at injury, and postinjury interval, $F(1,270)$ = 4.86, p = .03, indicating a slower recovery of word fluency for younger children with severe CHI. The growth curves in this figure show that younger children with severe CHI made less postinjury improvement than younger children with mild CHI children and older children with severe CHI. Three main effects were significant: CHI severity: $F(1,270)$ = 20.46, p = .0001; interval: $F(1,118)$ = 27.71, p = .0001; and age at injury: $F(1,270)$ = 80.69, p = .0001

sustained their head injury in late childhood or adolescence, the trajectories for verbal fluency in severely injured children are diminished relative to those of the mildly injured groups. The curves converge for the groups who sustained their head trauma during adolescence. In contrast, the word fluency growth curves for children who had severe injuries at the youngest age did not follow this pattern. The gap in word fluency between the youngest patients with mild and severe CHI persisted throughout the 3-year follow-up period. Consistent with the slower recovery from severe CHI depicted for young children in Figure 11-3, we found a triple interaction of injury severity, age at injury, and postinjury interval. The main effects for injury severity, postinjury interval, and age at injury were also significant.

To summarize, analysis of the growth curves for verbal fluency indicates that development of word fluency is impaired to a greater degree when severe injury occurs in young children relative than when it occurs in older children. Although word generation improves and continues to develop across the injury severity and age spectrums, the persistence of deficit after severe CHI contrasts with resolution of the left frontal lesion effect.

Implications for Reorganization of Function

The transient effect of a left frontal lesion on word fluency could be explained on the basis of reorganization of function, but it is also conceivable that viability of some tissue at the site of the contusion or hematoma is sufficient to support development. Functional brain imaging, particularly fMRI, could examine the neural mechanisms involved in recovery of function (Buckner et al., 1996). Transfer of word generation to homotopic regions of the right hemisphere would produce right frontal activation during testing, whereas increased participation by adjacent left anterior structures would potentially shift the site of activation while preserving asymmetric left hemisphere activation. Chronometric measures, such as magneto-encephalography, could be useful in characterizing slowing of word generation at various intrahemispheric sites that might also reflect the effects of reduced corticocortical connectivity.

In summary, our findings for recovery and development of verbal fluency indicate that severe diffuse brain insult has more devastating effects than focal frontal lesions. Although the effects of left frontal lesions in young children are compatible (albeit more transient) with observations in adults with corresponding lesion sites, the consequences of severe diffuse brain injury appear to be comparable or worse in young children. The growth curve analysis of word fluency produced a pattern of findings that concurs with the findings of a study by our group (Thompson et al., 1994) indicating that sensorimotor skills are more impaired in young children following severe CHI than in older children sustaining comparable injuries. Further research is necessary to determine the extrapolation of these findings to other domains of neurobehavioral development after early brain injury.

ACKNOWLEDGMENTS
Preparation of this chapter was supported by grant NS-21889 from the NIH/NINDS. We are indebted to Gilda Warren and Angela Williams for their assistance with word processing and editing.

References

Adams, J.H., Graham, D.I., Scott, G., Parker, L.S., and Doyle, D. (1980) Brain damage in fatal non-missile head injury. Journal of Clinical Pathology 33:1132–1145.

Aram, D.M., Meyers, S.C., and Ekelman, B.L. (1990) Fluency of conversational speech in children with unilateral brain lesions. *Brain and Language,* 38:105–121.

Bates, E., Thal, D., Trauner, D., Fenson, J., Aram, D., Eisele, J., and Nass, R. (1997) From first words to grammar in children with focal brain injury. *Developmental Neuropsychology,* 13:275–344.

Benton, A.L. (1968) Differential behavioral effects in frontal lobe disease. *Neuropsychologia,* 6:53–60.

Benton, A.L., Hamsher, K., and Sivan, A.B. (1993) *Manual for the Multilingual Aphasia Examination,* 3rd ed. Iowa City, IA: AJA Associates.

Buckner, R.L., Corbetta, M., Schatz, J., Raichle, M.E., and Petersen, S.E. (1996) Preserved speech abilities and compensation following prefrontal damage. *Proceedings of the National Academy of Sciences of the USA,* 93:1249–1253.

Carlsson, G., and Hugdahl, K. (1998) Cerebral reorganization in children with congenital hemiplegia: Evidence from Dichotic Listening Test. In H.S. Levin and J. Grafman (eds.) *Cerebral Reorganization of Function after Brain Injury.* New York: Oxford University Press, pp.

Chugani, H.T. (1997) Developmental brain plasticity studied with positron emission tomography. Presented at the Seventh International Symposium on Neural Regeneration, Asilomar Conference Center, Pacific Grove, CA.

Chugani, H.T., Phelps, M.E., and Mazziotta, J.C. (1987) Positron emission tomography study of human brain functional development. *Annals of Neurology,* 22:487–497.

Ewing-Cobbs, L., Levin, H.S., Eisenberg, H.M., and Fletcher, J.M. (1987) Language functions following closed-head injury in children and adolescents. *Journal of Clinical and Experimental Neuropsychology,* 9:575–592.

Feldman, H.M., Holland, A.L., Kemp, S.S., and Janosky, J.E. (1992) Language development after unilateral brain injury. *Brain and Language,* 42:89–102.

Francis, D.J., Fletcher, J.M., Stuebing, K.K., Davidson, K.C., and Thompson, N.M. (1991) Analysis of change: Modeling individual growth. *Journal of Consulting and Clinical Psychology,* 59:27–37.

Kraus, J.F., Rock, A., and Hemyari, P. (1990) Brain injuries among infants, children, adolescents, and young adults. *American Journal of Diseases of Children,* 144:684–691.

Levin, H.S., Culhane, K.A., Hartmann, J., Evankovich, D., Mattson, A.J., Harward, H., Ringholz, G., Ewing-Cobbs, L., and Fletcher J.M. (1991) Developmental changes in performances on tests of purported frontal lobe functioning. *Developmental Neuropsychology,* 7:377–395.

Levin, H.S., Gary, H.E., Jr., and Eisenberg, H.M. (1989) NIH Traumatic Coma Data Bank Research Group: Duration of impaired consciousness in relation to lateralization of intracerebral lesion after severe head injury. *Lancet,* 1:1001–1003.

Levin, H.S., Grossman, R.G., and Kelly, P.J. (1976) Aphasia disorder in patients with closed head injury. *Journal of Neurology, Neurosurgery, and Psychiatry,* 39:1062–1070.

Levin H.S., Mendelsohn, D., Lilly, M.A., Yeakley, J., Song, J, Scheibel, R.S., Harward, H, Fletcher, J.H., Kufera, JA, Davidson, KC, Bruce, D (1997) Magnetic resonance imaging in relation to functional outcome of pediatric closed head injury: A test of the OMMAYA-Gennarellimodel-Neurosurgery 40:432–441.

Levin, H.S., Scheller, J., Rickard, T., Grafman, J., Martinkowski, K., Winslow, M., and Mirvis, S. (1996) Dyscalculia and dyslexia after right hemisphere injury in infancy. *Archives of Neurology,* 53:88–96.

McIntosh, T.K., Smith, D.H., Meaney, D.F., Kotapka, M.J., Gennarelli, T.A., and Graham, D.I. (1996) Neuropathological sequelae of traumatic brain injury: Relationship to neurochemical and biochemical mechanisms. *Laboratory Investigation,* 74:315–342.

Papanicolaou, A.C., Moore, B.D., Deutsch, G., Levin, H.S., and Eisenberg, H.M. (1988) Evidence for right-hemisphere involvement in recovery from aphasia. *Archives of Neurology,* 45:1025–1029.

Phelps, E.A., Hyder, F., Blamire, A.M., and Shulman, R.G. (1997) fMRI of the prefrontal cortex during overt verbal fluency. *NeuroReport* 8:561–565.

Satz, P., Strauss, E., Hunter, M., and Wada, J. (1994) Re-examination of the crowding hypothesis: Effects of age at onset. *Neuropsychology,* 8:255–262.

Simpson, D.A., Cockington, R.A., Hanieh, A., Raftos, J., and Reilly, P.L. (1991) Head injuries in infants and young children: The value of the Paediatric Coma Scale: Review of the literature and report on a study. *Child's Nervous System,* 7:183–190.

Stiles, J., Stern, C., Trauner, D., and Nass, R. (1996) Developmental change in spatial grouping activity among children with early focal brain injury: Evidence from a modeling
task. *Brain and Cognition,* 31:46–62.

Strauss, E., Satz, P., and Wada, J. (1990) An examination of the crowding hypothesis in
epileptic patients who have undergone the carotid amytal test. *Neuropsychologia,* 28:
1221–1227.

Teasdale, G., and Jennett, B. (1974) Assessment of coma and impaired consciousness: A
practical scale. *Lancet,* 2:81–84.

Teuber, H.L. (1974) Why two brains? In F.O. Schmitt and F.G. Worden (eds.), *The Neurosciences: Third Study Program.* Cambridge, MA: MIT Press, pp. 71–74.

Thal, D.J., Marchman, V., Stiles, J., Aram, D., Trauner, D., Nass, R., and Bates, E. (1991)
Early lexical development in children with focal brain injury. *Brain and Language,* 40:
491–527.

Thompson, N.M., Francis, D.J., Stuebing, K.K., Fletcher, J.M., Ewing-Cobbs, L., Miner,
M.E., Levin, H.S., and Eisenberg, H. (1994) Motor, visual-spatial, and somatosensory
skills after traumatic brain injury in children and adolescents: A study of change. *Neuropsychology,* 8:333–342.

Weiller, C., Isensee, C., Rijntijes, M., Huber, W., Muller, S., Bier, D., Dutschka, K., Woods,
R.P., Noth, J., and Diener, H.C. (1995) Recovery from Wernicke's aphasia: A positron
emission tomographic study. *Annals of Neurology,* 37:723–732.

Woods, B.T. (1980) The restricted effects of right-hemisphere lesions after age one: Wechsler
test data. *Neuropsychologia,* 18:65–70.

Woods, B.T. and Carey, S. Language deficits after apparent clinical recovery from childhood
aphasia. *Ann Neurol,* 1979 6:405–409.

Warburton, E., Price, C.J., Swinburn, K., Wise, R.J. Mechanisms of recovery from aphasia:
evidence from positron emission tomography studies. *J Neurol Neurosurg Psychiatry,*
1999 66:155–161.

12

Cerebral Reorganization in Children with Congenital Hemiplegia: Evidence from the Dichotic Listening Test

GÖRAN CARLSSON AND KENNETH HUGDAHL

The best evidence of cerebral reorganization in humans includes the amazingly well-spared language functions after early left-sided brain lesions. Although clinical and experimental studies have revealed that language functions are lateralized to the left hemisphere and nonverbal, visuospatial functions are controlled by the right hemisphere (Bogen, 1969, 1985; Rasmussen & Milner, 1977; Sperry, 1974), language functions may shift to the right intact hemisphere after an early left-sided brain lesion (e.g., Milner, 1974). It has been confirmed that language functions are generally spared in cases of early unilateral brain lesions regardless of the cause or location of the lesion (Aram & Eisele, 1992; Dennis & Whitaker, 1977). However, nonverbal functions are generally impaired regardless of the location of the lesion (LeVere et al., 1988; Nass et al., 1989).

The new language areas may perform the same function as the damaged areas, although not necessarily in the same manner (Chelune & Edwards, 1981). Reorganization of language functions may not be complete, but rather may leave qualitative linguistic deficits, that is delayed acquisition of syntactic awareness (Dennis & Whitaker, 1976) or selective problems in the rate, strategy, and mastery of discrete language functions (Dennis, 1980a, 1980b; Dennis & Kohn, 1975).

The acquisition of language functions by the intact right hemisphere may also interfere with nonverbal functions in this hemisphere through the "crowding effect" (Nass et al., 1989; Rasmussen & Milner, 1977; Satz, et al., 1994; Strauss, et al., 1990; Teuber, 1974, 1975). This effect is restricted largely to nonverbal, nonlinguistic ability. It occurs in right hemisphere speech dominance only after early left hemisphere lesions (Satz et al., 1994), probably because language functions develop earlier than nonverbal functions and thus seem to occupy the intact hemisphere first and deny the later-developing nonverbal functions access to these areas (Teuber, 1975). This may explain the preserved linguistic skills and impaired nonverbal functions in children with congenital hemiplegia (Carlsson, 1994).

By contrast, right hemisphere lesions at any age consistently impair performance IQ and nonverbal functions (Glos & Pavlovkin, 1985; Glos et al., 1987; Ichiba, 1991; Levine et al., 1987; Nass et al., 1989; Riva et al., 1989). This is in accordance with lateralized nonverbal functions in the right hemisphere.

Recovery of cognitive functions after brain injury depends on a variety of factors, such as stage of brain maturity when the damage occurred, lesion size, lesion location, and gender differences. The broad variations in the literature regarding the critical periods for language acquisition (about 1 to 8 years) after early unilateral brain damage may be due to the heterogeneity of the groups studied in terms of lesion location, bilateral brain involvement, and the presence of confounding impairments (e.g., seizures), among other factors.

Cerebral Dominance

Knowing a patient's hemispheric speech dominance is considered a prerequisite for drawing a reliable conclusion as to which hemisphere is impaired and for understanding mechanisms behind the reorganization of cognitive functions (Satz et al., 1994). Speech and handedness are the two best-known examples of cerebral dominance. The universality and specificity of right-handedness in all human cultures imply that there must be a biologically based explanation for these phenomena (Annett, 1985; McManus & Bryden, 1992).

Pathological Handedness and Speech Lateralization

According to the concept of *pathological handedness* (Satz, 1972, 1973; Satz et al., 1985b), there should be an increased incidence of left-handedness in children with early brain damage to the left hemisphere. A left hemisphere lesion causes a shift in hand preference in otherwise genotypic right-handers, thus increasing the overall percentage of left-handers in these children. Children with hemiplegia, that is, lost or impaired motor function on the right or left side of the body due to prenatal or perinatal damage to either the left or right cerebral hemisphere, should be particularly prone to pathological handedness (Hiscock & Hiscock, 1990; Orsini, 1984). This should imply not only the well-known phenomenon of proneness to pathological left-handedness, but also the possible existence of an over representation of pathological right-handedness.

If early left hemisphere damage causes a shift in handedness, it should also affect hemispheric language control, with a shift to the other hemisphere. This can be predicted from studies using the intracarotid sodium amytal test (Rasmussen &

Milner, 1977) which show that brain lesions producing a shift in handedness also affect hemispheric language control. Furthermore, Dennis and Whitaker (1976) have shown that left hemispherectomies in the first year of life do not lead to obvious aphasia in right-handed children. It should be noted, however, that not all cases of early left brain injury lead to a shift in language function, as pointed out by Satz et al. (1988).

In general, the probability of speech representation in the intact hemisphere is high, especially when the lateral preference changes (Rasmussen & Milner, 1977).

Dichotic Listening

The dichotic listening technique is probably the most frequently used experimental method to assess lateralization of language function (Bryden, 1988; Hugdahl, 1995). Dichotic listening for consonant-vowel (CV) presentations has the unique ability to probe one hemisphere directly and to inhibit or block the other hemisphere simultaneously (Kimura, 1967).

Dichotic listening involves listening to two simultaneously presented sounds, one in each ear. The stimulus materials used consist of six CV syllables, for example /ba/, /ta/, and /ka/, presented through earphones, so that /ba/, for example, can be heard through the right earphone and /ta/ simultaneously through the left one. The subject is instructed to report immediately what he or she hears.

Subjects with lateralization of language to the left hemisphere are faster and more accurate in reporting items that are presented to the right ear. This right-ear advantage (REA) in normal individuals has often been taken as evidence of left hemisphere language dominance. Conversely, subjects showing a left ear advantage (LEA) for verbal material are assumed to have right hemisphere language dominance (see Bryden, 1988, and Hugdahl, 1995, for reviews).

Most studies have been performed with either dichotic words or digits presented in sequence or with fused words (Wexler & Halwes, 1983; Zatorre, 1989). A second characteristic of dichotic listening (DL) validation studies is that they typically have been conducted in adult patient populations.

The CV syllables are consistently found to produce the most robust right-ear advantages in right-handed individuals (Hugdahl & Andersson, 1984; Shankweiler & Studdert-Kennedy, 1967; Studdert-Kennedy & Shankweiler, 1970). The validity of CV syllables in revealing lateralization of speech was believed to be about 0.8 for adults with the intracarotid amobarbital procedure (Strauss, 1988). The perception of CV syllables is also dependent on the functional integrity of the contralateral temporal (Kimura, 1961) and frontal lobes, including the basal ganglia (Eslinger & Damasio, 1988).

Hugdahl and his group recently also validated the CV syllable technique against position emission tomography (PET) blood flow measurements (Hugdahl et al., 1999. The perception of CV syllables increased cortical blood flow in the superior temporal gyrus, particularly on the left side.

Dichotic Listening and the Wada Test

The dichotic listening (DL) test we used was validated against the gold standard, the Wada test, an invasive test in which phenobarbital is injected into the carotid artery, the so-called intracarotid amobarbital procedure (IAP). The Wada test is typically used to evaluate speech dominance before surgery for epilepsy. Our variation on the Wada test was similar to that used at the Montreal Neurological Institute, Canada, and at the Sahlgren University Hospital, Göteborg, Sweden, when adult patients were tested (Malmgren et al., 1992). However, in a few cases, our procedure had to be adapted because children were tested.

Thirteen children and adolescents between 10 and 19 years of age with partial seizures were assessed with the DL test and the Wada test. A catheter was placed into the carotid artery via the femoral artery. Angiography was used to make sure that the arterial blood flow was unilaterally distributed and to determine to what extent overflow occurred from one hemisphere to the other. Electroencephalography (EEG) was performed to ensure that the injected hemisphere was sedated and to determine to what extent seizure activity was present in the awake hemisphere.

Ten of the subjects were left hemisphere dominant for language, as determined by the Wada test (Wada, 1949; Wada & Rasmussen, 1960), and three subjects were right hemisphere dominant. All ten of the left hemisphere dominant subjects were right-handed, and the three right hemisphere dominant subjects were left-handed. There was a significant REA in the left hemisphere dominant group (Tukey's LSD: $p < .03$ and a correspondingly significant LEA in the right hemisphere dominant group (Tukey's LSD: $p < .003$).

As can be seen in the scatterplots (Fig. 12-1) of individual data split for the right and left hemisphere dominant groups in the preoperative test, the dichotic listening data mimics the amobarbital data quite well. The plots in Figure 12-1a, b are called a *response space* (Hugdahl, 1995) based on the responses from both the right and left ears. Note the 45°-symmetry line that divides the response-space into an REA half and an LEA half.

Each circle in the scatterplots represents an individual subject. As Figure 12-1b shows, all three right hemisphere dominant subjects displayed on LEA both pre- and post-operatively. Of the ten subjects with left hemisphere dominance, eight showed an REA, one showed an LEA, and one subject showed no ear advantage (NEA) preoperatively.

We concluded that the DL CV syllables method is fairly robust with regard to speech dominance, as determined by the intracarotid amobarbital procedure in an adolescent sample (Hugdahl et al. 1997). However, the overall percentage of correct classifications for left and right hemisphere dominant subjects was only 92%; thus caution is necessary when using the DL method in clinical practice since 8% of all subjects still were not correctly classified.

Dichotic Listening in Monozygotic Twins

The validity of DL in determining speech lateralization can also be illustrated by the study of monozygotic twin pair with congenital hemiplegia, one right-sided

(A)

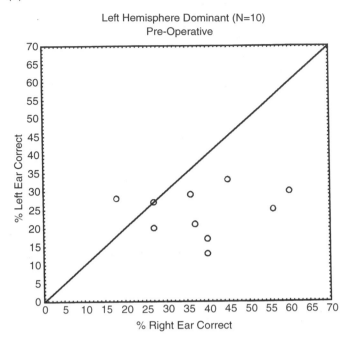

Left Hemisphere Dominant (N=10)
Pre-Operative

(B)

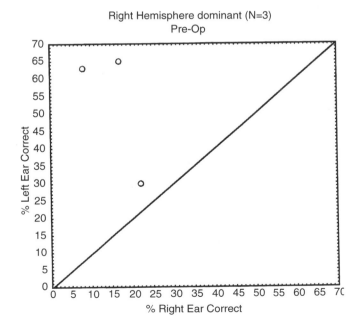

Right Hemisphere dominant (N=3)
Pre-Op

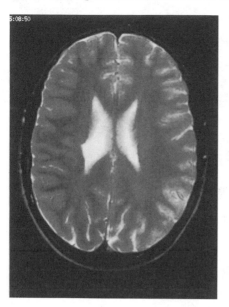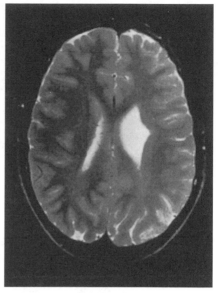

Figure 12-2. Magnetic resonance imaging scans of the two twins showing the lesions in the periventricular areas. Note that the left side is on the right in the figures, and vice versa, according to standard neurological imaging conventions.

and the other left-sided (Hugdahl & Carlsson, 1996). Monozygotism was demonstrated by conventional markers including a DNA analysis. Magnetic resonance imaging (MRI) revealed identical lesions (in size and onset) between the twin brothers. However, one twin retained a lesion in the left hemisphere and the other twin a corresponding lesion in the right hemisphere (Fig. 12-2). Thus, the brothers represented two highly comparable cases without seizures or mental retardation.

The two brothers were assessed with a DL (CV) test. As can be seen in Figure 12-3, the left hemisphere–impaired (LHI) twin preferred the left ear. This boy could not modulate his LEA by focusing attention on the right ear. In addition, he preferred his left hand and left foot.

The right hemisphere–impaired (RHI) twin showed a mirror-reversed picture. He preferred the right ear (i.e., REA) and could not modulate this ear advantage by focusing his attention on the left ear. He also preferred his right hand and right foot. The DL results and lateral preferences showed a clear discrepancy between the two twins, which implies speech lateralization in the intact hemisphere (Hugdahl & Carlsson, 1994). This is in line with previous group data (Carlsson et al., 1992;

Figure 12-1. Scatterplots of DL results showing the individual data. Each point represents one of the 13 subjects in the study. The diagonal line is the 45° "no ear advantage" (NEA) symmetry line. (A) Findings in the left hemisphere speech dominant subjects (n = 10). (B) Findings in the right hemisphere speech dominant subjects (n = 3).

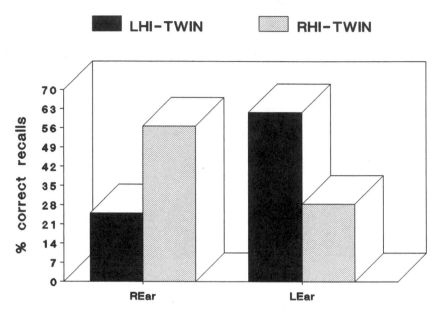

Figure 12-3. Dichotic listening results for the right (REar) and left (LEar) ear input and for the left (LHI) and right (RHI) twins.

Korkman & von Wendt, 1995) in that the RHI children were right-handed, right-footed, and right-eyed. Left hemisphere–impaired children, by contrast, were left-handed and left-footed and preferred the left eye.

Cerebral Reorganization of Language in Children with Congenital Hemiplegia

Many neuropsychological studies of children with unilateral brain lesions have been published but only a few studies of well-defined early unilateral brain lesions in children without, for example, seizures (Aram & Eisele, 1992) have been carried out. Our clinical and experimental neuropsychological approach was chosen to describe and understand the cognitive impairments in hemiplegic children. Well-defined unilateral lesions were used to comprehend the neurobiological mechanisms behind the cognitive impairments. This approach also provided the opportunity to study functional or behavioral plasticity, that is, how the brain (re)organizes cognitive functions after an early injury. However, to determine specific effects of unilateral brain lesions, it is crucial to select two homogeneous groups with congenital hemiplegia of pre- or perinatal origin, one group with a left-sided and the other with a right-sided brain lesion.

Population-based findings in children with congenital hemiplegia are very heterogeneous. In one such study of 194 patients (Uvebrant, 1988), from which the main part of our sample was selected, there were several associated impairments among the subjects, often occurring in combination. Large brain lesions and severe motor and sensory impairments were associated with epilepsy, language impediments, hearing and visual deficits, and mental retardation.

Children with exclusively unilateral brain lesions of pre- and perinatal origin who had slight to moderate hemiparesis were included in our study, without the confounding effects of mental retardation, epilepsy, and visual and hearing impairments. A population of 2–3 million inhabitants was required to gather the sample of 31 children included in our study.

The LHI group consisted of 18 children with right-sided hemiplegia, and the RHI group consisted of 13 children with left-sided hemiplegia. The hemiplegia was classified as slight to moderate in both groups. A sex- and age-matched control group of 19 children (10–16 years old) without known brain impairments was selected.

Lateral Preferences

In Carlsson's (1994) study, 16 subjects (84%) in the control group were right-handers, as were 13 (100%) of the RHI subjects. However, only two (11%) of the LHI subjects were right-handed. The difference was statistically significant ($p < .05$) when the chi-square test was used. The same trend was seen for footedness, with 84% and 100% of right-foot preference for the normal controls and RHI subjects, respectively, but 0% for the LHI subjects. The difference between the hemiplegic groups was statistically significant. Thus, about 15% of the subjects in the control group were left-handed and left-footed. This was in clear contrast to the children with hemiplegia. None of these children were left-handed or left-footed in the RHI group, but as many as about 89% were left-handed and 100% were left-footed in the LHI group.

Dichotic Listening Performance in Children
with Congenital Hemiplegia

The DL (CV) test was used to disclose speech dominance. The DL measures revealed superiority for the ear contralateral to the intact hemisphere. That is, the LHI children preferred the left ear, and the RHI children preferred the right ear. The control group also preferred the right ear.

In Figure 12-4 the individual results in the LHI group are shown. Every circle represent a subject. The majority of the LHI children (78%) showed a LEA and were considered to have a right hemisphere dominance for speech, while the majority of the RHI children (69%) and normal controls (68%) displayed a REA indicating a left hemisphere dominance for speech. These findings are corroborated by those of other studies in congenital hemiplegia (Korkman & von Wendt, 1995; Nass et al., 1992).

(A)

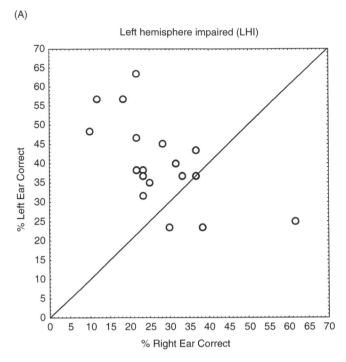

(B)

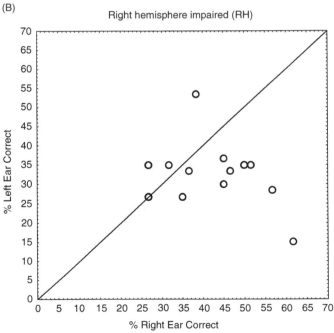

Figure 12-4. Frequency distribution of subjects with REA and LEA for the (LHI) group (A), the RHI group (B), and the NC group (C). *(Continued)*

240

(C)

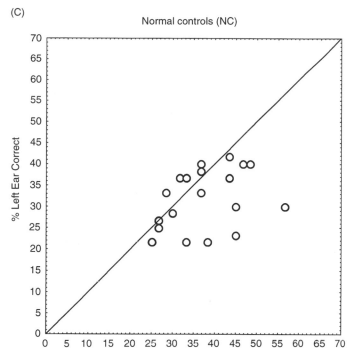

Figure 12-4. (*Continued*)

Thus, the DL data showed a large difference between the LHI group and the RHI and normal controls in terms of both magnitude and direction of ear advantage. This difference was not due to a hearing impairment because all subjects had normal audiometry (see the inclusion criteria). This does not mean that hemispheric speech dominance was correctly identified in all cases. Since no Wada test was employed, subjects with bilateral speech could not be entirely ruled out.

Cognitive Consequences of Language Reorganization

Most of the hemiplegic children we studied seemed to allocate speech and language functions to the intact hemisphere, as indicated by lateral preferences and DL performances. With regard to the cognitive consequences of the reallocation of language functions in children with left-sided brain lesions, the development of verbal and nonverbal functions provided some additional information about the mechanisms behind the reorganization of cognitive functions. The LHI group showed preserved speech but with deficient verbal function compared with the RHI group and normal controls (Carlsson et al., 1994).

Interestingly, the whole difference represented inadequate verbal quality of performance by the girls in the LHI group. The boys in the LHI group showed average verbal functions and the girls impaired verbal functions. There may be indirect evidence for the assumption that girls are more "committed" to process language in the left hemisphere (cf. Bishop, 1981; Strauss et al., 1990) because girls were less impaired in nonverbal functions than LHI boys, implying more sparing of nonverbal functions and less crowding of right hemisphere functions.

Furthermore, both hemiplegic groups showed impaired nonverbal functions compared with the normal controls (Carlsson et al., 1994). These findings are corroborated by a large body of empirical evidence from children with both right- and left-sided hemiplegia (Glos & Pavlovkin, 1985; Aram & Ekelman, 1986; Riva & Cazzaniga, 1986; Levine et al., 1987; Nass et al., 1989; Banich et al., 1990). Thus there are considerable similarities in nonverbal impairments between children and adults with right hemisphere lesions, whereas LHI children differ from adults with respect to their relatively preserved verbal functions and impaired nonverbal functions. We argue that the impaired nonverbal functions were caused by (1) a primary lesion in the right hemisphere (RHI), which interferes with the presumably preprogrammed right hemisphere nonverbal functions, and (2) a relocation of verbal functions after a left-sided brain lesion (LHI) was presumed to "crowd" the nonverbal functions of the right hemisphere. Concerning the first point: in the RHI group the nonverbal functions were considered impaired due to a primary lesion in the right hemisphere because these functions cannot effectively be retained in the impaired hemisphere or relocated to the intact left hemisphere since the left hemisphere is already committed to language functions. The intact left hemisphere, although capable of basic visuospatial perception, may not contribute significantly to complex visuospatial and visuoconstructive functions. Concerning the second point: language functions seem to have priority in cognitive development, perhaps because they develop earlier than nonverbal functions and thereby deny the nonverbal functions full access to the same regions. This idea is in line with the "crowding hypothesis" (Satz et al., 1990, 1994; Strauss et al., 1990; Teuber, 1974).

Conclusion

The DL test was used to determine speech dominance in children with early unilateral brain injuries. The validity of this test is high, but predictions of hemispheric dominance were substantially improved when DL performances were combined with lateral preferences and the cognitive outcome in children with well-defined, homogeneous unilateral brain lesions. However, handedness and the DL findings do not convincingly disclose speech lateralization in every single case, presumably because the DL test does not identify individuals with bilateral speech.

Without access to well-defined, homogeneous groups with unilateral brain lesions (site, size, and onset) and knowledge of hemispheric speech dominance, it is hard to draw valid conclusions about cerebral reorganization of cognitive functions after early brain lesions. Insufficient knowledge about speech dominance may obscure the consequences of unilateral brain lesions in childhood.

Neuropsychological studies of children with congenital hemiplegia support the general observation that there is a remarkable preservation of verbal skills after lesions in the immature brain. However, this may reflect sparing and compensation of a cognitive function rather than recovery of an initially deficient function (Chelune & Edwards, 1981). Language functions are believed to be spared in children with RHI. In children with LHI, language functions may be compensated for by inter- or intrahemispheric reorganization due to functional plasticity. Thus, the new language areas may perform the same functions as the damaged areas, although not necessarily in the same manner.

The reallocation of language functions seems to be most efficient after early lesions, but this reorganization may cause at least as much impairment of nonverbal functions as a primary lesion in the right hemisphere due to the "crowding effect."

Right-sided brain-injured children revealed impairments in nonverbal functions corresponding to the impairments found in children with left-sided lesions, which may imply that nonverbal functions are neither spared nor relocated.

Thus, even under the most favorable conditions of early unilateral brain lesions in childhood (i.e., without associated impairments), functional plasticity appears to be of limited advantage to the individual with regard to total cognitive capacities (LeVere et al., 1988; Norsell, 1988). It appears that there are serious restrictions on cerebral reorganization even after early unilateral brain lesions, as in congenitally hemiplegic children.

ACKNOWLEDGMENT

We want to thank our collaborators in this research: Paul Uvebrant, and L.-M. Wiklund, Department of Pediatrics, Sahlgren, University Hospital of Göteborg, and Jan Arvidsson, Ryhov Hospital, Jönköping, Sweden

References

Annett, M. (1985) *Left, Right, Hand and Brain: The Right Shift Theory.* London: Erlbaum.

Aram, D.M., and Eisele, J.A. (1992) Plasticity and recovery of higher cognitive functions following early brain injury. In I. Rapin and S.J. Segalowitz (eds.), *Handbook of Neuropsychology,* Vol. 6. Amsterdam: Elsevier, pp. 73–92.

Aram, D.M., and Ekelman, B.L. (1986) Cognitive profiles of children with early onset of unilateral lesions. *Developmental Neuropsychology,* 2:155–172.

Banich, M.T., Levine, S.C., Kim, H., and Huttenlocher, P. (1990) The effects of developmental factors on IQ in hemiplegic children. *Neuropsychologia,* 28:35–47.

Bishop, D.V.M. (1981) Plasticity and specificity of language localization in the developing brain. *Developmental Medicine and Child Neurology,* 23:251–255.

Bishop, D.V.M. (1990) *Handedness and Developmental Disorder.* Philadelphia: J.B. Lippinicott.

Bogen, J.E. (1969) The other side of the brain II: An appositional mind. *Bulletin of the Los Angeles Neurological Societies,* 3:135–162.

Bogen, J.E. (1985) The callosal syndromes. In K.M. Heilman and E. Valenstein (eds.), *Clinical Neuropsychology.* New York: Oxford University Press, pp. 295–322.

Bryden, M.P. (1988) An overview of the dichotic listening procedure and its relation to cerebral organization. In K. Hugdahl (ed.), *Handbook of Dichotic Listening: Theory, methods, and research.* Chichester, UK: Wiley, pp. 1–43.

Carlsson, G. (1994) *Children with Hemiplegic Cerebral Palsy: Neuropsychological Consequences of Early Unilateral Brain Lesions.* Göteborg: Academic Dissertation, pp. 1–148.

Carlsson, G., Hugdahl, K., Uvebrant, P., Wiklund, L.-M., and von Wendt, L. (1992) Pathological left-handedness revisited: Dichotic listening in children with left vs. right congenital hemiplegia. *Neuropsychologia,* 30:471–481.

Carlsson, G., Uvebrant, P., Hugdahl, K., Wiklund, L.-M., Arvidsson, J., and von Wendt, L.
(1994) Verbal and non-verbal function of children with right- versus left-hemiplegic
cerebral palsy of pre- or perinatal origin. *Developmental Medicine and Child Neurology,* 36:503–512.

Chelune, G.J., and Edwards, P. (1981) Early brain lesions: Ontogenetic environmental and
considerations. *Journal of Consulting and Clinical Psychology,* 49:777–790.

Dennis, M. (1980a) Language acquisition in a single hemisphere: Semantic organization.
In D. Caplan (ed.), *Biological Studies of Mental Processes.* Cambridge, MA: MIT Press,
pp. 159–185.

Dennis, M. (1980b) Capacity and strategy for syntactic comprehension after left or right
hemidecortication. *Brain and Language,* 10:287–317.

Dennis, M., and Kohn, B. (1975) Comprehension of syntax in infantile hemiplegics after
cerebral hemidecortication. Left hemisphere superiority. *Brain and Language,* 2:472–
482.

Dennis, M., and Whitaker, H.A. (1976) Language acquisition following hemidecortication:
Linguistic superiority of the left over the right hemisphere. *Brain and Language,* 3:404–
433.

Dennis, M., and Whitaker, H.A. (1977) Hemispheric equipotentiality and language acquisition. In S.J. Segalowitz and F.A. Gruber (eds.), *Language Development and Neurological Theory.* New York: Academic Press, pp. 93–106.

Eslinger, P.J., and Damasio, H. (1988) Anatomical correlates of paradoxic ear extinction.
In K. Hugdahl (ed.), *Handbook of Dichotic Listening: Theory, Methods and Research.*
Chichester, UK: Wiley, pp. 139–160.

Glos, J., and Pavlovkin, M. (1985) Profile of intellectual achievements in the WISC of
children with hemiplegic form of cerebral palsy. *Studia Psychologica,* 27:37–46.

Glos, J., Pavlovkin, M., Dianiskova, O., Javorova, J., and et, al. (1987) Intellectual performance of hemiplegic children with cerebral palsy in WISC. *Psychologia a Patopsy-
chologia Dietata,* 22:307–318 (Abstract).

Hiscock, M., and Hiscock, C.K. (1990) Laterality in hemiplegic children: Implications for
the concept of pathological left-handedness. In S. Coren (ed.), *Left-Handedness: Behavioral Implications and Anomalies.* Amsterdam: North-Holland, pp. 131–152.

Hugdahl, K. (1995) Dichotic listening: Probing temporal lobe functional integrity. In
R.J. Davidson and K. Hugdahl (eds.), *Brain Asymmetry.* Cambridge, MA: MIT Press,
pp. 123–156.

Hugdahl, K., and Andersson, L. (1984) A dichotic listening study of differences in cerebral
organization in dextral and sinistral subjects. *Cortex,* 20:135–141.

Hugdahl, K., and Carlsson, G. (1994) Dichotic listening and focused attention in children
with hemiplegic cerebral palsy. *Journal of Clinical and Experimental Neuropsychology,*
16:84–92.

Hugdahl K., and Carlsson G. (1996) Dichotic Listening Performance in a Monozygotic
Twin-pair with Left-and Right-sided Hemiplegia. *Neurocase,* 2:141–147.

Hugdahl, K., Bronnick, K., Kyllingbaeck, S., Law, I., Gade, A., and Paulson, O.B. (1999)
Brain activation during presentations of consonant-vowel and musical instruments stimuli: A^{5}O-PET study, *Neuropsychologia,* 37, 431–440.

Hugdahl, K., Carlsson, G., Uvebrant, P., and Lundervold, A.J. (1997) Dichotic listening performance and intracarotid amobarbital injections in children/adolescents: Comparisons pre- and post-operatively. *Archives of Neurology,* 54:7494–1500

Ichiba, N. (1991) A study of functional plasticity of the brain in childhood. I. Critical period dislodging lateralization of language in the brain. *No To Hattatsu,* 23:548–554 (Abstract).

Kimura, D. (1961) Some effects of temporal-lobe damage on auditory perception. *Canadian Journal of Psychology,* 15:156–165.

Kimura, D. (1967) Functional asymmetry of the brain in dichotic listening. *Cortex,* 3:163–168.

Korkman, M., and von Wendt, L. (1995) Evidence of altered dominance in children with congenital spastic hemiplegia. *Journal of the International Neuropsychological Society,* 1:261–270.

LeVere, N.D., Gray-Silva, S., and LeVere, T.E. (1988) Infant brain injury: The benefit of relocation and the cost of crowding. In S. Finger, T.E. LeVere, C.R. Almli, and D.G. Stein (eds.), *Brain Injury and Recovery—Theoretical and Controversial Issues.* New York: Plenum Press, pp. 133–150.

Levine, S.C., Huttenlocher, P., Banich, M.T., and Duda, E. (1987) Factors affecting cognitive functioning of hemiplegic children. *Developmental Medicine and Child Neurology,* 29:27–35.

Malmgren, K., Bilting, M., Hagberg, I., Hedström, A., Silfvenius, H., and Starmark, J.E. (1992) A compound score for estimating the influence of inattention and somnolence during the intracarotid amobarbital test. *Epilepsy Research,* 12:253–259.

McManus, I.C., and Bryden, M.P. (1992) The genetics of handedness, cerebral dominance, and lateralization. In I. Rapin and S.J. Segalowitz (eds.), *Handbook of Neuropsychology,* Vol. 6. Amsterdam: Elsevier, pp. 115–144.

Milner, B. (1974) *Hemispheric Specialization: Scope and Limits.* The Neurosciences: Third Study Program. Cambridge, MA: MIT Press, pp. 75–89.

Nass, R., deCoudres-Peterson, H.D., and Koch, D. (1989) Differential effects of congenital left and right brain injury on intelligence. *Brain and Cognition,* 9:258–266.

Nass R., Sadler A., E, Sidtis J. and J (1992) Differential effects of congenital versus acquired unilateral brain injury on dichotic listening performance—evidence for sparing and asymmetric crowding. *Neurology,* 42:1960–1965.

Norsell, U. (1988) Arguments against redundant brain structures. In S. Finger, T.E. LeVere, C.R. Almli, and D.G. Stein (eds.), *Brain Injury and Recovery: Theoretical and Controversial Issues.* New York: Plenum Press, pp. 151–163.

Orsini D. (1984) Early brain injury and lateral development. Early brain injury and lateral development. Doctoral dissertation. State University of New York Stony Brook.

Rasmussen, T., and Milner, B. (1977) The role of early left-brain injury in determining lateralization of cerebral speech function. In S.J. Dimond and D.A. Blizzard (eds.), *Evolution and Lateralization of the Brain,* Vol. 229, pp. 355–369.

Riva, D., and Cazzaniga, L. (1986) Late effects of unilateral brain lesions sustained before and after age one. *Neuropsychologia,* 24:423–428.

Riva, D., Dal Brun, A., Pantaleoni, C., Milani, N., and Fedrizzi, E. (1989) Emiplegia spastica congenita: evoluzione neuropsicologica. *Neuropsich Etàa Evol,* 4:73–82.

Satz, P. (1972) Pathological left-handedness: An explanatory model. *Cortex,* 8:121–135.

Satz, P. (1973) Left-handedness and early brain insult. *Neuropsychologia,* 11:115–117.

Satz, P., Orsini, D., Saslow, E., and Henry, R. (1985a) Early brain injury and pathological left-handedness: Clues to a syndrome. In D.F. Benson and E. Zaidel (eds.), *The Dual*

Brain—Hemispheric Specialization in Humans. New York: Guilford Press, pp. 117–125.

Satz, P., Orsini, D.L., Saslow, E., and Henry, R. (1985b) The pathological left-handedness syndrome. *Brain and Cognition,* 4:27–46.

Satz, P., Strauss, E., Hunter, M., and Wada, J. (1994) Re-examination of the crowding hypothesis: Effects of age of onset. *Neuropsychology,* 8:255–262.

Satz, P., Strauss, E., Wada, J., and Orsini, D.L. (1988) Some correlates of intra- and inter-hemispheric speech organization after left focal brain injury. *Neuropsychologia,* 26:245–350.

Satz, P., Strauss, E., and Whitaker, H. (1990) The ontogeny of hemispheric specialization: Some old hypothesis revisited. *Brain and Language,* 38:596–614.

Shankweiler, D. and Studdert-Kennedy, M. (1967) Identification of consonants and vowels presented to left and right ears. *Quarterly Journal of Experimental Psychology,* 19:59–63.

Sperry, R.W. (1974) *Lateral Specialization in the Surgically Separated Hemispheres.* The Neurosciences: Third Study Program. Cambridge, MA: MIT Press, pp. 5–19.

Strauss, E. (1988) Dichotic listening and sodium amytal: Functional and morphological aspects of hemispheric asymmetry. In K. Hugdahl (ed.), *Handbook of Dichotic Listening: Theory, Methods and Research.* Chichester, UK: Wiley, pp. 117–138.

Strauss, E., Satz, P., and Wada, J. (1990) An examination of the crowding hypothesis in epileptic patients who have undergone the carotid amytal test. *Neuropsychologia,* 28:1221–1227.

Studdert-Kennedy, M., and Shankweiler, D. (1970) Hemipsheric specialization for speech perception. *Journal of the Acoustical Society of America,* 48:579–594.

Teuber, H.L. (1974) Recovery of function following lesions of the central nervous system: History and prospect. *Neuroscience's Research Program Bulletin,* 12:197–209.

Teuber, H.L. (1975) Recovery of function after brain injury in man. In R. Porter and D.W. Fitzsimons (eds.), *Outcomes of Severe Damage to the Nervous System.* Ciba Foundation Symposium 34. Amsterdam: Elsevier-North Holland, pp. 159–186.

Uvebrant, P. (1988) Hemiplegic cerebral palsy: Aetiology and outcome. Hemiplegic cerebral palsy: Aetiology and outcome. *Acta Paediatrica Scandinavica,* Supplement 345.

Wada, J. (1949) A new method for the determination of the side of cerebral speech dominance. A preliminary report on the intracarotid injection of sodium amytal in man. *Medical Biology,* 14:221–222.

Wada, J., and Rasmussen, T. (1960) Intracarotid injections os sodium amytal for the lateralization of cerebral speech dominance. *Journal of Neurosurgery,* 17:266–282.

Wexler, B.E., and Halwes, T. (1983) Increasing the power of dichotic listening methods: The fused rhymed words test. *Neuropsychologia,* 21:59–66.

Zatorre, R.J. (1989) Perceptual asymmetry on the dichotic fused words test and cerebral speech lateralization determined by the carotid amytal test. *Neuropsychologia,* 27:1207–1219.

13

Reorganization of Motor Function in Cerebral Palsy

L.J. CARR

Cerebral palsy is a descriptive term for the persistent disorder of movement or posture secondary to nonprogressive pathology of the immature brain. The Etiology and outcome of cerebral palsy are diverse. The functional motor outcome cannot be simply predicted by the size and site of the central nervous system (CNS) lesion (Bouza et al., 1994; Kotlarek et al., 1981; Wiklund & Uvebrant, 1991); other factors including additional functional impairments are also important. There is clinical evidence that the outcome is strongly influenced by the age at which the damage occurred; it is generally better when damage is sustained early in development. This has been attributed to the plasticity of the developing CNS and its ability to reorganize. This chapter will discuss the current evidence of such plasticity in children and young adults with cerebral palsy. Some key clinical and neurophysiological studies will be reviewed. Data will be presented to support the view that reorganization of descending motor pathways may occur in humans following early damage and that this reorganization may be functionally significant.

Clinical Evidence of Central Nervous System Reorganization in Humans

The functional effects of acquired stroke contrast markedly with those of a congenital lesion. For example, the effects of a large left-sided stroke on speech production appear to be critically age-related. When stroke occurs in adult life, the resulting aphasia is usually severe and permanent, whereas a young child with a similar lesion is never left with permanent aphasia (Vargha-Khadem et al., 1985; Woods, 1980). Uvebrant (1988) conducted a population-based study in South West Sweden, reviewing 169 cases of hemiplegic cerebral palsy. He found that sensory and motor impairments tended to be mildest in preterm infants and most severe in

247

A   B

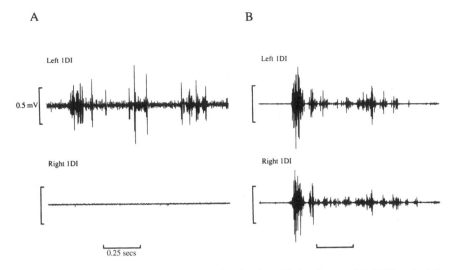

Figure 13-1. Subjects attempted to oppose the thumb and index finger of the left hand while the right hand was relaxed. Surface EMG activity was recorded from the left and right 1DI muscles. (a) Recording from a healthy 8-year-old child; EMG activity is restricted to the left hand. (b) Recording from a 5-year-old child with congenital right-sided hemiplegia and strong mirror movements (grade 4, group A) shows simultaneous and symmetrical EMG activity in the left and right 1DI muscles.

those who became hemiplegic postnatally. The results of surgical hemispherectomy provide further evidence of the importance of the time of lesion in determining the outcome. Gardner et al., (1955) examined the residual function of adults after hemispherectomy, comparing those with tumor to those with intractable epilepsy and infantile hemiplegia (i.e., within the first year of life). They noted that the group with infantile hemiplegia never showed complete hemiparalysis preoperatively and that, following surgery, only a transient deterioration in motor function was seen; useful hand function was often preserved. This was not the case in those with tumor, who always showed severe impaiment of distal function. Gardner et al. suggested that when one hemisphere was impaired early in life, other parts of the brain take over, to some extent, the function of the destroyed parts.

Alteration of neuronal connections is further suggested by the anomalous sensory and motor functions sometimes seen after early brain injury: some children with cerebral palsy show hyperaesthesia (Rudel et al., 1966), and children with infantile hemiplegia show a high incidence of persistent mirror movements (Woods & Teuber, 1978). When voluntary movements of one limb are made, mirror movements describe the symmetrical but unintentional movements that may be seen in the opposite limb. These movements may occur during normal development but are usually weak (Lazarus & Todor, 1987). They are pathological if they are pronounced and persistent. An electromyographic (EMG) recording of mirror movements in intrinsic hand muscles is shown in Figure 13-1.

Neurophysiological and Neuroradiological Evidence of
Central Nervous System Reorganization in Humans

More recent studies have used modern techniques to elucidate some of the possible mechanisms underlying these clinical observations. Farmer, working with Stephens and his group (Farmer et al., 1990), explored mirror movements in a subject with the Klippel Feil syndrome using a battery of neurophysiological tests. They concluded that these movements were a clinical marker of abnormally branched, bilaterally distributed corticospinal (CS) axons. Similar findings occured in a subsequent study of four children with congenital hemiplegic cerebral palsy and strong mirror movements (Farmer et al., 1991). It was suggested that in these subjects the undamaged hemisphere was controlling movements bilaterally, as Woods and Teuber (1978) had also proposed. This work was extended in our study, which investigated 33 subjects with hemiplegic cerebral palsy (see below and Carr et al., 1993).

A number of studies have used transcortical magnetic stimulation (TCMS) to explore the disruptive effects of disease on functional CS projections and motor maps in humans (Beradelli et al., 1991; Boniface et al., 1991; Cohen et al., 1991). These studies are described in detail in Chapter 15. Abnormal CS projections have been demonstrated after early CNS damage; Benecke et al., (1991) found abnormal ipsilateral responses to TCMS in the upper limb muscles of two subjects after hemispherectomy, both of whom had had hemiplegia since infancy. The amplitude and latency of the ipsilateral response was directly related to residual motor function. Transcortical magnetic stimulation may evoke abnormal coactivation of the gastrocnemius and soleus muscles in subjects with congenital spastic diplegia (Brouwer & Ashby, 1990). It was suggested that these misdirected CS fibers may account for the impaired motor control seen in the lower limbs of these subjects. A more recent study has suggested that motor output may also be altered in adults following ischemic stroke; ipsilateral responses were often evoked from the undamaged hemisphere (Netz et al., 1997). However, in contrast to the findings of Benecke et al., this reorganization had no clear functional benefits.

Functional imaging may give further insight into motor recovery after early brain damage. Sabatini et al., (1994) studied regional cerebral blood flow in a subject with an early left-sided hemiplegia and good functional recovery. Voluntary activation of either hand led to a similar increase in the left premotor and sensorimotor cortices; there was no detectable change in flow in the right hemisphere. Nirkko et al. (1997) performed TCMS and functional magnetic resonance imaging (fMRI) in a woman with infantile hemiplegia and strong mirror movements. Transcortical magnetic stimulation over the damaged hemisphere did not elicit any motor responses in intrinsic hand muscles, whereas stimulation over the healthy hemisphere evoked symmetrical bilateral responses. With movement of either hand, functional imaging showed activation only of the motor area of the healthy left hemisphere and the right cerebellum. These studies all support the view that the immature CNS may be capable of reorganization of function following damage.

Histological Evidence of Central Nervous System Reorganization in Humans

To date there is no histological evidence of remodeled CS projections in humans.

Animal Evidence of Central Nervous System Reorganization

Lesion experiments in animals suggest that, as in humans, the motor consequences of CNS damage are influenced by the age at which the damage occurs. The Kennard principle describes the functional "benefits" of early lesions (Kennard, 1942). Cortical reorganization and novel CS projections have been demonstrated histologically following such early damage. In hemispherectomized infant rats, a novel CS projection may develop from the intact cortex (Hicks & D'Amato,1970; Leong & Lund, 1973). Tracing studies indicate that a further ipsilateral contribution may be made by decussated CS axons recrossing at spinal levels (Barth & Stanfield, 1990; Rouiller et al., 1991). This remodeling of CS pathways is associated with sparing of forelimb stride and some aspects of forelimb placing (Barth & Stanfield, 1990; Hicks & D'Amato, 1970). It is not seen in adult lesioned rats. Similarly, studies in the hamster showed that after neonatal pyramidotomy, axons from the intact CS tract may sprout into denervated spinal cord, with arbors branching bilaterally (Kuang & Kalil, 1990). Hamsters with the earliest lesions showed superior forelimb skills when manipulating seeds (Reh & Kalil, 1982). In both rats and hamsters the CS tract decussates postnatally (at days 1 and 3, respectively). The brain is small compared to its final adult size, so that at the time of birth the brains of these animals are analogous to that of a 16-week-human fetus.

Studies in young cats and monkeys can be more closely related to humans, since in these species the CS tract decussates before birth. In cats following neonatal hemispherectomy, CS projections from the intact hemisphere may develop into ipsilateral spinal cord (Gomez-Pinilla et al., 1986). These cats perform significantly better than adult lesioned cats on a range of movement, posture, and sensory functions (Villablanca et al., 1986). This preservation of motor function is critically dependent on the time of the lesion (Armand & Kably, 1993). In primates there is no histological evidence of the remodeling of CS tracts following CNS damage. Anomalous projections have not been demonstrated after unilateral removal of the sensorimotor cortex in the infant rhesus monkey (Sloper et al., 1983). While initially these lesions had a less disruptive effect on the infant monkey (in agreement with Kennard's observations), the long-term effects appeared to be similar in both infant and adult lesioned monkeys (Passingham et al., 1983). Goldman and Galkin (1978) found that prenatal cortical resection may be associated with preservation of function; following prenatal removal of the association cortex bilaterally, one rhesus monkey performed delayed-response tasks with the competence of surgically unaltered animals. The thalami, the main source of projections to the prefrontal cortex, did not show the characteristic degeneration seen following postnatal resection, and ectopic sulci were noted in the frontal, temporal, and occipital lobes. This suggests that anatomical and behavioral reorganization may occur in primates, but this depends critically on the maturity of the brain at the time of damage.

With this human clinical and animal experimental background in mind, my colleagues and I used an electrophysiological approach to determine whether anatomical reorganization after early brain damage could be demonstrated in humans (Carr et al., 1993).

A Study of Patterns of Central Motor Reorganization in Hemplegic Cerebral Palsy

Subjects and Methods

Thirty-three subjects with hemiplegic cerebral palsy were studied with local ethical approval. At the time of the study, the subjects were between 2 and 26 years of age; CNS damage had occurred at least 1 year earlier. In 24 subjects the hemiplegia was congenital, with damage occurring before the end of the neonatal period (28 days). In nine subjects the hemiplegia was acquired later in life, between 4 months and 23 years of age. The hemiplegia was right-sided in 22 subjects and left-sided in 11 subjects. For comparison, 17 healthy subjects 2 to 21 years of age were also studied.

Neurological and electrophysiological assessment was undertaken in all subjects, with particular attention to the upper limbs. Two particular aspects of hand function were noted. The first was the ability to perform relatively independent finger movements (RIFM) with either hand. There is evidence that this skill reflects the presence of direct corticomotoneuronal connections, normally derived entirely from the contralateral motor cortex (Kuypers, 1973; Lawrence & Hopkins, 1976; Phillips & Porter, 1964). Second, the presence and intensity of any mirror movements were assessed and graded from 0 to 4, as described by Woods and Teuber (1978), where 0 indicates no clear imitative movement and 4 indicates that movement is equal to that expected for the intended hand. As discussed above, earlier work had suggested that these movements may reflect underlying abnormalities of CS tracts (Farmer et al., 1990, 1991). Subjects with mirror movements were actively recruited for the study.

Three techniques were used to examine projections to motoneuron pools from cortex and at the spinal cord level:

1. To assess functional CS projections,TCMS of each motor cortex was performed using a Magstim 200 stimulator and a focal coil (double 70 mm). Electromyographic responses were recorded from the first dorsal interossei (1DI) of the left and right hands using surface electrodes.
2. Cross-correlation analysis of multiunit EMG was performed by comparing the times of occurrence of motor unit spikes when the left and right 1DI muscles were coactivated. Motoneuron pools sharing a common drive will show short-term synchronization of their motor unit discharges. A narrow central peak in the cross-correlation histogram may represent the

simultaneous arrival of monosynaptic excitatory postsynaphic potentials (EPSPs), reflecting activity in branched last-order neurons (Kirkwood & Sears, 1978; Moore et al., 1970; Sears & Stagg, 1976). However, a contribution from oligosynaptic EPSPs as a result of presynaptic synchronization cannot be excluded (Kirkwood & Sears, 1991; Kirkwood et al., 1982).

3. Cutaneomuscular reflexes were recorded from 1DI or forearm extensor muscles following stimulation of the digital nerves of the index finger. The filtered, rectified EMG was averaged, time locked to the stimulus. In healthy adults this leads to a triphasic modulation of ongoing EMG; an initial increase (E1) is followed by a decrease (I1), followed by a second increase (E2). While the early components are thought to be spinal in origin, there is evidence that the E2 component has a transcortical pathway analogous to the M2 of the stretch reflex (Farmer et al., 1990; Jenner & Stephens, 1982; Matthews, 1991). The configuration of the reflex undergoes maturational changes; the later components are not initially present (Evans et al., 1990; Issler & Stephens, 1983).

Results

Control Subjects. All control subjects performed RIFM with ease. Mirror movements were absent or weak (less than three). Focal magnetic stimulation of either motor cortex evoked EMG responses only in contralateral 1DI muscles ($n = 12$). Electromography recorded from coactivated left and right 1DI muscles did not show correlogram peaks in any subject when cross-correlation analysis was performed (see Fig. 13-3). Cutaneomuscular reflexes were always restricted to the stimulated side, there was no modulation of EMG activity in the homologous muscle of the nonstimulated side (see Fig. 13-4).

Hemiplegic Subjects. Clinical and electrophysiological results distinguished four groups of subjects; A, B, C, and D. The findings are summarized in Table 13-1.

In groups C and D, TCMS evoked only contralateral responses; ipsilateral responses were never seen. Cross-correlation analysis of EMG responses recorded from coactivated left and right 1DI muscles did not show any correlogram peaks; thus, there was no evidence of branched last-order synaptic inputs to the motoneuron pools of these muscles. Cutaneomuscular reflexes were always restricted to the stimulated side.

The subjects in group C were clinically the most severely affected; all had acquired their hemiplegia after 2 years of age. Stimulation of either cortex failed to evoke EMG responses in the hemiplegic hand. In adults with unilateral stroke this finding is associated with severe clinical deficits (Homberg et al., 1991). The subjects in group D all had mild hemiplegia. The results of TCMS were indistinguishable from those of the control subjects. In adults, such results are associated with mild clinical deficits (Homberg et al., 1991).

In contrast, TCMS demonstrated novel CS projections in subjects from groups A and B. In both groups, stimulation of the undamaged motor cortex evoked short

Table 13-1. Summary of Clinical and Neurophysiological Findings in Subjects and Controls

| Group | N | RIFM | Strong MM | Peak in L/R Correlogram | I1, E2 on Nonstim Side | Response to Stimulation of: | | | |
| | | | | | | Undamaged MC | | Damaged MC | |
						Ipsi	Contra	Ipsi	Contra
A	11	5	11	11	7/7	10/10	10/10	0/10	0/10
B	10	3	0	0	0/7	10/10	10/10	0/10	4/10
C	3	0	0	0	0/3	0/3	3/3	0/3	0/3
D	9	9	0	0	0/8	0/9	9/9	0/9	9/9
						Left MC		Right MC	
Control	17	N/A	0	0	0/10	0/12	2/12	0/12	12/12

Abbreviations: RIFM, ability to make relatively independent finger movements with the hemiplegic hand; Strong MM, grade 3–4 mirror movements; I1, E2 nonstim, I1, E2 components of cutaneomuscular reflex recorded on the nonstimulated side following stimulation of digital nerves of the unaffected hand, stated as a fraction of the number of subjects with a mature reflex on the stimulated side; MC, motor cortex; Ipsi/Contra, ipsilateral/contralateral 1DI muscle.

latency responses in both ipsilateral and contralateral 1DI muscles, as illustrated in Figure 13-2. In subjects from group A, these ipsilateral and contralateral responses were of similar size and latency, whereas in subjects from group B, the ipsilateral responses were significantly smaller and later than the contralateral responses (paired t-test; $p < .05$), occurring 0.4 to 13.8 milliseconds (ms) after the contralateral response (mean, 4 ms later; SD, 4.2 ms).

Further clinical and neurophysiological differences distinguished groups A and B, suggesting that there were at least two patterns of reorganization. As shown in Table 13-1, all subjects in group A had strong mirror movements. In these subjects, cross-correlograms constructed between EMG responses of left and right 1DI showed short-duration central peaks (mean duration, 18.1 ms; range, 12.5–24.3 ms). An example is shown in Figure 13-3. This finding indicates the likely presence of common last-order inputs to the motoneuron pools of the left and right 1DI. Together with the results of TCMS, this suggests that in subjects in group A, CS axons from the undamaged motor cortex have branched and are distributed bilaterally to the motoneuron pools of the upper limbs. This conclusion is further supported by the results of cutaneomuscular reflex testing; when the unaffected hand was stimulated, the late components of the reflex were recorded simultaneously from the nonstimulated side. This is shown in Figure 13-4. It was never seen when the hemiplegic hand was stimulated.

The ipsilateral motor cortex was the only demonstrable source of CS inputs to the hemiplegic hand in subjects in group A. Electromyographic responses were never evoked by TCMS of the damaged motor cortex. Five of these subjects were able to perform RIFM with the hemiplegic hand. This suggests that in these subjects the ipsilateral tract may make direct corticomotoneuronal connections.

(1) AB: 14 years. Left sided hemiplegia, pronounced mirror movements.

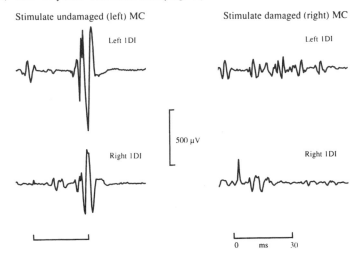

(2) JA: 16 years. Left sided hemiplegia, no mirror movements.

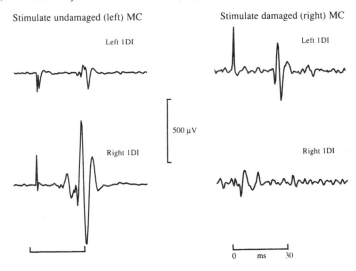

Figure 13-2. Results of TCMS in two subjects with hemiplegia. Electromyographic responses were recorded from preactivated left and right 1DI muscles as single sweeps, time locked to the stimulus at time 0. (1) Results in a 14-year-old subject from group A with a congenital left-sided hemiplegia and strong mirror movements. Stimulation of the undamaged motor cortex (MC) evokes simultaneous responses in the contralateral (right) and ipsilateral (left) 1DI muscles that are similar in size. No EMG response is seen following stimulation of the damaged MC, only ongoing EMG. (2) Results in a 16-year-old subject from group B with congenital left-sided hemiplegia but no mirror movements. Stimulation of the undamaged MC evokes a response in the ipsilateral left 1DI muscle that is later and smaller than the response in the contralateral right 1DI muscle. Stimulation of the damaged MC evokes a contralateral response.

Control.

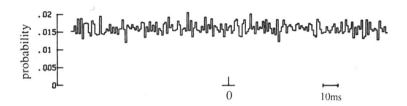

Group A.

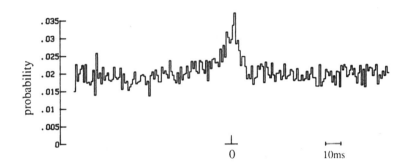

Group B.

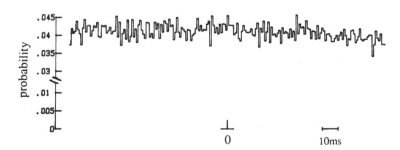

Figure 13-3. Cross-correlograms constructed from motor unit spikes of multiunit EMG recorded from the left and right 1DI while both hands were active. Each cross-correlogram was constructed from at least 3500 spikes for each side. In a 17-year-old subject from group A, there is a central peak of around 15 ms in duration. In contrast, no peaks are present in the correlograms of a healthy 10-year-old control subject or of a 16-year-old subject from group B; neither of these subjects showed strong mirror movements.

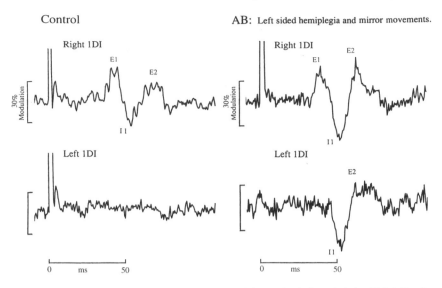

Figure 13-4. Cutaneomuscular reflexes recorded from the left and right 1DI following stimulation of the digital nerves of the right index finger at a rate of 3 per second and at twice threshold for perception. (A) The reflex in a healthy control subject averaged from 775 sweeps of rectified EMG. A triphasic response (E1, I1 and E2) is seen in the right 1DI. There is no modulation of ongoing EMG in the left 1DI. (B) The reflex in a 14-year-old subject from group A with congenital left-sided hemiplegia and strong mirror movements averaged from 975 sweeps of rectified EMG. Stimulation of the unaffected right hand evokes a triphasic response in the right 1DI. The I1 and E2 components are seen simultaneously in the left 1DI. Stimulation of the left index finger evokes only an E1 component, which is restricted the left 1DI.

In subjects in group B branched last-order presynaptic inputs were not detected between the left and right motoneuron pools to 1DI using cross-correlation analysis (Fig. 13-3). Cutaneomuscular reflexes were restricted to the stimulated hand. Together with the results of TCMS, this finding suggests that in these subjects, while CS axons from the undamaged cortex are again distributed bilaterally, these projections are separate and not branched. Furthermore, the functional effects appear less marked than those described in group A. Subjects in group B did not have strong mirror movements (graded <3). Only three subjects could perform RIFM, and in these subjects TCMS of the damaged motor cortex evoked short-latency EMG responses in the contralateral hemiplegic hand. Thus, the ipsilateral tract described in group B is not associated with the ability to perform RIFM.

Discussion

The main conclusion of the present study is that reorganization of CS projections may be demonstrated after early unilateral CNS damage. Reorganization of descending motor pathways was found in 64% of the hemiplegic subjects studied, namely, the subjects in groups A and B. In these subjects, a novel ipsilateral CS tract arising from the undamaged motor cortex was demonstrated. These projections appear to have functional significance, with strong mirror movements (as seen in group A), a clinical marker of one pattern of reorganization.

The subjects in groups C and D did not show evidence of reorganization of motor pathways. Presumably, in these subjects, CNS damage either occurred too late (group C) or was too mild (group D) to promote detectable reorganization of CS pathways.

The pathophysiology of the reorganization in groups A and B is not known. The hemiplegia was congenital in all subjects from group A and in eight of the ten subjects in group B. However, clinical history and neuroimaging indicated that CNS injury had generally occurred earlier in subjects in group A than in those in group B, namely, before the 32nd week of gestation. Two subjects in group B had acquired their hemiplegia postnatally, at 9 months and 7 years, respectively. The two groups were further differentiated by the presence or absence of strong mirror movements and by the results of the neurophysiological tests. The results suggest that in the subjects in group A, CS axons from the undamaged motor cortex have branched bilaterally to supply the left and right motoneuron pools of the distal upper limb muscles. In the subjects in group B, CS axons appear to be distributed bilaterally as separate nonbranched projections. In the subjects in group A, the underlying mechanism is likely to involve remodeling and axonal sprouting. Some possible models are suggested by animal studies (see the discussion at the beginning of the chapter), in which the most robust axonal sprouting is generally seen after the earliest lesions. While aberrant CS projections may be seen transiently during normal development, under normal circumstances they are retracted (Alisky & Swink, 1992) and do not make functional connections (Kuang & Kalil, 1994). It is possible, however, that early CNS lesions may alter this process.

Concerning the subjects in group B, one hypothesis is that rather than remodeling of axons, preexisting ipsilateral CS pathways were unmasked. This was the conclusion of the Netz et al. study (1997), in which 15 adults were examined after stroke using TCMS. Ipsilateral thenar responses were evoked by TCMS of the undamaged hemisphere in 11 subjects. These responses were of significantly longer latency than the contralateral responses (mean, 6 ms) and of higher threshold (mean, 64% versus 27%). Contralateral responses from the damaged motor cortex were evoked in all but one subject, but at a higher threshold than contralateral responses from the undamaged motor cortex (mean 45% versus 27%). These ipsilateral pathways were a feature of the "poor recovery" group. Of the ten subjects in this group, only three could make some selective finger movements; interestingly, they tended to show the lower thresholds to TCMS over the damaged motor cortex. Clearly there may be similarities between this adult study and our subjects in group B, particularly the two subjects with postnatally acquired hemiplegia. Compared to the other subjects in group B, these two subjects showed the greatest discrepancy between ipsilateral and contralateral response latency (at 7.6 and 13.8 ms, respectively). However, these two subjects did not show markedly raised thresholds to TCMS either for the ipsilateral response or for the damaged motor cortex ($\leq$ 10% higher than the contralateral threshold). The unmasking of ipsilateral pathways is difficult to prove. While CS projections are most numerous to distal contralateral muscles (Palmer & Ashby, 1992; Phillips & Porter, 1964) clinical studies have demonstrated some ipsilateral muscle weakness following unilateral stroke, particularly in proximal muscles (Colebatch & Gandevia, 1989). Primate studies confirm that ipsilateral CS degeneration occurs after unilateral cortical lesions (Kuypers & Brinkman, 1970; Liu & Chambers, 1964). In our study, TCMS failed to elicit ipsilateral responses in 12 healthy children and 12 hemiplegic children. Ipsilateral excitatory responses are occasionally demonstrated in healthy adult subjects (Netz et al., 1997; Wasserman et al., 1994). However, the optimal position for evoking ipsilateral responses in healthy subjects usually differs from the optimal position for contralateral responses. In our study, only limited mapping of the motor cortex was possible; however, in no hemiplegic subject was a discrete ipsilateral stimulating position found, and responses were usually evoked bilaterally. This was also the case in the study of Netz et al. (1997). This observation contrasts with that of healthy controls and does not support unmasking of preexisting projections; rather, it suggests that the mechanism of ipsilateral responses differs in healthy controls and subjects with hemiplegia.

Another possibility is that other rapidly conducting brain stem pathways, such as the reticulospinal tract, may be involved. They are known to be bilaterally distributed and are in close proximity to the CS tract (Nathan et al., 1997).

Cerebral palsy may offer unique insights into neuroplasticity and reorganization of function in humans. With the refinement of neuroradiological techniques, lesions can now be defined accurately with respect to timing and site. Combining functional imaging with neurophysiological tests enables more accurate localization of function. In addition to motor functions, sensory functions such as vision, hearing, and speech are all amenable to study (see the introductory discussion). There is evidence that following an early unilateral lesion, speech may be relocated to the contralateral hemisphere and language preserved, albeit at some cost to performance skills (Vargha-Khadem et al., 1985; Woods, 1980). There is also evidence that certain behavioral phenotypes, such as hyperactivity, are more common in hemiplegic cerebral palsy and that this is a direct result of the underlying brain damage rather than of environmental factors (Goodman, 1997).

When neuroplasticity is investigated in humans, controlled studies are difficult. In contrast to animal studies, the etiology, site, and size of lesions cannot be standardized. The natural history of cerebral palsy is still not fully understood, and other confounding variables such as intelligence and environmental factors will influence the outcome. For example, epilepsy is one of the most significant determinants of the cognitive outcome (Vargha-Khadem et al., 1992). This makes evaluation of theraputic interventions very difficult. Ongoing studies are currently attempting to measure the benefits of physiotherapy programs in cerebral palsy.

In evaluating possible pharmacological interventions, one must first consider the range of etiological factors. Clearly, no single intervention is appropriate for the range of pathologies that may result in cerebral palsy; compare a migration defect that occurs in the early stages of pregnancy with perinatal asphyxia. Interventions aimed at preventing ischemic cell death are being evaluated. N-methyl-D-aspartate receptors are likely to be important factors in neurotoxicity, and the possibility of conferring protection using anatagonists has been studied in animal models (Butcher et al., 1997). More important, neurotrophic factors (particularly nerve growth factor and brain-derived neurotrophic factor) are likely to be involved in promoting neuronal plasticity. It is already established that they actively regulate the survival, differentiation, and maintenance of specific populations of neurons, principally by synaptic stabilization (Thoenen, 1995). Their expression varies according to physiological activity and following brain injury. There is increasing evidence that these neurotrophic factors may induce plasticity in both developing and adult animals. For example, brain-derived neurotrophic factor induces plasticity when exogenously applied to the visual cortex of a monocularly deprived kitten (Cellerino & Maffei, 1996) and in adult mice it may induce neuronal hypertrophy (Guilhem et al., 1996). However, under physiological conditions, its action is less clear, and at present, none of these agents are in clinical use in adults or children.

It is likely that continuing medical advances will clarify the critical determinants underlying plasticity and patterns of reorganization of function in humans after early CNS damage. Enhancement of these naturally occurring processes with effective therapeutic interventions may then be possible.

ACKNOWLEDGMENTS

I would like to thank my colleagues: Professor J.A. Stephens, Dr. L.M. Harrison, Dr. A.L. Evans, and Dr. S.F. Farmer. Also, thank you to all the children who participated in the study, and to the staff of the London Hemiplegia Register and of the Bobath Centre for the Treatment of Children with Cerebral Palsy. L.J. Carr was supported by an MRC Training Fellowship.

References

Alisky, J.M., Swink, T.D., and Tolbert, D.L. (1992) The postnatal spatial and temporal development of corticospinal projections in cats. *Experimental Brain Research,* 88:265–276.

Armand, J., and Kably, B. (1993) Critical timing of sensorimotor cortex lesions for the recovery of motor skills in the developing cat. *Experimental Brain Research,* 93:73–88.

Barth, T.M., and Stanfield, B.B. (1990) The recovery of forelimb placing behavior in rats with neonatal cortical damage involves the remaining hemisphere. *Journal of Neuroscience,* 10:3449–3559.

Benecke, R., Meyer, B.-U., and Freund, H.-J. (1991) Reorganisation of descending motor pathways in patients after hemispherectomy and severe hemispheric lesions demonstrated by magnetic stimulation. *Experimental Brain Research,* 83:419–426.

Berardelli, A., Inghilleri, M., Cruccu, G., Mercuri, B., and Manfredi, M. (1991) Electrical and magnetic transcranial stimulation in patients with corticospinal damage due to stroke or motor neurone disease. *Electroencephalography and clinical Neurophysiology,* 81:389–396.

Boniface, S.J., Mills, K.R., and Schubert, M. (1991) Responses of single spinal motoneurons to magnetic brain stimulation in healthy subjects and patients with multiple sclerosis. *Brain,* 114:643–662.

Bouza, H., Dubowitz, L.M.S., Rutherford, M., and Pennock, J.M. (1994) Prediction of outcome in children with congenital hemiplegia: a magnetic resonance imaging study. *Neuropediatrics,* 25:60–66.

Brouwer, B., and Ashby, B. (1990) Do injuries to the developing human brain alter corticospinal projections. *Neuroscience Letters,* 108:225–230.

Butcher, S.P., Henshall, D.C., Teramura, Y., Iwasaki, K., and Sharkey, J. (1997) Neuroprotective action of FK506 in experimental stroke: In vivo evidence against an antiexcitotoxic mechanism. *Journal of Neuroscience,* 17:6939–6946.

Carr, L.J., Harrison, L.M., Evans, A.L., and Stephens, J.A. (1993) Patterns of central motor reorganization in hemiplegic cerebral palsy. *Brain,* 116:1223–1247.

Cellerino, A., and Maffei, L. (1996) The action of neurotrophins in the development of plasticity of the visual cortex. *Progress in Neurobiology,* 49:53–71.

Cohen, L.G., Roth, B.J., Wasserman, E.M., Topka, H., Fuhr, P., Schultz, J., and Hallett, M. (1991) Magnetic stimulation of the human cerebral cortex, an indicator of reorganization in motor pathways in certain pathological conditions. *Journal of Clinical Neurophysiology,* 8:56–65.

Cohen, M.E., and Duffner, P.K. (1981) Prognostic indicators in hemiparetic cerebral palsy. *Annals of Neurology,* 9:353–357.

Colebatch, J.G., and Gandevia, S.C. (1989) The distribution of muscular weakness in upper motor neuron lesions affecting the arm. *Brain,* 112:749–763.

Evans, A.L., Harrison, L.M., and Stephens, J.A. (1990) Maturation of the cutaneomuscular reflex recorded from the first dorsal interosseus muscle in man. *Journal of Physiology (London),* 428:425–440.

Farmer, S.F., Harrison, L.M., Ingram, D.A., and Stephens, J.A. (1991) Plasticity of central motor pathways in children with hemiplegic cerebral palsy. *Neurology (Cleveland),* 41: 1505–1510.

Farmer, S.F., Ingram, D., and Stephens, J.A. (1990) Mirror movements studied in a patient with Klippel-Feil syndrome. *Journal of Physiology (London),* 428:467–484.

Gardner, W.J., Karnosh, L.J., McClure, C.C., and Gardner, A.K. (1955) Residual function following hemispherectomy for tumour and for infantile hemiplegia. *Brain,* 78:487–502.

Goldmann, P.S., and Galkin, T.W. (1978) Prenatal removal of frontal association cortex in the fetal rhesus monkey: Anatomical and functional consequences in postnatal life. *Brain Research (Amsterdam),* 152:451–485.

Gomez-Pinilla, F., Villablanca, J.R., Sonnifer, B.J., and Levine, M.S. (1986) Rorganization of pericruciate cortical projections to the spinal cord and dorsal column nuclei after neonatal or adult cerebral hemispherectomy in cats. *Brain Research (Amsterdam),* 385:343–355.

Goodman, R. (1997) Psychological aspects of hemiplegia. *Archives of Disease in Childhood,* 76:177–178.

Guilhem, D., Dreyfus, P.A., Makiura, Y., Suzuki, F., and Onteniente, B. (1996) Short increase of BDNF messenger RNA triggers kainic acid–induced neuronal hypertrophy in adult mice. *Neuroscience,* 72:923–931

Hicks, S.P., and D'Amato, C.J. (1970) Motor-sensory and visual behavior after hemispherectomy in newborn and mature rats. *Experimental Neurology,* 29:416–438.

Homberg, V., Stephan, K.M., and Netz, J. (1991) Transcranial stimulation of motor cortex in upper motoneurone syndrome: Its relation to the motor deficit. *Electroencephalography and Clinical Neurophysiology,* 81:379–388.

Issler, H., and Stephens, J.A. (1983) The maturation of cutaneous reflexes studied in the upper limb in man. *Journal of Physiology (London),* 335:643–654.

Jenner, J.R., and Stephens, J.A. (1982) Cutaneous reflex responses and their central nervous pathways studied in man. *Journal of Physiology (London),* 333:405–419.

Kennard, M.A. (1942) Cortical reorganization of motor function: Studies on series of monkeys of various ages from infancy to maturity. *Archives of Neurology and Psychiatry (Chicago),* 48:227–240.

Kirkwood, P.A., and Sears, T.A. (1978) The synaptic connections to intercostal motoneurons as revealed by the average common excitation potential. *Journal of Physiology (London),* 275:103–134.

Kirkwood, P.A., and Sears, T.A. (1991) Cross-correlation analyses of motoneuron inputs in a coordinated motor act. In J. Kruger (ed.), *Neuronal Cooperativity.* Berlin and Heidelberg: Springer-Verlag, pp. 225–248.

Kirkwood, P.A., Sears, T.A., Tuck, D.L., and Westgaard, R.H. (1982) Variations in the time course of the synchronization of intercostal motoneurons in the cat. *Journal of Physiology (London),* 327:105–135.

Kotlarek, F., Rodewig, R., and Brull, D. (1981) Computed tomographic findings in congenital hemiparesis in childhood and their relation to etiology and prognosis. *Neuropediatrics,* 12:101–109.

Kuang, R.Z., and Kalil, K. (1990) Specificity of corticospinal axon arbors sprouting into denervated spinal cord. *Journal of Comparative Neurology,* 302:461–472

Kuang, R.Z., and Kalil, K. (1994) Development of specificity in corticospinal connections by axon collaterals branching selectively into appropriate spinal targets. *Journal of Comparative Neurology,* 344:270–282

Kuypers, H.G. (1973) The anatomical organization of the descending pathways and their contributions to motor control especially in primates. In J.E. Desmedt (ed.), *New Developments in Electromyography and Clinical Neurophysiology,* Vol. 3. Basel: Karger, pp. 36–68.

Kuypers, H.G., and Brinkman, J. (1970) Precentral projections to different parts of the spinal intermedial zone in the rhesus monkey. *Brain Research,* 24:29–48.

Lawrence, D.G., and Hopkins, D.A. (1976) The development of motor control in the rhesus monkey: Evidence concerning the role of corticomotoneurone connectons. *Brain,* 99:235–254.

Lazarus, J.A.C., and Todor, J.L. (1987) Age differences in the magnitude of associated movement. *Developmental Medicine and Childhood Neurology,* 29:726–733.

Leong, S.K., and Lund, R.D. (1973) Anomalous bilateral corticofugal pathways in albino rats after neonatal lesions. *Brain Research,* 62:218–221.

Liu, C.N., and Chambers, W.W. (1964) An experimental study of the cortico-spinal system in the monkey (*Macaca mulatta*). *Journal of Comparative Neurology,* 123:257–284.

Matthews, P.B.C. (1991) The human stretch reflex and the motor cortex. *Trends in Neurosciences,* 14:87–91.

Moore, G.P., Segundo, J.P., Perkel, D.H., and Levitan, H. (1970) Statistical signs of synaptic interaction in neurons. *Biophysical Journal,* 10:876–900.

Nathan, P.W., Smith, M., and Deacon, P. (1997) Vestibulospinal, reticulospinal and descending propriospinal nerve fibers in man. *Brain,* 119:1809–1833.

Netz, J., Lammers, T., and Homberg, V. (1997) Reorganization of motor output in the non-affected hemisphere after stroke. *Brain,* 120:1579–1586.

Nirkko, A.C., Rosler, K.M., Ozdoba, M.D., Heid, M.D., Schroth, M.D., and Hess, M.D. (1997) Human cortical plasticity: Functional recovery with mirror movements. *Neurology,* 48:1090–1095.

Palmer, E., and Ashby, P. (1992) Corticospinal projections to upper limb motoneurons in humans. *Journal of Physiology (London),* 448:397–412.

Passingham, R.E., Perry, V.H., and Wilkinson, F. (1983) The long-term effects of removal of sensorimotor cortex in infant and adult rhesus monkeys. *Brain,* 106:675–705.

Phillips, C.G., and Porter, R. (1964) The pyramidal projections to motoneurons of some groups of the baboon's forelimb. *Progress in Brain Research,* 12:222–245.

Reh, T.A., and Kalil, K. (1982) Functional role of regrowing pyramidal tract fibers. *Journal of Comparative Neurology,* 211:276–283.

Rouiller, E.M., Laing, F., Moret, V., and Weisendanger, M. (1991) Trajectory of redirected corticospinal axons after unilateral lesion of the sensorimotor cortex in neonatal rat; a Phaseolus Vulgaris-Leucoagglutinin (PHLA-L) tracing study. *Experimental Neurology,* 114:53–65.

Rudel, R.G., Teuber, H.-L., and Twitchell, T.E. (1966) A note on hyperaesthesia in children with early brain damage. *Neuropsychologia,* 4:351–356.

Sabatini, U., Toni, D., Pantano, P., Brughitta, G., Padovani, A., Bozza, L., and Lenzi, L.L. (1994) Motor recovery after early brain damage: a case of brain plasticity. *Stroke,* 25:514–517.

Sears, T.A., and Stagg, D. (1976) Short-term synchronization of intercostal motoneuron activity. *Journal of Physiology (London),* 263:357–381.

Sloper, J., Brodal, P., and Powell, T.P.S. (1983) An anatomical study of the effects of unilateral removal of the sensorimotor (SM) cortex in infant monkeys on subcortical projections of the contralateral SM cortex. *Brain,* 106:707–716.

Thoenen, H. (1995) Neurotrophins and neuronal plasticity. *Science,* 270:593–598.

Uvebrant, P. (1988) Hemiplegic cerebral palsy: Aetiology and outcome. *Acta Paediatrica Scandinavica,* Supplement 345.

Vargha-Khadem, F., Isaacs, E., van der Werf, S., Rob, S., and Wilson, J. (1992) Development of intelligence and memory in children with hemiplegic cerebral palsy. The deleterious effect of early seizures. *Brain,* 115:315–329.

Vargha-Khadem, F., O'Gorman, A.M., and Watters, G.V. (1985) Aphasia and handedness in relation to hemispheric side, age at injury and severity of cerebral lesion during childhood. *Brain,* 108:677–696.

Villablanca, J.R., Burgess, J.W., and Olmstead, C.E. (1986) Recovery of function after neonatal or adult hemispherectomy in cats: 1. Time course, movement, posture and sensorimotor tests. *Behavioral Brain Research,* 19:205–226.

Wasserman, E.M., Pascual-Leone, A., and Hallett, M. (1994) Cortical motor representation of the ipsilateral hand and arm. *Experimental Brain Research,* 100:121–132.

Wiklund, L.-M., and Uvebrant, P. (1991) Hemiplegic cerebral palsy: Correlation between CT morphology and clinical findings. *Developmental Medicine and Child Neurology,* 33:512–523.

Woods, B.T. (1980) The restricted effects of right-hemisphere lesions after age one; Wechsler test data. *Neuropsychologia,* 18:65–70.

Woods, B.T., and Teuber, H.-L. (1978) Mirror movements after childhood hemiparesis. *Neurology (Cleveland),* 28:1152–1158.

III

Techniques for Studying Neuroplasticity in Humans

14

The Developmental Disorders:
Does Plasticity Play a Role?

PAULINE A. FILIPEK

The term *plasticity* generally refers to the brain's ability to recover function that was lost as the result of a defined insult that produced a discrete lesion. It is generally accepted that the brain of a child is more plastic, and therefore has a potentially greater capacity for recovery, than does the brain of an adult. The same premise holds for the brain of an infant relative to the brain of an older child. In adults, both large and small lesions can produce large behavioral deficits, while in the child many very large lesions result in relatively small behavioral deficits, presumably due to the greater capacity of plasticity (Nass & Gazzaniga, 1987).

Cognitive neuroscientists have traditionally looked at a given lesion—size, location, age at onset, acute versus chronic state—and subsequentally at the resulting behavioral deficit as the means for localization of function (Damasio & Damasio, 1989; Heilman & Valenstein, 1985; Mesulam, 1985). The child or adult with a behavioral deficit resulting from a lesion is presumed to have had normal behavior (or the capacity thereof) before the insult. Therefore, any behavioral deficits present after the onset of a given lesion are assumed to have been caused by that lesion. The neural systems responsible for the resulting deficient behaviors are then localized within or adjacent to that lesion. Discrete focal lesions are relatively rare in childhood, so that relatively little is known about lesion-based brain–behavior correlations or cerebral reorganization within the developmental realm (Filipek, 1996; Filipek et al., 1992, 1995a.

But now let us reverse this approach to begin not with the discrete lesion, but rather with a large spectrum of abnormal behaviors occurring within the developmental trajectory of childhood, whether normal or abnormal, but nontheless one that is continually evolving. These so-called developmental disorders include deficits in the traditional behavioral domains of cognition, language, visual-spatial function, attention, and socialization. However, none of the developmental disorders—autistic spectrum, developmental language, attention deficit hyperactivity, or reading

265

disorders—has characteristic discrete focal lesions or recognized encephaloclastic processes. In fact, the vast majority of the neuroimaging or gross neuropathologic studies of these disorders demonstrate normal gross neuroanatomy.

Developmental cognitive neuroscientists must therefore begin with the spectrum of behaviors occurring within these disorders and work backward in an attempt to identify the developmentally anomalous neural systems that are responsible for the large behavioral deficits. Since there is no distinct "insult onset" in these developmental disorders, the effects of plasticity are also little understood. This chapter will review what is currently known about the anomalous structure of the brain in the developmental disorders.

The magnetic resonance imaging (MRI) studies that will be reviewed in the following sections involved markedly differing qualitative or quantitative imaging methods, as well as differing subject characteristics. It is therefore not surprising that the results obtained from one-dimensional (e.g., length on a single slice), two-dimensional (e.g., area on a single slice), and three-dimensional (e.g., volume on all slices) methods are not necessarily concordant across collective studies. Regardless of these previous findings, current neuroimaging techniques give us for the first time the opportunity to develop a cognitive approach to the developmental disorders with the ability to image the entire brain in vivo within an acceptable imaging time for children.

Autistic Spectrum and Developmental Language Disorders: Too Much of a Good Thing or Plasticity at Work?

Autistic Spectrum Disorders

The autistic spectrum or pervasive developmental disorders consist of a spectrum of deficits in the behavioral domains of social interaction, verbal and nonverbal communication, and restrictive, repetitive patterns of behaviors (Table 14-1) (American Psychiatric Association, 1994). Although Kanner first described the syndrome of autism in 1943, the term *autism* did not appear in the *Diagnostic and Statistical Manual of Mental Disorders* until the Third Edition, (DSM-III) was published in 1980, having been referenced as "childhood schizophrenia" in previous editions. In DSM-IV (1994), pervasive developmental disorders is an umbrella diagnosis that includes autistic disorder, Asperger's disorder, childhood disintegrative disorder, Rett's disorder, and pervasive developmental disorder—not otherwise specified (Table 14-2). As of this writing, much controversy remains in the field about the existence of Asperger's disorder as a distinct syndrome, other than representing high-functioning autistic disorder. More and more clinicians in the field are beginning to consider the five diagnostic entities as one continuum on the autistic spectrum. However, this discussion will be limited to autistic disorder (AD) unless otherwise noted.

Neuropathologic Findings in Autistic Disorder. There have been only a few comprehensive neuropathologic studies of the autistic brain, and many of the findings

Table 14-1. Diagnostic Criteria for Autistic Disorder

A. A total of six (or more) items from (1), (2), and (3), distributed as noted across A1–A3:
  1. *Qualitative impairment in social interaction,* manifested by at least two of the following:
     • Marked impairment in the use of multiple nonverbal behaviors, such as eye-to-eye gaze, facial expression, body postures, and gestures to regulate social interaction
     • Failure to develop peer relationships appropriate to the developmental level
     • Lack of spontaneous seeking to share enjoyment, interests, or achievements with other people (e.g., by lack of showing, bringing, or pointing out objects of interest)
     • Lack of social or emotional reciprocity
  2. *Qualitative impairment in communication,* as manifested by at least one of the following:
     • Delay in or total lack of the development of spoken language (not accompanied by an attempt to compensate by alternative modes of communication such as gesture or mime)
     • In individuals with adequate speech, marked impairment in the ability to initiate or sustain a conversation with others
     • Stereotyped and repetitive use of language or idiosyncratic language
     • Lack of varied, spontaneous make-believe or social imitative play appropriate to the developmental level
  3. *Restrictive, repetitive, and stereotypic patterns of behavior, interests, and activities,* as manifested by at least one of the following:
     • Encompassing preoccupation with one or more stereotyped and restricted patterns of interest that is abnormal in either intensity or focus
     • Apparently inflexible adherence to specific nonfunctional routines or rituals
     • Stereotyped and repetitive motor mannerisms (e.g., hand or finger flapping or twisting or complex whole-body movements)
     • Persistent preoccupation with parts of objects
B. Delays or abnorrmal functioning in at least one of the following areas, with onset prior to age 3 years: (1) social interaction, (2) language as used in social communication, or (3) symbolic or imaginative play.
C. The disturbance is not better accounted for by Rett's disorder or Childhood Disintegrative Disorder.

Source: Adapted from American Psychiatric Association (1994).

are also inconsistent across studies. Most studies have reported normal-appearing gross neuroanatomy without evidence of neuronal migration anomalies or other abnormalities. Neuronal cell counts were similar in the cerebral cortex from one autistic subject (Coleman et al., 1985). Bauman and Kemper (1985, 1994) performed microscopic studies of the cerebral cortex and found only mild cytoarchitectonic abnormalities, which were confined to the anterior cingulate gyrus in five subjects, without evidence of abnormalities in the basal forebrain, thalamus, hypothalamus,

Table 14-2. The Pervasive Developmental Disorders

Autistic disorder
Asperger's disorder
Childhood disintegrative disorder
Rett's disorder
Pervasive developmental disorder—not otherwise specified (PDD-NOS), atypical autism

Source: Adapted from American Psychiatric Association (1994).

or basal ganglia. The only forebrain abnormalities were found in the limbic system, where reduced neuron size and increased cell-packing density were found in the hippocampus, subiculum, entorhinal cortex, amygdala, mammillary bodies, anterior cingulate, and septum.

In the cerebellar hemispheres, a decreased density (up to a 50% to 60% reduction) in the number of Purkinje and granular cells in the cerebellar hemispheres (mostly posteriorly and inferiorly) has been reported, without significant gliosis or other evidence of an atrophic or degenerative process (Arin et al., 1991; & Kemper Bauman, 1994; Ritvo et al., 1986; Williams et al., 1980). In the posterior vermis, a milder (~25%) reduction in Purkinje cells was also noted, without gross hypoplasia (Bauman & Kemper, 1994; Ritvo et al., 1986). The inferior olivary nuclei also had small, pale neurons, without the retrograde cell loss and atrophy usually seen with perinatal or postnatal Purkinje cell loss (Bauman & Kemper, 1994). Therefore, the available postmortem data provide evidence of microscopic pathology, predominantly localized to the cerebellar hemispheres and, to a lesser extent, to the cerebellar vermis, but not to the degree sufficient to account for the hypoplasia reported in some neuroimaging studies.

Anatomic Magnetic Resonance Imaging Studies in Autistic Disorder. In support of the grossly normal anatomy noted by the pathology studies above, a review of neuroimaging studies revealed a relatively small prevalence of focal lesions in subjects with autism (approximately 5%). None of the lesions was located in consistent regions of the brain (Filipek et al., 1992), for example, left Brodmann areas 6, 8, and 9 (Damasio et al., 1980), left occipital heterotopia (Gaffney et al., 1987), right lateral geniculate nucleus infarct (Gillberg & Svandsen, 1983), and agenesis of the corpus callosum (Caparulo et al., 1981). In a subsequent study, the prevalence of lesions on MRI in childhood AD was equal to that of normal control volunteers (Filipek et al., 1992).

However, cortical migration malformations have been noted on MRI in high-functioning subjects with AD or Asperger's including polymicrogyria, schizencephaly, and macrogyria, with no collective preference for a particular lobe or hemisphere (Berthler 1994, Berthier et al., 1990; Piven et al., 1990). It is unclear whether these findings of cortical dysplasias are more prevalent in autism than is currently recognized, as another study of 63 developmentally disabled children did not note any dysplasias (Filipek et al., 1992). Additional systematic evaluations of cortical architecture in larger cohorts will be needed to address this issue.

It is now generally recognized that head size and brain/cerebral volumes are larger in children with AD than in control children. This finding is based on studies of head circumference (Davidovitch et al., 1996; Lainhart et al., 1997; Woodhouse et al., 1996), autopsy studies (Bailey et al., 1993; ML Bauman, personal communication), and quantitative MRI (Filipek et al., 1992; Piven et al., 1992, 1996). In contrast, qualitative parietal lobe atrophy was reported on MRI scans based on apparently enlarged sulcal widths (Courchesne et al., 1993).

The lateral ventricles of some subjects with AD were wider or larger than those of control subjects (Campbell et al., 1982; Gaffney et al., 1989) that were not associated with birth weight, head circumference, language development scores, adaptive behavior scores, congenital anomalies, or severity of asocial symptoms (Campbell et al., 1982). Other investigators have reported normal ventricular size (Creasey et al., 1986; Filipek et al., 1992; Garber et al., 1989; Nowell et al., 1990; Prior, 1984; Rosenbloom et al., 1984). Enlarged ventricles are a nonspecific indication of possible cerebral injury or maldevelopment and cannot be related specifically to the neuroanatomic basis of AD.

The limbic system has often been implicated in the pathogenesis of autism, particularly in microscopic neuroanatomic studies (Bauman, 1991; Bauman & Kemper, 1985, 1990, 1994). Nowell et al. (1990) noted the qualitatively normal amygdala and limbic systems. More recently, on MRI scans, the cross-sectional area of the posterior hippocampus, including the subiculum and the dentate gyrus (Saitoh et al., 1995), as well as the volumes of the amygdala and hippocampus (Filipek et al., 1992), were similar in subjects with AD and in controls. In addition, the corpus callosum has been variably reported as being either smaller posteriorly in some subjects with AD (Egaas et al., 1995), with signal intensities similar to those in controls (Belmonte et al., 1995), or as being similar in area to normal controls (Filipek et al., 1992).

Much attention has been paid to the posterior fossa and cerebellar vermis since the initial report of smaller 2D areas of vermal lobules VI and VII in AD (Courchesne et al., 1988), a finding also replicated in a larger cohort that included the original 1988 subjects (Courchesne, 1994a). The authors felt that these findings represented a consistent anatomic abnormality in most autistic subjects, and believed that they might be responsible for the characteristic behavioral deficits. However, eight subsequent studies (Garber & Rittvo, 1992; Filipek et al., 1992; Hashimoto, 1992a, 1993a, 1993b; Holttum et al., 1992; Kleinman et al., 1992; Piven et al., 1992), using similar techniques, reported finding no differences in area measures of vermal lobules VI and VII in a total of 111 male and 21 female autistic subjects collectively aged 2 to 53 years old.

Subsequently, two apparent subtypes of vermal lobules VI and VII sizes in AD was reported: 86% with hypoplasia and 7% with hyperplasia (Courchesne et al., 1994a), the combination of which produced the apparently normal mean vermal areas noted in the other studies (Filipek et al., 1992; Garber & Rittvo, 1992; Holttum et al., 1992; Kleinman et al., 1992; Piven et al., 1992). To test this hypothesis further, the investigators (Courchesne, 1994) statistically reanalyzed the measures of vermal lobules VI and VII from their two previous studies (Courchesne et al., 1988, 1994a), plus two of the discordant studies (Kleinman et al., 1992; Piven et al., 1992). The collective vermis area measures were statistically smaller when compared with the normal controls used in three of the autism studies (Courchesne, 1988, 1994a; Piven et al., 1992) and a fourth study composed of only normal volunteers (Raz et al., 1992). A bimodal distribution across the collective autistic subjects was also noted: 87% with vermal hypoplasia and 13% with vermal hyperplasia, which correlated highly with "verbal or social intelligence" (Courchesne, 1994b p. 220).

In contrast to their previous findings, another imaging group recently reported that *all* the cerebellar vermal lobules (not just VI and VII) were significantly smaller in area in 102 AD subjects aged 3 months to 20 years (Hashimoto et al., 1995). However, the majority of the childhood controls were *medical* controls imaged by medical necessary, rather than normal children, and therefore were not IQ matched to the AD cohort (IQ = 60 ± 25). This further implicates IQ as contributing to size of vermal lobules VI and VII (Piven & Arndi, 1995) and supports the need for IQ-matched subjects and controls in morphometric analyses (Filipek, 1995).

Normal cerebellar hemisphere sulcal widths and the absence of cerebellar atrophy have been noted, in accord with the gross neuropathologic findings (Murakami et al., 1989; Rumsey et al., 1988). Smaller cerebellar hemispheres have been reported in AD by 2D area measures on MRI (Gaffney, 1987; Gaffney, Tsai, Kuperman & Minchin Murakami et al., 1989). However, it cannot yet be concluded that the smaller cerebellar hemisphere areas reported in these studies are indicative of generalized cerebellar hypoplasia in autism. The brain stem has also been a focus of numerous conflicting neuroimaging studies attempting to identify correlates of potential functional disturbances in autistic subjects (Courchesne et al., 1985; Ornitz et al., 1985). These studies used variably matched control groups and differing MRI methods and suggest potential dependence of these measures on IQ (Gaffney et al., 1988; Hashimoto et al., 1991, 1992a, 1992b, 1993a, 1993b, 1995; Hsu et al., 1991). Therefore, no definitive conclusions can be drawn concerning the presence of midbrain, pontine, or medullary structural anomalies by MRI as being characteristic in autism.

Unresolved issues persist concerning differing imaging and study methods and the matching of autistic and control subjects for age, IQ, handedness, and socioeconomic status. To date, all of the neuropathologic abnormalities in the cerebellum have been noted only by microscopic analyses. Therefore, the jury is still out concerning the presence of characteristic cerebellar structural anomalies, as visualized by neuroimaging studies, in all subjects with autism. The interested reader is referred to a recent review for further details (Filipek, 1995b).

Developmental Language Disorders

Developmental Language Disorders (DLD), also called *Specific Language Impairment,* refer to the inadequate acquisition of one or more aspects of language despite adequate hearing, sensorimotor, and cognitive skills (Table 14-3) (Allen, 1989; Rapin, 1996; Rapin & Allen, 1987; Tuchman et al., 1991). This developmental disorder should be considered as distinct from *language delay,* a term that should be reserved for those children who demonstrate a simple delay resulting from chronic ear infections, which resolves (with or without speech and language therapy) once tympanostomy tubes are placed.

Neuropathological Findings in Developmental Language Disorders. Very few postmortem studies have been performed in patients with developmental language disorders. In a young boy with probable verbal auditory agnosia, which is analogous to word deafness in adults (Rapin & Allen, 1987), Landau and colleagues (1960) originally reported bilateral perisylvian cystic lesions with surrounding cortical dys-

Table 14-3. Diagnostic Criteria for Communication Disorders
(Developmental Language Disorders)

A. The scores obtained from a battery of standardized, individually administered tests of receptive
and/or expressive language development are substantially below those obtained on standardized
tests of nonverbal intellectual capacity. Symptoms of both receptive (difficulty understanding
words, sentences, or specific types of words) and expressive (markedly limited vocabulary, errors
in tense, difficulty recalling words or producing sentences with developmentally appropriate
length or complexity) deficits may be present (Mixed Receptive-Expressive Language Disorder),
or only expressive deficits may occur (Expressive Language Disorder).
B. The difficulties with receptive and/or expressive language significantly interfere with academic
or occupational achievement or with social communication.
C. Criteria are not met for a Pervasive Developmental Disorder.
D. If Mental Retardation, a speech-motor or sensory deficit, or environmental deprivation is present,
the language difficulties are in excess of those usually associated with these problems.

Source: Adapted from American Psychiatric Association (1994), pp. 58, 60.

plasias. In a 7-year-old girl with developmental dysphasia, Cohen and colleagues
(1989) found a single dysplastic microgyrus in the left insular cortex.

Anatomic Magnetic Resonance Imaging Studies in Developmental Language Disorders. Neuroimaging studies have reported few additional anomalies, including
lesions in the left inferomedial temporal and left anterior temporal regions (Hier
& Rosenberger, 1980), bilateral encephalomalacia adjacent to caudate nuclei and
isolated white matter "bright spots" (Jernigan et al., 1991), and atypical perisylvian
gyral configurations in a set of twins (Plante et al., 1989). Recently, a less common
sylvian fissure morphology was found to occur more frequently in both hemispheres
of ten children with DLD, their parents, and their siblings (Jackson & Plante, 1996;
Plante et al., 1991).

Several groups of investigators have measured MRI-based en bloc hemispheric
brain regions in language-disordered children. The right perisylvian regions have
been noted to be larger in some children with DLD (Plante et al., 1991), and the
left perisylvian regions have been reported to be either smaller (Jernigan et al.,
1991) or similar in volume (Plante et al., 1991) to the controls. In only right-handed
subjects, both posterior perisylvian language areas were reduced in volume (Jernigan et al., 1991). In addition, the right diencephalic (thalamic) volume was smaller
in the combined cohort, whereas the volumes of both caudate nuclei were reduced
in only the right-handed subjects (Jernigan et al., 1991). The corpus callosum in
children with DLD has also be found to be similar to that of controls but significantly larger in area in the familial cases (Njiokiktjien et al., 1994).

*Morphometric Analysis in a Mixed Autistic Disorder and Developmental Language
Disorder Cohort.* Magnetic resonance imaging–based morphometry was performed on developmentally disordered school-age children diagnosed with AD (by
DSM III-R criteria; DSM III-R, 1987), developmental language disorder, or non-autistic, low IQ as preschoolers. The normal control children had headaches or

Table 14-4. Characteristics of Subjects with Autistic Disorder, Developmental Language Disorder, and Nonautistic Low IQ

Subjects	NVIQ Criteria[a]	N	NVIQ	Males/Females	Mean Age ± SD
High AD	≥80	13	98 ± 17^b	11/2	9.3 ± 1.0
Low AD	<80	16	49 ± 19^c	14/2	8.8 ± 1.6
DLD	≥80	25	101 ± 23^b	17/8	8.1 ± 1.6^d
NALIQ	<80	9	42 ± 26^c	4/5	8.1 ± 2.2
Controls	—	30	—	15/15	9.1 ± 1.2

NALIQ, Nonautistic, low IQ.

[a]Based on the traditional nonverbal IQ (NVIQ) criteria for DLD in preschoolers (Aram, 1992).

[b,c]No group differences in NVIQ.

[d]Group difference in age ($p < .01$).

Source: Data from Filipek (1992).

were volunteers with normal histories, examination findings, and school achievement. See Table 14-4 for characteristics of the cohort.

Anatomic segmentation was performed on specifically adapted coronal MRI scans to extract individual structures using algorithms that have been described in detail elsewhere (Caviness et al., 1996; Filipek, 1989, 1991, 1992, 1994, 1997; Kennedy & Nelson, 1987; Kennedy et al., 1987). Subsequently, *hemispheric regions* (Filipek et al., 1992, 1997) were defined for additional morphometric analyses. *Precallosal* (prefrontal) and *retrocallosal* (posterior parietal/occipital) *regions* included those coronal slices anterior and posterior to the corpus callosum, respectively. The *pericallosal regions* included the coronal slices surrounding the corpus callosum in continuum, and were divided into *anterior pericallosal* (frontal/anterior temporal, anterior to the anterior commissure) and *posterior pericallosal regions* (anterior parietal/posterior temporal, including and posterior to the anterior commissure). The anterior and posterior pericallosal regions were further divided into *superior, inferior,* and *temporal pericallosal* sections by hand-drawn lines connecting the sylvian fissure, superior circular insular sulcus, and superolateral lateral ventricle, and the sylvian fissure, inferior circular insular sulcus, and optic tract/amygdala/hippocampus. (Specific details of the hemispheric regions can be found in Filipek et al., 1997). For clarity in this discussion, the hemispheric regions will be referred to primarily by their lobar names, e.g., *prefrontal* (*precallosal*).

Cerebral hemispheres in both AD and DLD were larger in volume than in the normal controls, as a result of larger volumes of diencephalon and white matter, with a corpus callosum that was similar in size to that of the normal controls. In the subjects with both AD and DLD, the volumes of the hippocampus (in accord with M.L. Bauman, personal communication, and Saitoh, 1995), amygdala, and ventricular system were similar to those of the normal controls. In contrast, all nonautistic, low IQ (NALIQ) structures were smaller than those of controls except for the hippocampus and, surprisingly, the ventricular system.

In both high and low AD, the larger hemispheric volumes were due to dispro-portionately larger volumes of white matter in the anterior and posterior temporal hemispheric regions (which include the primary auditory and auditory association cortices) and, in high AD, to the prefrontal and posterior parietal-occipital regions (which includes the parietal association regions). In the children with DLD, who have language deficits similar to those of children with AD, the larger white matter volumes also localized to the anterior and posterior temporal and posterior parietal-occipital hemispheric regions, as seen in the children with high AD. In contrast, despite significantly smaller hemispheric volumes, children with NALIQ had rela-tively preserved prefrontal, temporal and parietal association regions, which differed considerably from those with the high and low AD volumetric profile.

In the children with AD, the volumes of the cerebellar hemispheres and areas of vermal lobules I–V were larger than those of the controls, while the areas of lobules VI and VII were similar to those of controls. There was no evidence of a bimodal distribution of vermal area measures in this AD cohort, as suggested by Courchesne et al. (1994a) as the cause of apparently normal mean areas of vermal lobules VI and VII.

Reading Disorder or Developmental Dyslexia: Too Little of a Good Thing?

The term *reading disorder* (RD) refers to a disorder of accuracy, speed, or com-prehension of the written word, independent of age, intelligence, education, and any sensory deficits (Table 14-5). It is a common developmental disorder in which the development of reading and spelling skills is disrupted, usually by an underlying phonological deficit (Shaywitz et al., 1995). Reading disorder affects approximately 5% of the population and is almost equally prevalent in males and females, with a gender ratio (M:F) of around 1.52 (Shaywitz et al., 1990; Wadsworth et al., 1992). Genetic influences have been documented in the etiology of RD (Pennington, 1995), and RD has been linked to genetic markers on the short arm of chromosome 6 (Cardon et al., 1994). More recently, two distinct RD phenotypes, reflecting dif-ferent levels in the hierarchy of reading skills, have been linked to two different chromosomes: phonological awareness to chromosome 6 and single-word reading

Table 14-5. Diagnostic Criteria for Reading Disorder

A. Reading achievment, as measured by individually administered standardized tests of reading accuracy or comprehension, is substantially below that expected given the person's chronological age, measured intelligence, and age-appropriate education.

B. The disturbance in Criterion A significantly interferes with academic achievement or activities of daily living that require reading skills.

C. If a sensory deficit is present, the reading difficulties are in excess of those usually associated with it.

Source: Adapted from American Psychiatric Association (1994), p. 50.

to chromosome 15 (Grigorenko et al., 1997). However, we know less about the neuroanatomical basis for RD than we do about its genetics.

Neuropathological Findings in Reading Disorder

Galaburda et al. (1985) and Humphreys et al. (1990) performed the only comprehensive postmortem studies in severe adult dyslexics. They found a very high frequency of microdysgenesis, particularly in the frontal and temporal opercula and more prominent in the left hemisphere than in the right hemisphere. They also measured the planum temporale, a triangular landmark (*not* a distinct structure) located on the superior surface of the temporal lobes just posterior to Heschl's gyrus. In approximately 65% of normal brains, the left planum is larger than the right, while the right is larger than the left ("reversed" asymmetry) in 11%, with the remaining 24% symmetric (Geschwind & Levitsky, 1968). Galaburda et al. (1985) and Humphreys et al. (1990) reported larger areas of the right plana temporale, producing symmetric plana in all the subjects with RD (100% prevalence in this RD sample vs. 24% prevalence in normals). These findings in dyslexic brains suggested anomalous brain development during the late stages of corticogenesis, potentially leading to improved neuronal survival, and subsequent redefinition of cortical architecture underlying asymmetry and cerebral dominance (Galaburda, 1988, 1992).

Anatomic Magnetic Resonance Imaging Studies in Reading Disorder

Areas of the corpus callosum were found to be larger posteriorly (isthmus and splenium) in male subjects with RD (Rumsey et al. 1996) and in the splenium in both male and female RD subjects with a codiagnosis of attention deficit/hyperactivity disorder of (ADHD) (Duara et al., 1991). The female subjects with RD-ADHD also had larger anterior (genu) regions as well (Duara et al., 1991). Male subjects with RD have been reported to have larger posterior regions (isthmus and splenium). In contrast, the corpus callosum has been reported to be similar in total area (Larsen et al., 1992), and to be smaller anteriorly (genu) relative to that of normal controls (Hynd et al., 1995) in some subjects with RD. Each of these studies used a different method to define callosal subregions. The interested reader is referred to Filipek (1995) for a review of this topic.

The insula was shorter bilaterally in RD (Hynd et al., 1990), which may be associated with the decreased glucose use noted in these subjects during reading tasks (Gross-Glenn et al., 1991). The surface area of the temporal lobe was smaller posteriorly and superiorly in the left hemisphere in RD (Kushch, et al., 1993). This produced symmetric surface area measures that correlated inversely with reading comprehension abilities in this cohort.

Although the planum temporale does not have clearly defined boundaries (Filipek et al., 1992, 1995a; Galaburda, 1988, Galaburda, 1993), it nevertheless is the most prevalent landmark in neuroanatomical studies of RD, both in vivo and in vitro. Sometimes even on postmortem examination (Galaburda, 1988), and def-

Table 14-6. The Planum Temporale in Reading Disorders

Authors	Measurement	Finding	Lateralization
Galaburda (1988)	Surface area	Symmetry	Larger right
Hynd et al. (1990)	Length	Right ≥ left	Shorter left
Larsen et al. (1990)	Length	Symmetry	Longer right
Leonard et al. (1993)	Length, temporal/parietal banks	—	—
Schultz et al. (1994)	Convolutional surface area, including temporal/parietal banks	Left > right	Normal pattern

initely on MRI (Filipek, et al., 1995, 1996), accurate identification of the planum boundaries is extremely difficult. This structural ambiguity has led to neuroimaging measurements of only unidimensional lengths, to the creation of often discrepant criteria for plana boundaries, or to the avoidance of this landmark altogether (Jernigan et al., 1991). Therefore, despite its popularity, direct comparisons cannot be made at present across the published studies of the plana temporale in dyslexia (Hynd et al., 1990; Larsen et al., 1990; Leonard et al. 1993; Schultz et al., 1994), which are summarized in Table 14-6 (Filipek, 1995a).

Morphometric Analyses in Dyslexic Twins

Full MRI-based morphometric analyses were performed on the brains of monozygotic and dizygotic twin pairs with RD (Filipek et al., 1995). Significantly smaller volumes were seen in for female subjects with RD in the amygdala, frontal (anterior-superior), and posterior parietal-occipital (retrocallosal) cortices and, for male subjects with RD, in the insula, diencephalon, and smaller areas of the corpus callosum, implicating both cortical and subcortical systems, respectively. Significantly greater monozygotic than dizygotic correlations were noted for all structures except for frontal (anterior-superior) cortex and amygdala, suggesting a genetic influence, whereas greater dizygotic than monozygotic correlations were noted for the frontal (anterior-superior) cortex and insula, suggesting shared environmental influences on these structures (Table 14-7).

Attention Deficit/Hyperactivity Disorder: Too Little of a Good Thing Too?

Historical Perspective

The concept of attention-deficit/hyperactivity disorder (American Psychiatric Association, 1994) as a distinct disorder evolved considerably in the twentieth century. Initially described in 1902 as a "defect in moral control" (Still, 1902), it was later called *minimal brain damage* (Tredgold, 1908) and then *minimal brain dysfunction* (*MBD*) (Bax & MacKeith, 1963). With the appearance of DSM-III (1980), the formal diagnostic term was changed to *attention deficit disorder +/− hyperactivity,*

Table 14-7. Reading Disordered Twin Study

	RD	Controls
Total N	55	17
Monozygotic twins	28	6
Singletons	5	2
Dizygotic twins	14	8
Singletons	8	1
Gender	27 M/28 F	8 M/9 F
Age (years)	18.6 ± 4.0	17.7 ± 2.6
Full-scale IQ[a]	99.2 ± 9.3	120.8 ± 8.2
DISCR[a,b]	-1.22 ± 0.57	2.4 ± 0.66
Handedness[c]	1.16 ± 0.24	1.07 ± 9.12

[a]$p < 0.001$

[b]DISCR, discriminant weights analysis of the Peabody Individual Achievement Test scores of Reading Recongnition, Reading Comprehension, and Spelling (Dunn, 1970).

[c]Range, 1.0 (right-handed) to 2.0 (left-handed).

which focused for the first time on the attentional aspects of the disorder (Douglas, 1972). In the subsequent revision, DSM-III-R (1987) named it *attention-deficit/hyperactivity disorder (ADHD)*, so that the hyperactive symptomatology received greater emphasis. This was retained in DSM-IV (1994) with the addition of three clinical subtypes: predominantly hyperactive-impulsive, predominantly inattentive, and combined types (Table 14-8). An informative review of the historical perspectives can be found in Sandberg and Barton (1996).

Fronto-Striatal and Posterior Dysfunction in Attention Deficit/Hyperactivity Disorder

Attention deficit/hyperactivity disorder, a developmental disorder without related lesions, consists of variable degrees of hyperactivity, impulsivity, and inattention. (Barkley et al., 1990; Clements & Peters, 1962; Fletcher et al., 1994; Hynd et al., 1991; Lahey et al., 1994; Shaywitz et al., 1994.) Recent studies have implicated the caudate and frontal regions in the associated deficits of sustained attention to tasks (Chelune et al., 1986; Grodzinsky & Diamond, 1992; Hellman et al., 1991; Voeller, 1991). Chronic low-dose N-methyl-4-phenyl-A,2,3,6-tetrahydropyridine (MPTP) administration in monkeys results in cognitive dysfunction on tasks related to the frontostriatal circuits and behaviors similar to those in children with ADHD, such as delayed response, impersistence, frustration, need for redirection, restlessness, and fidgeting (Roeltgen & Schneider, 1991). Postmortem studies in these monkeys noted depleted dopamine and norepinephrine in the head of the caudate and norepinephrine in the prefrontal, frontal, and inferior temporal cortical regions (Roeltgen & Schneider, 1991; Schneider, 1990).

Table 14-8. Diagnostic Criteria for Attention Deficit/Hyperactivity Disorder

A. Six or more of the following symptoms of *either (A1) Inattention* or *(A2) Hyperactivity-Impulsivity* that have persisted for at least 6 months to a degree that is maladaptive and inconsistent with developmental level:

(1) Inattention	• Fails to pay attention to details or makes careless mistakes
	• Has difficulty sustaining attention
	• Does not seem to listen
	• Fails to complete tasks (without being oppositional)
	• Has difficulty organizing activities
	• Becomes bored easily
	• Often loses things
	• Is easily distracted or forgetful
(2) Hyperactivity	• Fidgets
	• Acts as if "driven by a motor"
	• Runs about or climbs excessively
	• Has difficulty playing quietly
	• Often talks excessively
	• Is unable to remain seated
Impulsivitiy	• Blurts out answers before the questions are complete
	• Has difficulty awaiting turn
	• Interrupts or intrudes on others

B. Some hyperactive or inattentive symptoms were present before 7 years of age.

C. Some impairment from the symptoms is present in two or more settings, such as at school or work and at home.

D. There must be clear evidence of clinically significant impairment in social, academic, or occupational functioning.

E. The symptoms do not occur within the course of a Pervasive Developmental Disorder, Schizophrenia, or other Psychotic Disorder or other mental disorder (e.g., Mood Disorder, Anxiety Disorder).

Attention Deficit/Hyperactivity Disorder, Combined Type
if Criteria A(1) and A(2) are both met

Attention Deficit/Hyperactivity Disorder, Predominantly Inattentive Type
if Criterion A(1) is met but Criterion A(2) is not met

Attention Deficit/Hyperactivity Disorder, Predominantly Hyperactive-Impulsive Type
if Criterion A(2) is met but Criterion A(1) is not met

Source: Adapted from American Psychiatric Association (1994), pp. 83–85.

Recent neural network theories of attention (Mesulam, 1990; Morecraft et al., 1993; Posner, 1990; Posner & Raichle, 1997) implicate parallel processing of both anterior (frontostriatal and executive) and posterior regions based on lesion and functional imaging studies in adults (Corbetta et al., 1993; Petersen et al., 1994). Specifically, Posner et al (1990, 1994) have postulated three attentional networks:

• The Alerting (vigilance) Network, localized to the right lateral prefrontal lobe, especially the superior region of Brodmann area 6, permits maintenance of the alert state.

- The Executive Network, localized to the anterior cingulate and basal ganglia, detects an object and brings it into conscious awareness.
- The Orienting (selective) Network, localized to both superior parietal lobules, thalamus, and midbrain, disengages and reorients attention to new targets.

Structural Neuroimaging (Anatomic Magnetic Resonance Imaging) in Attention Deficit/Hyperactivity Disorder

It currently appears that the cerebral hemispheres may be smaller in subjects with ADHD than in normal controls. Two-dimensional (2D) hemispheric area on a single selected MRI slice (Hynd et al., 1990) and volumes computed from three-dimensional (3D) MRI scans (Castellanos et al., 1996; Filipek et al., 1997) were approximately 5% smaller in the subjects with ADHD. In addition, the right frontal lobe was smaller in some subjects with ADHD on measurement of both 2D widths of the frontal lobe (Hynd et al., 1990) and 3D volumes of the prefrontal regions (Castellanos et al., 1996). However, despite being measured in essentially the same manner on the MRI scans, some ADHD subjects had a right frontal region that essentially paralleled that of the normal controls (right prefrontal $p = .86$; left prefrontal $p = .93$). These differences are probably due to differences in the ADHD cohorts rather than in the MRI morphometric methods.

Anatomic magnetic resonance imaging studies have found differences, albeit discordant, in the volume and asymmetry of the caudate in ADHD children and adolescents. The left caudate was smaller than the right in some studies (Filipek et al., 1997; Hynd et al., 1993), the right caudate was smaller in other studies (Castellanos et al., 1994, 1996), and both caudates were normal in yet another study (Aylward et al., 1996). However, the definition of what was included as "caudate" in each of these studies differs and is probably responsible for the discordant findings. The globus pallidus was also smaller in some ADHD boys, most predominantly on the left (Aylward et al., 1996) or right (Castellanos et al., 1996) side. Most recently, Casey et al. (1997a) reported that measures of response inhibition (sensory selection, response selection, and response execution tasks) correlated significantly with the volumetric measures of the right prefrontal region, right caudate, and left globus pallidus (Castellanos et al., 1996).

Smaller areas of the corpus callosum have also been reported in some ADHD children and adolescents, including smaller areas of the genu (Hynd, 1991b) and splenium (Hynd, 1991b; Semrud-Clikeman et al., 1994). The rostrum, genu, rostral body, and anterior midbody were also smaller, but not significantly so, in some of the ADHD subjects (Semrud-Clikeman et al., 1994). Those ADHD subjects who did not respond favorably to stimulant medication had the smallest splenial measures, so that for the first time a potential medication response effect was noted (Semrud-Clikeman et al., 1994). The anterior rostrum and rostral body, but not the genu or splenium, were also smaller in another ADHD cohort (Giedd et al., 1994). In addition, the rostral body areas (serving the premotor and supplementary motor cortical regions (Witelson, 1989) correlated negatively with impulsivity/hyperactivity scores from the Connors questionnaires (Goyette et al., 1978). These discordant findings are most likely due to significantly different methods used by each of the studies, which are reviewed in Filipek, 1995.

Anatomic Magnetic Resonance Imaging and Attentional Networks in Attention Deficit/Hyperactivity Disorder

On the basis of the cognitive models noted above, Filipek et al. (1997) analyzed hemispheric and structural volumes by MRI-based morphometry in a carefully diagnosed yet small cohort of 15 teenage boys with "pure" ADHD (without comorbid diagnoses). These subjects had received medication for at least 6 months prior to the study and were felt to be responding favorably at the time of the MRI scan. Five of the subjects had not previously responded favorably to stimulant medication (methylphenidate or dextroamphetamine) but responded favorably to other nonstimulant psychopharmacologic regimens. The MRI scans were analyzed as previously described for the AD and DLD cohorts.

Localized hemispheric developmental anomalies were noted in the ADHD subjects compared with the normal control subjects. Specifically, the ADHD subjects had smaller en bloc and white matter (but not cortex) volumes of the right frontal (anterior-superior) hemispheric region, smaller en bloc volumes of the bilateral peri-basal ganglia (anterior-inferior) hemispheric regions, and smaller white matter volumes of the bilateral posterior parietal-occipital (retrocallosal) hemispheric regions, as well as smaller left caudate and caudate head volumes (Table 14-9). The remainder of the measures were similar in the ADHD and control subjects.

The smaller caudate and retrocallosal region white matter volumes may be differentially related to the clinical response to stimulant medication. The stimulant responders had the smallest, symmetric caudate volumes and the smallest left anterior-superior (frontal) cortex volumes, while the non-responders had reversed caudate asymmetry and the smallest retrocallosal (parietal-occipital) white matter volumes. The finding of similar ventricular volumes in this ADHD cohort without enlarged external cerebrospinal fluid spaces indicates that the underlying pathophysiology is the result of a neurodevelopmental process that alters the neural system configuration in children with ADHD, particularly in the right hemisphere, rather than causing cerebral degeneration or atrophy.

The right frontal (anterior-superior) hemispheric region includes structures implicated in two of the three attentional networks: the right posterior prefrontal cortex, motor association area, including Brodmann area 6 (the *alerting network),* and the midanterior cingulate *(executive attention network).* In addition, the caudate is implicated in the *executive attention network* (Mesulam, 1990; Posner & Petersen, 1990, Posner & Raichle, 1997). The smaller right frontal (anterior-superior) en bloc and white matter, bilateral peribasal ganglia (anterior-inferior) en bloc, and left caudate volumes noted in ADHD may represent the structural correlate of compromised function of the right frontal-striatal circuits implicated in both the alerting and executive attention networks (Posner & Raichle, 1997). These anomalies are concordant with those found in previous lesion studies in adults or experimental animals Chelune et al., 1986; Grodzinsky & Diamond, 1992; Iversen, 1977); with

Table 14-9. Selected Brain and Hemisphere Regional Volumes in Attention Deficit/
Hyperactivity Disorder

	ADHD (Right)	ADHD (Left)	Control (Right)	Control (Left)
Global Measures (cm³)				
Cerebral hemispheres	627.9 ± 47.4	625.1 ± 46.9	659.4 ± 47.1	653.5 ± 46.0
Total caudatte[b]	5.1 ± 0.9	5.05 ± 0.9[a]	5.6 ± 0.9	5.7 ± 0.8
Caudate head[b]	3.8 ± 0.6	3.7 ± 0.6[b]	4.1 ± 0.6	4.3 ± 0.7
Hemispheric Regions (cm³)				
En bloc frontal (anterior- superior) region[a]	64.9 ± 9.0[b]	63.4 ± 9.2	73.6 ± 11.8	71.2 ± 11.9
Frontal (anterior-superior) white matter[c]	26.1 ± 3.7[d]	23.9 ± 3.4	31.3 ± 6.4	27.1 ± 5.2
En bloc peribasal ganglia (anterior-inferior) region[b]	31.5 ± 4.5[c]	31.4 ± 4.0[a]	34.9 ± 3.8	34.4 ± 3.6

Posterior parietal-occipital
    (retrocallosal) white
    matter[c]
	61.6 ± 12.7[c]	58.7 ± 11.4[b]	70.9 ± 8.9	67.8 ± 9.1

Asymmetry Coefficients				
Total caudate[c]	-0.020 ± 0.06		0.024 ± 0.03	
Caudate head[b]	-0.023 ± 0.06		0.026 ± 0.05	
En bloc frontal (anterior- superior) region[b]	-0.09 ± 0.05		-0.14 ± 0.08	
En bloc posterior parietal- occipital (retrocallosal) region	0.03 ± 0.04		0.04 ± 0.06	

Notes:

All values reported as group means $\pm$ standard deviation.

All posthoc comparisons used Scheffe's method to maintain $\alpha = 0.05$.

[a]$p < 0.04$.

[b]$p < 0.03$.

[c]$p < 0.02$.

[d]$p < 0.01$.

Source: Adapted from Filipek (1997).

the known extensive corticostriatal-thalamic interconnections (Alexander et al., 1986; Goldman-Rakic, 1987, 1988); with the role of dopamine and the caudate in ADHD (Heilman et al., 1991; Roeltgen & Schneider, 1991; Voeller, 1991a); and with the normal development of attentional constructs in children (Casey et al., 1997b). Anomalous development of fiber connections between these regions may produce compromised but not total lack of function (Alexander et al., 1986; Goldman-Rakic, 1987, 1988). Interestingly, the anterior regions of the corpus callosum, corresponding to the prefrontal/premotor/supplementary motor/frontal motor cortices (Witelson, 1989) were smaller, but not significantly so, in these subjects with ADHD relative to the normal controls (Semrud-Clikeman et al., 1994).

The bilaterally smaller white matter volumes in ADHD in the retrocallosal regions were very interesting, as this finding also implicates the *orienting network* (Posner & Raichle, 1997). Neuropsychological deficits of the posterior attentional systems have not been demonstrated by some investigators (Bloomingdale & Swanson, 1989; Shaywitz et al., 1994; Swanson et al., 1991; Sergeant & Scholten, 1983; Taylor, 1986; van der Meere & Sergeant, 1988) but have been noted by others (e.g., Heilman et al., 1991; Posner, 1997; Voeller, 1991b). The smaller white matter volumes are concordant with the findings of smaller area measures of the splenium of the corpus callosum in two previous studies of children and adolescents with ADHD (Hynd et al., 1991b; Semfud-Clikeman et al., 1994). Fewer ipsilateral and reciprocal contralateral interconnections between the posterior parietal-occipital regions of the brain may result in less activation in the frontal regions (Cavada & Goldman-Rakic, 1989a, 1989b; Graziano et al., 1994; Jones & Powell, 1970; Mesulam, 1990, 1994; Morecraft et al., 1993).

Since the arbitrary frontal (anterior-superior) hemispheric region applied in the present analyses includes not only the posterior prefrontal and midanterior cingulate cortices, but also the anterior primary motor, motor association, and supplementary motor cortices, this region encompasses multiple neural systems that subserve both attentional and motoric symptoms, which cannot be differentiated by the present analyses. Regardless, the results noted in this study, however preliminary, support the conceptual framework of anomalous neural systems in ADHD, with the possibility of differential morphologic substrates based predominantly on hyperactive/impulsive versus inattentive symptoms.

In summary, the MRI-based findings in ADHD have not been consistent across studies, but taken together these studies indicate that persons with ADHD have, at minimum, frontostriatal developmental anomalies when compared with non-ADHD control subjects. These collective studies provide support for the further investigation of frontostriatal, executive/cingulate, and posterior parietal brain–behavior correlations in ADHD using functional and structural neuroimaging techniques.

ACKNOWLEDGMENTS

This work was supported in part by HD 27802 and HD 28202 from the National Institute of Child Health and Human Development and by NS 35896 from the National Institute of Neurological Disorders and Stroke, National Institutes of Health, Bethesda, Maryland.

References

Alexander, G.E., DeLong, M.R., and Strick, P.L. (1986) Parallel organization of functionally segregated circuits linking basal ganglia and cortex. *Annual Review of Neuroscience,* 9:357–381.

Allen, D.A. (1989) Developmental language disorders in preschool children: Clinical subtypes and syndromes. *School Psychology Review,* 18:442–451.

American Psychiatric Association. (1980) *Diagnostic and Statistical Manual of Mental Disorders,* 3rd ed. Washington, DC: American Psychiatric Association.

American Psychiatric Association. (1987) *Diagnostic and Statistical Manual of Mental Disorders,* 3rd ed. rev. Washington, DC: American Psychiatric Association.

American Psychiatric Association. (1994) *Diagnostic and Statistical Manual of Mental Disorders,* 4th ed. Washington, DC: American Psychiatric Association.

Aram, D.M., Morris, R., and Hall, N.E. (1992) The validity of discrepancy criteria for identifying children with developmental language disorders. *Journal of Learning Disabilities,* 25:549–554.

Arin, D.M., Bauman, M.L., and Kemper, T.L. (1991) The distribution of Purkinje cell loss in the cerebellum in autism. *Neurology,* 41(Suppl 1):307.

Aylward, E.H., Reiss, A.L., Reader, M.J., Singer, H.S., Brown, J.E., and Denckla, M.B. (1996) Basal ganglia volumes in children with attention-deficit hyperactivity disorder. *Journal of Child Neurology,* 11:112–115.

Bailey, A., Luthert, P., Bolton, P., Le Couteur, A., Rutter, M., and Harding, B. (1993) Autism and megalencephaly. *Lancet,* 341:1225–1226.

Barkley, R.A., DuPaul, G.J., and McMurray, M.B. (1990) A comprehensive evaluation of attention deficit disorder with and without hyperactivity as defined by research criteria. *Journal of Consulting and Clinical Psychology,* 58:775–789.

Bauman, M.L. (1991) Microscopic neuroanatomic abnormalities in autism. *Pediatrics,* 87:791-796.

Bauman, M.L., and Kemper, T.L. (1985) Histoanatomic observations of the brain in early infantile autism. *Neurology,* 35:866–874.

Bauman, M.L., and Kemper, T.L. (1990) Limbic and cerebellar abnormalities are also present in an autistic child of normal intelligence [abstract]. *Neurology,* 40(Suppl 1):359.

Bauman, M.L., and Kemper, T.L. (1994) Neuroanatomic observations of the brain in autism. In M.L. Bauman and T.L. Kemper (eds.), *The Neurobiology of Autism* Baltimore: Johns Hopkins University Press, pp. 119–145.

Bax, M.C.O., and MacKeith, R.C. (1963) Minimal brain damage—a concept discarded. In R.C. MacKeith and M.C.O. Bax (eds.), *Minimal Cerebral Dysfunction. Little Club Clinics in Developmental Medicine, No. 10.* London: Heinemann.

Belmonte, M., Egaas, B., Townsend, J., and Courchesne, E. (1995) NMR intensity of corpus callosum differs with age but not with diagnosis of autism. *NeuroReport,* 6:1253–1256.

Berthier, M.L. (1994) Corticocallosal anomalies in Asperger's syndrome [letter]. *American Journal of Roentgenology,* 162:236–237.

Berthier, M.L., Starkstein, S.E., and Leiguarda, R. (1990) Developmental cortical anomalies in Asperger's syndrome: Neuroradiological findings in two patients. *Journal of Neuropsychiatry and Clinical Neurosciences,* 2:197–201.

Bloomingdale, L.M., and Swanson, J.M. (1989) *Attention Deficit Disorder: Current Concepts and Emerging Trends in Attentional and Behavioral Disorders of Childhood.* New York: Pergamon Press.

Campbell, M., Rosenbloom, S., Perry, R., George, A., Kricheff, I., Anderson, L., Small, A., and Jennings, S. (1982) Computerized axial tomography in young austistic children. *American Journal of Psychiatry,* 139:510–512.

Caparulo, B.K., Cohen, D.J., Rothman, S.L., Young, J.G., Katz, J.D., Shaywitz, S.E., and Shaywitz, B.A. (1981) Computed tomographic brain scanning in children with developmental neuropsychiatric disorders. *Journal of the American Academy of Child and Adolescent Psychiatry,* 20:338–257.

Cardon, L.R., Smith, S.D., Fulker, D.W., Kimberling, W.J., Pennington, B.F., and DeFries, J.C. (1994) Quantitative trait locus for reading disability on chromosome 6. *Science,* 266:276–279.

Casey, B.J., Castellanos, F.X., Giedd, J.N., Marsh, W.L., Hamburger, S.D., Schubert, A.B., Vauss, Y.C., Vaituzis, A.C., Dickstein, D.P., Sarfatti, S.E., and Rapoport, J.L. (1997a) Implication of right frontostriatal circuitry in response inhibition and attention-deficit/

hyperactivity disorder. *Journal of the American Academy of Child and Adolescent Psychiatry,* 36:374–383.

Casey, B.J., Trainor, R., Giedd, J., Vauss, Y., Vaituzis, C.K., Hamburger, S., Kozuch, P., and Rapoport, J.L. (1997b) The role of the anterior cingulate in automatic and controlled processes: A developmental neuroanatomical study. *Developmental Psychobiology,* 30: 61–69.

Castellanos, F.X., Giedd, J.N., Eckburg, P., Marsh, W.L., Vaituzis, A.C., Kaysen, D., Hamburger, S.D., and Rapoport, J.L. (1994) Quantitative morphology of the caudate nucleus in attention deficit hyperactivity disorder. *American Journal of Psychiatry,* 151:1791–1796.

Castellanos, F.X., Giedd, J.N., Marsh, W.L., Hamburger, S.D., Vaituzis, A.C., Dickstein, D.P., Sarfatti, S.E., Vauss, Y.C., Snell, J.W., Lange, N., Kaysen, D., Krain, A.L., Ritchie, G.F., Rajapakse, J.C., and Rapoport, J.L. (1996) Quantitative brain magnetic resonance imaging in attention-deficit hyperactivity disorder. *Archives of General Psychiatry,* 53:607–616.

Cavada, C., and Goldman-Rakic, P.S. (1989a) Posterior parietal cortex in rhesus monkey: I. Parcellation of areas based on distinctive limbic and sensory corticocortical connections. *Journal of Comparative Neurology,* 287:393–421.

Cavada, C., and Goldman-Rakic, P.S. (1989b) Posterior parietal cortex in rhesus monkey: II. Evidence for segregated corticocortical networks linking sensory and limbic areas with the frontal lobe. *Journal of Comparative Neurology* 287:422–445.

Caviness, V.S., Kennedy, D.N., Richelme, C., Rademacher, J., and Filipek, P.A. (1996) The human brain age 7–11 years. A volumetric analysis based upon magnetic resonance images. *Cerebral Cortex,* 6:726–736.

Chelune, G.J., Ferguson, W., Koon, R., and Dickey, T.O. (1986) Frontal lobe disinhibition in attention deficit disorder. *Child Psychiatry and Human Development, 16:*221–234.

Clements, S.D., and Peters, J.E. (1962) Minimal brain dysfunctions in the school-aged child. *Archives of General Psychiatry,* 6:185–187.

Cohen, M., Campbell, R., and Yaghmai, F. (1989) Neuropathological abnormalities in developmental dysphasia. *Annals of Neurology,* 25:567–570.

Coleman, P.D., Romano, J., Lapham, L., and Simon, W. (1985) Cell counts in cerebral cortex of an autistic patient. *Journal of Autism and Developmental Disorders,* 15:245–255.

Corbetta, M., Miezin, F.M., Shulman, G.L., and Petersen, S.E. (1993) A PET study of visuospatial attention. *Journal of Neuroscience,* 13:1202–1226.

Courchesne, E., Press, G.A., and Yeung-Courchesne, R. (1993) Parietal lobe abnormalities detected with MR in patients with infantile autism. *American Journal of Roentgenology,* 160:387–393.

Courchesne, E., Saitoh, O., Yeung-Courchesne, R., Press, G.A., Lincoln, A.J., Haas, R.H., and Schreibman, L. (1994a) Abnormalities of cerebellar vermian lobules VI and VII in patients with infantile autism: Identification of hypoplastic and hyperplastic subgroups by MR imaging. *American Journal of Roentgenology,* 162:123–130.

Courchesne, E., Townsend, J., and Saitoh, O. (1994b) The brain in infantile autism: Posterior fossa structures are abnormal. *Neurology,* 44:214–223.

Courchesne, E., Yeung-Courchesne, R., Hicks, G., and Lincoln, A. (1985) Functioning of the brainstem auditory pathway in non-retarded autistic individuals. *Electroencephalography and Clinical Neurophysiology,* 61:491–501.

Courchesne, E., Yeung-Courchesne, R., Press, G.A., Hesselink, J.R., and Jernigan, T.L. (1988) Hypoplasia of cerebellar vermal lobules VI and VII in autism. *New England Journal of Medicine,* 318:1349–1354.

Creasey, H., Rumsey, J., Schwartz, M., Duara, R., Rapoport, J., and Rapoport, S. (1986) Brain morphometry in autistic men as measured by volumetric computed tomography. *Archives of Neurology,* 43:669–672.

Damasio, H., and Damasio, A.R. (1989) *Lesion Analysis in Neuropsychology.* New York: Oxford University Press.

Damasio, H., Maurer, R., Damasio, A.R., and Chui, H. (1980) Computerized tomographic scan findings in patients with autistic behavior. *Archives of Neurology,* 37:504–510.

Davidovitch, M., Patterson, B., and Gartside, P. (1996) Head circumference measurements in children with autism. *Journal of Child Neurology,* 11:389–393.

Douglas, V.I. (1972) Stop, look and listen: The problem of sustained attention and impulse control in hyperactive and normal children. *Canadian Journal of Behavioural Science,* 4:259–282.

Duara, R., Kushch, A., Gross-Glenn, K., Barker, W.W., Jallad, B., Pascal, S., Loewenstein, D.A., Sheldon, J., Rabin, M., Levin, B., and Lubs, H. (1991) Neuroanatomic differences between dyslexic and normal readers on magnetic resonance imaging scans. *Archives of Neurology,* 48:410–416.

Dunn, L.M., and Markwardt, F.C. (1970) *Peabody Individual Achievement Test.* Circle Pines, MN: American Guidance Service.

Egaas, B., Courchesne, E., and Saitoh, O. (1995) Reduced size of corpus callosum in autism. *Archives of Neurology,* 52:794–801.

Filipek, P.A. (1995a) Neurobiological correlates of developmental dyslexia—What do we know about how the dyslexics' brains differ from those of normal readers? *Journal of Child Neurology,* 10(Suppl 1):S62–S69.

Filipek, P.A. (1995b) Quantitative magnetic resonance imaging in autism: The cerebellar vermis. *Current Opinion in Neurology,* 8:134–138.

Filipek, P.A. (1996) Structural variations in measures of developmental disorders. In R.W. Thatcher, G.R. Lyon, J. Rumsey, and N. Krasnegor (eds.), *Developmental Neuroimaging: Mapping the Development of Brain and Behavior.* San Diego, CA: Academic Press, pp. 169–186.

Filipek, P.A. (1999) Neuroimaging in the developmental disorders: The state of the science. *Journal of Child Psychology and Psychiatry,* 40:113–128.

Filipek, P.A., Kennedy, D.N., and Caviness, V.S., Jr. (1991) Volumetric analysis of central nervous system neoplasm based on MRI. *Pediatric Neurology,* 7:347–351.

Filipek, P.A., Kennedy, D.N., and Caviness, V.S., Jr. (1992) Neuroimaging in child neuropsychology. In I. Rapin and S. Segalowitz (eds.), *Handbook of Neuropsychology. Volume 6: Child Neuropsychology.* Amsterdam: Elsevier, pp. 301–329.

Filipek, P.A., Kennedy, D.N., Caviness, V.S., Rossnick, S.L., Spraggins, T.A., and Starewicz, P.M. (1989) MRI-based brain morphometry: Development and application to normal subjects. *Annals of Neurology,* 25:61–67.

Filipek, P.A., Pennington, B.F., Holmes, J.F., Lefly, D., Kennedy, D.N., Meyers, J.M., Lang, J.E., Gayan, J., Galaburda, A.M., Simon, J.M., Filley, C.M., Caviness, V.S., and DeFries, J.C. (1995) Developmental dyslexia: Cortical and subcortical anomalies by MRI-based morphometry [abstract]. *Annals of Neurology,* 38:509.

Filipek, P.A., Richelme, C., Kennedy, D.N., and Caviness, V.S. (1994) The young adult human brain: An MRI-based morphometric analysis. *Cerebral Cortex,* 4:344–360.

Filipek, P.A., Richelme, C., Kennedy, D.N., Rademacher, J., Pitcher, D.A., Zidel, S.Y., and Caviness, V.S. (1992b) Morphometric analysis of the brain in developmental language disorders and autism. *Annals of Neurology,* 32:475.

Filipek, P.A., Semrud-Clikeman, M., Steingard, R.J., Renshaw, P.F., Kennedy, D.N., and Biederman, J. (1997) Volumetric MRI analysis comparing attention-deficit hyperactivity disorder and normal controls. *Neurology,* 48:589–601.

Fletcher, J.M., Shaywitz, B.A., and Shaywitz, S.E. (1994) Attention as a process and as a disorder. In G.R. Lyon (ed.), *Frames of References for the Assessment of Learning Disabilities.* New York: Guilford Press, pp. 103–116.

Gaffney, G.R., Kuperman, S., Tsai, L.Y., and Minchin, S. (1988) Morphological evidence for brainstem involvement in infantile autism. *Biological Psychiatry,* 24:578–586.

Gaffney, G.R., Kuperman, S., Tsai, L.Y., and Minchin, S. (1989) Forebrain structure in infantile autism. *Journal of the American Academy of Child and Adolescent Psychiatry,* 28:534–537.

Gaffney, G.R., and Tsai, L.Y. (1987) Brief report: Magnetic resonance imaging of high level autism. *Journal of Autism and Developmental Disorders,* 17:433–438.

Gaffney, G.R., Tsai, L.Y., Kuperman, S., and Minchin, S. (1987) Cerebellar structure in autism. *American Journal of Diseases of Children,* 141:1330–1332.

Galaburda, A.M. (1988) The pathogenesis of childhood dyslexia. *Research Publications—Association for Research in Nervous and Mental Disease,* 66:127–138.

Galaburda, A.M. (1992) Neurology of developmental dyslexia. *Current Opinion in Neurology and Neurosurgery,* 5:71–76.

Galaburda, A.M. (1993) The planum temporale [editorial]. *Archives of Neurology,* 50:457.

Galaburda, A.M., Sherman, G.F., Rosen, G.D., Aboitiz, F., and Geschwind, N. (1985) Developmental dyslexia: Four consecutive patients with cortical anomalies. *Annals of Neurology,* 18:222–233.

Garber, H.J., Ritvo, E.R., Chiu, L.C., Griswold, V.J., Kashanian, A., Freeman, B.J., and Oldendorf, W.H. (1989) A magnetic resonance imaging study of autism: Normal fourth ventricle size and absence of pathology. *American Journal of Psychiatry,* 146:532–534.

Garber, J.H., and Ritvo, E.R. (1992) Magnetic resonance imaging of the posterior fossa in autistic adults. *American Journal of Psychiatry,* 149:245–247.

Geschwind, N., and Levitsky, W. (1968) Human brain: Left-right asymmetry in temporal speech region. *Science,* 161:186–187.

Giedd, J.N., Castellanos, F.X., Casey, B.J., Kozuch, P., King, A.C., Hamburger, S.D., and Rapoport, J.L. (1994) Quantitative morphology of the corpus callosum in attention deficit hyperactivity disorder. *American Journal of Psychiatry,* 151:665–669.

Gillberg, C., and Svendsen, P. (1983) Childhood psychosis and computed tomographic brain scan findings. *Journal of Autism and Developmental Disorders,* 13:19–32.

Goldman-Rakic, P.S. (1987) Development of cortical circuitry and cognitive function. *Child Development,* 58:60–622.

Goldman-Rakic, P.S. (1988) Topography of cognition: Parallel distributed networks in primate association cortex. *Annual Review of Neuroscience,* 11:137–156.

Goyette, C.H., Connors, C.K., and Ulrich, R.F. (1978) Normative data on revised Connors parent and teacher rating scales. *Journal of Abnormal Child Psychology,* 6:221–236.

Graziano, M.S., Yap, G.S., and Gross, C.G. (1994) Coding of visual space by premotor neurons. *Science,* 266:1054–1057.

Grigorenko, E.L., Wood, F.B., Meyer, M.S., Hart, L.A., Speed, W.C., Shuster, A., and Pauls, D.L. (1997) Susceptibility loci for distinct components of developmental dyslexia on chromosomes 6 and 15. *American Journal of Human Genetics,* 60:27–39.

Grodzinsky, G.M., and Diamond, R. (1992) Frontal lobe functioning in boys with attention-deficit hyperactivity disorder. *Developmental Neuropsychology,* 8:427–445.

Gross-Glenn, K., Duara, R., Barker, W.W., Loewenstein, D., Chang, J.Y., Yoshii, F., Apicella, A.M., Pascal, S., Boothe, T., Sevush, S., Jallad, B.J., Novoa, L., and Lubs, H.A. (1991) Positron emission tomographic studies during serial word reading by normal and dyslexic adults. *Journal of Clinical and Experimental Neuropsychology,* 13:531–544.

Hashimoto, T., Murakawa, K., Miyazaki, M., Tayama, M., and Kuroda, Y. (1992a) Magnetic resonance imaging of the brain structures in the posterior fossa in retarded autistic children. *Acta Paediatrica,* 81:1030–1034.

Hashimoto, T., Tayama, M., Miyazaki, M., Murakawa, K., and Kuroda, Y. (1993a) Brainstem and cerebellar vermis involvement in autistic children. *Journal of Child Neurology,* 8:149–153.

Hashimoto, T., Tayama, M., Miyazaki, M., Murakawa, K., Sakurama, N., Yoshimoto, T., and Kuroda, Y. (1991) Reduced midbrain and pons size in children with autism. *Tokushima Journal of Experimental Medicine,* 38:15–18.

Hashimoto, T., Tayama, M., Miyazaki, M., Murakawa, K., Shimakawa, S., Yoneda, Y., and Kuroda, Y. (1993b) Brainstem involvement in high functioning autistic children. *Acta Neurologica Scandinavica,* 88:123–128.

Hashimoto, T., Tayama, M., Miyazaki, M., Sakurama, N., Yoshimiti, T., Murakawa, K., and Kuroda, Y. (1992b) Reduced brainstem size in children with autism. *Brain and Development,* 14:94–97.

Hashimoto, T., Tayama, M., Murakawa, K., Yoshimoto, T., Miyazaki, M., Harada, M., and Kuroda, Y. (1995) Development of the brainstem and cerebellum in autistic patients. *Journal of Autism and Developmental Disorders,* 25:1–18.

Heilman, K.M., and Valenstein, E. (eds.). (1985) *Clinical Neuropsychology.* New York: Oxford University Press.

Heilman, K.M., Voeller, K.K.S., and Nadeau, S.E. (1991) A possible pathophysiological substrate of attention deficit hyperactivity disorder. *Journal of Child Neurology,* 6 (Suppl):S76–S81.

Hier, D.B., and Rosenberger, P.B. (1980) Focal left temporal lobe lesions and delayed speech acquisition. *Developmental and Behavioral Pediatrics,* 1:54–56.

Holttum, J.R., Minshew, N.J., Sanders, R.S., and Phillips, N.E. (1992) Magnetic resonance imaging of the posterior fossa in autism. *Biological Psychiatry,* 32:1091–1101.

Hsu, M., Yeung-Courchesne, R., Courchesne, E., and Press, G.A. (1991) Absence of magnetic resonance imaging evidence of pontine abnormality in infantile autism. *Archives of Neurology,* 48:1160–1163.

Humphreys, P., Kaufmann, W.E., and Galaburda, A.M. (1990) Developmental dyslexia in women: Neuropathological findings in three patients. *Annals of Neuroology,* 28:727–738.

Hynd, G.W., Hall, J., Novey, E.S., Eliopulos, D., Black, K., Gonzalez, J.J., Edmonds, J.E., Riccio, C., and Cohen, M. (1995) Dyslexia and corpus callosum morphology. *Archives of Neurology,* 52:32–38.

Hynd, G.W., Hern, K.L., Novey, E.S., Eliopulos, D., Marshall, R., Gonzalez, J.J., and Voeller, K.K. (1993) Attention deficit-hyperactivity disorder and asymmetry of the caudate nucleus. *Journal of Child Neurology,* 8:339–347.

Hynd, G.W., Lorys, A.R., Semrud-Clikeman, M., Nieves, N., Huettner, M.I.S., and Lahey, B.B. (1991a) Attention-deficit disorder without hyperactivity: A distinct behavioral and neurocognitive syndrome. *Journal of Child Neurology,* 6 (Suppl):S37–S43.

Hynd, G.W., Semrud-Clikeman, M., Lorys, A.R., Novey, E.S., and Eliopulos, D. (1990) Brain morphology in developmental dyslexia and attention deficit disorder/hyperactivity. *Archives of Neurology,* 47:919–926.

Hynd, G.W., Semrud-Clikeman, M., Lorys, A.R., Novey, E.S., Eliopulos, D., and Lyytinen, H. (1991b) Corpus callosum morphology in attention-deficit hyperactivity disorder (ADHD): Morphometric analysis of MRI. *Journal of Learning Disabilities,* 24:141–146.

Iversen, S.D. (1977) Behavior after neostriatal lesions in animals. In I. Divac and R.G.E. Oberg (eds.), *The Neostriatum.* Elmsford, NY: Pergamon Press, pp. 195–210.

Jackson, T., and Plante, E. (1996) Gyral morphology in the posterior Sylvian region in families affected by developmental language disorder. *Neuropsychology Review,* 6: 81–94.

Jernigan, T.L., Hesselink, J.R., Sowell, E., and Tallal, P.A. (1991) Cerebral structure on magnetic resonance imaging in language- and learning-impaired children. *Archives of Neurology,* 48:539–545.

Jones, E.G., and Powell, T.P. (1970) An anatomical study of converging sensory pathways within the cerebral cortex of the monkey. *Brain,* 93:793–820.

Kanner, L. (1943) Autistic disturbances of affective contact. *The Nervous Child,* 2:217–250.

Kennedy, D.N., Filipek, P.A., and Caviness, V.S., Jr. (1989) Anatomic segmentation and volumetric calculations in nuclear magnetic resonance imaging. *IEEE Transactions on Medical Imaging,* TMI-8:1–7.

Kennedy, D.N., and Nelson, A.C. (1987) Three-dimensional display from cross-sectional tomographic images: An application to magnetic resonance imaging. *IEEE Transactions on Medical Imaging,* TMI-6:134–140.

Kleinman, M.D., Neff, S., and Rosman, N.P. (1992) The brain in infantile autism: Are posterior fossa structures abnormal? *Neurology,* 42:753–760.

Kushch, A., Gross-Glenn, K., Jallad, B., Lubs, H., Rapin, M., Feldman, E., and Duara, R. (1993) Temporal lobe surface area measurements on MRI in normal and dyslexic readers. *Neuropsychologia,* 31:811–821.

Lahey, B.B., Applegate, B., McBurnett, K., Biederman, J., Greenhill, L., Hynd, G.W., Barkley, R.A., Newcorn, J., Jensen, P., Richters, J., Garfinkel, B., Kerdyk, L., Frick, P.J., Ollendick, T., Perez, D., Hart, E.L., Waldman, I., and Shaffer, D. (1994) DSM-IV field trials for attention deficit hyperactivity disorder in children and adolescents. *American Journal of Psychiatry,* 151:1673–1685.

Lainhart, J.E., Piven, J., Wzorek, M., Landa, R., Santangelo, S.L., Coon, H., and Folstein, S.E. (1997) Macrocephaly in children and adults with autism. *Journal of the American Academy of Child and Adolescent Psychiatry,* 36:282–290.

Landau, W., Goldstein, R., and Kleffner, F. (1960) Congenital aphasia: A clinico-pathologic study. *Neurology,* 10:915–921.

Larsen, J.P., Høien, T., and Ödegaard, H. (1990) MRI evaluation of the size and symmetry of the planum temporale in adolescents with developmental dyslexia. *Brain and Language,* 39:289–301.

Larsen, J.P., Høien, T., and Ödegaard, H. (1992) Magnetic resonance imaging of the corpus callosum in developmental dyslexia. *Cognitive Neuropsychology,* 9:123–134.

Leonard, C.M., Voeller, K.K.S., Lombardino, L.J., Morris, M.K., Hynd, G.W., Alexander, A.W., Andersen, H.G., Garofalakis, M., Honeyman, J.C., Mao, J., Agee, O.F., and Staab, E.V. (1993) Anomalous cerebral structure in dyslexia revealed with magnetic resonance imaging. *Archives of Neurology,* 50:461–469.

Mesulam, M.-M. (1985) Patterns in behavioral neuroanatomy: Association areas, the limbic system, and hemispheric specialization. In M.-M. Mesulam (ed.), *Principles of Behavioral Neurology.* Philadelphia: FA Davis, pp. 1–70.

Mesulam, M.-M. (1990) Large-scale neurocognitive networks and distributed processing for attention, language, and memory. *Annals of Neurology,* 28:597–613.

Mesulam, M.-M. (1994) Neurocognitive networks and selectively distributed processing. *Review Neurologique,* 150:564–569.

Morecraft, R.J., Geula, C., and Mesulam, M.M. (1993) Architecture of connectivity within a cingulo-fronto-parietal neurocognitive network for directed attention. *Archives of Neurology,* 50:279–284.

Murakami, J.W., Courchesne, E., Press, G.A., Yeung-Courchesne, R., and Hesselink, J.R. (1989) Reduced cerebellar hemisphere size and its relationship to vermal hypoplasia in autism. *Archives of Neurology,* 46:689–694.

Nass, R.D., and Gazzaniga, M.S. (1987) Cerebral lateralization and specialization in human central nervous system. In V.B. Mountcastle, F. Plum, and S.R. Geiger (eds.), *Handbook of Physiology—The Nervous System: Higher Functions of the Brain.* Baltimore: Waverly Press, pp. 701–762.

Njiokiktjien, C., de Sonneville, L., and Vaal, J. (1994) Callosal size in children with learning disabilities. *Behavioral Brain Research,* 64:213–218.

Nowell, M.A., Hackney, D.B., Muraki, A.S., and Coleman, M. (1990) Varied MR appearance of autism: Fifty-three pediatric patients having the full autistic syndrome. *Magnetic Resonance Imaging,* 8:811–816.

Ornitz, E.M., Atwell, C.W., Kaplan, A.R., and Westlake, J.R. (1985) Brain-stem dysfunction in autism. Results of vestibular stimulation. *Archives of General Psychiatry,* 42: 1018–1025.

Pennington, B.F. (1995) Genetics of learning disabilities. *Journal of Child Neurology,* 10 (Suppl 1):S69–S77.

Petersen, S.E., Corbetta, M., Miezin, F.M., and Shulman, G.L. (1994) PET studies of parietal involvement in spatial attention: Comparison of different task types. *Canadian Journal of Experimental Psychology,* 48:319–338.

Piven, J., and Arndt, S. (1995) The cerebellum and autism [letter]. *Neurology,* 45:398–399.

Piven, J., Arndt, S., Bailey, J., and Andreasen, N. (1996) Regional brain enlargement in autism: A magnetic resonance imaging study. *Journal of the American Academy of Child and Adolescent Psychiatry,* 35:530–536.

Piven, J., Berthier, M.L., Starkstein, S.E., Nehme, E., Pearlson, G., and Folstein, S.E. (1990) Magnetic resonance imaging evidence for a defect of cerebral cortical development in autism. *American Journal of Psychiatry,* 147:734–739.

Piven, J., Nehme, E., Simon, J., Barta, P., Pearlson, G., and Folstein, S.E. (1992) Magnetic resonance imaging in autism: Measurement of the cerebellum, pons, and fourth ventricle. *Biological Psychiatry,* 31:491–504.

Plante, E. (1991) MRI findings in the parents and siblings of specifically language-impaired boys. *Brain and Language,* 41:67–80.

Plante, E., Swisher, L., and Vance, R. (1989) Anatomical correlates of normal and impaired language in a set of dizygotic twins. *Brain and Language,* 37:643–655.

Plante, E., Swisher, L., Vance, R., and Rapcsak, S. (1991) MRI findings in boys with specific language impairment. *Brain and Language,* 41:52–66.

Posner, M.I., and Petersen, S.E. (1990) The attention system of the human brain. *Annual Review of Neuroscience,* 13:25–42.

Posner, M.I., and Raichle, M.E. (1997) Networks of attention. In M.I. Posner and M.E. Raichle (eds.), *Images of Mind.* New York: Scientific American Library, pp. 153–179.

Prior, M., Tress, B., Hoffman, W., and Boldt, D. (1984) Computed tomographic study of children with classic autism. *Archives of Neurology,* 41:482–484.

Rapin, I. (ed.). (1996) *Preschool Children with Inadequate Communication: Developmental Language Disorder, Autism, Low IQ.* London: MacKeith Press.

Rapin, I., and Allen, D.A. (1987) Syndromes in developmental dysphasia and adult aphasia. *Research Publications—Association for Research in Nervous and Mental Disease,*
66:57–75.

Raz, N., Torres, I.J., Spencer, W.D., White, K., and Acker, J.D. (1992) Age-related regional differences in cerebellar vermis observed *in vivo. Archives of Neurology,* 149:
412–416.

Ritvo, E.R., Freeman, B.J., Scheibel, A.B., Duong, T., Robinson, H., Guthrie, D., and Ritvo,
A. (1986) Lower Purkinje cell counts in the cerebella of four autistic subjects: Initial
findings of the UCLA-NSAC Autopsy Research Report. *American Journal of Psychiatry,* 143:862–866.

Roeltgen, D.P., and Schneider, J.S. (1991) Chronic low-dose MPTP in nonhuman primates:
A possible model for attention deficit disorder. *Journal of Child Neurology,* 6(Suppl):
S82–S89.

Rosenbloom, S., Campbell, M., George, A., Kricheff, I., Taleporos, E., Anderson, L.,
Reuben, R., and Korein, J. (1984) High resolution CT scanning in infantile autism: A
quantitative approach. *Journal of the American Academy of Child and Adolescent Psychiatry,* 23:72–77.

Rumsey, J.M., Casanova, M., Mannheim, G.B., Patronas, N., De Vaughn, N., Hamburger,
S.D., and Aquino, T. (1996) Corpus callosum morphology, as measured with MRI, in
dyslexic men. *Biological Psychiatry,* 39:769–675.

Rumsey, J.M., Creasey, H., Stepanek, J., Dorwart, R., Patronas, N., Hamburger, S., and
Duara, R. (1988) Hemispheric asymmetries, fourth ventricular size, and cerebellar morphology in autism. *Journal of Autism and Developmental Disorders,* 18:127–137.

Saitoh, O., Courchesne, E., Egaas, B., Lincoln, A.J., and Schreibman, L. (1995) Cross-
sectional area of the posterior hippocampus in autistic patients with cerebellar and corpus callosum abnormalities. *Neurology,* 45:317–324.

Sandberg, S., and Barton, J. (1996) Historical development. In S. Sandberg (ed.), *Hyperactivity Disorders of Childhood.* New York: Cambridge University Press, pp. 1–25.

Schneider, J.S. (1990) Chronic exposure to low doses of MPTP. II. Neurochemical and
pathological consequences in cognitively-impaired, motor asymptomatic monkeys.
Brain Research, 534:25–36.

Schultz, R.T., Cho, N.K., Staib, L.H., Kier, L.E., Fletcher, J.M., Shaywitz, S.E., Shankweiler, D.P., Katz, L., Gore, J.C., Duncan, J.S., and Shaywitz, B.A. (1994) Brain morphology in normal and dyslexic children: The influence of sex and age. *Annals of
Neurology,* 35:732–742.

Semrud-Clikeman, M., Filipek, P.A., Biederman, J., Steingard, R., Kennedy, D.N., Renshaw, P., and Bekken, K. (1994) Attention-deficit hyperactivity disorder: Magnetic
resonance imaging morphometric analysis of the corpus callosum. *Journal of the American Academy of Child and Adolescent Psychiatry,* 33:875–881.

Sergeant, J., and Scholten, C.A. (1983) A stages-of-information approach to hyperactivity.
Journal of Child Psychology and Psychiatry and Allied Disciplines, 24:49–60.

Shaywitz, B.A., Fletcher, J.M., and Shaywitz, S.E. (1995) Defining and classifying learning disabilities and attention-deficit/hyperactivity disorder. *Journal of Child Neurology,*
10 (Suppl 1):S50–S57.

Shaywitz, S.E., Fletcher, J.M., and Shaywitz, B.A. (1994) Issues in the definition and classification of attention deficit disorder. *Topics in Language Disorders,* 14:1–25.

Shaywitz, S.E., Shaywitz, B.A., Fletcher, J.M., and Escobar, M.D. (1990) Prevalence of
reading disability in boys and girls. Results of the Connecticut Longitudinal Study.
Journal of the American Medical Association, 264:998–1002.

Still, G.F. (1902) The Coulstonian Lectures on some abnormal physical conditions in children. *Lancet,* 1:1008–1012, 1077–1082, 1163–1168.

Swanson, J.M., Posner, M., Potkin, S., Bonforte, S., Youpa, D., Fiore, C., Cantwell, D., and Crinella, F. (1991) Activating tasks for the study of visual-spatial attention in ADHD children: A cognitive anatomic approach. *Journal of Child Neurology,* 6(Suppl):S119–S127.

Taylor, E.T. (1986) *The Overactive Child.* London: MacKeith.

Tredgold, C.H. (1908) *Mental Deficiency (Amentia).* New York: W. Wood.

Tuchman, R.F., Rapin, I., and Shinnar, S. (1991) Autistic and dysphasic children. I: Clinical characteristics. *Pediatrics,* 88:1211–1218.

van der Meere, J.J., and Sergeant, J.A. (1988) Controlled processing and vigilance in hyperactivity: Time will tell. *Journal of Abnormal Child Psychology,* 16:641–655.

Voeller, K.K.S. (1991a) Toward a neurobiologic nosology of attention deficit hyperactivity disorder. *Journal of Child Neurology,* 6(Suppl):S2–S8.

Voeller, K.K.S. (1991b) What can neurological models of attention, inattention, and arousal tell us about attention-deficit hyperactivity disorder? *Journal of Neuropsychiatry and Clinical Neurosciences,* 3:209–216.

Wadsworth, S.J., DeFries, J.C., Stevenson, J., Gilger, J.W., and Pennington, B.F. (1992) Gender ratios among reading-disabled children and their siblings as a function of parental impairment. *Journal of Child Psychology and Psychiatry,* 33:1229–1239.

Williams, R.S., Hauser, S.L., Purpura, D.P., DeLong, G.R., and Swisher, C.N. (1980) Autism and mental retardation: Neuropathologic studies performed in four retarded persons with autistic behavior. *Archives of Neurology,* 37:749–753.

Witelson, S.F. (1989) Hand and sex differences in the isthmus and genu of the human corpus callosum: A postmortem morphological study. *Brain,* 112:799–835.

Woodhouse, W., Bailey, A., Rutter, M., Bolton, P., Baird, G., and Le Couteur, A. (1996) Head circumference in autism and other pervasive developmental disorders. *Journal of Child Psychology and Psychiatry,* 37:665–671.

15

Transcranial Magnetic Stimulation as a Tool for Detecting Changes in the Organization of the Human Motor System After Central and Peripheral Lesions

ERIC M. WASSERMANN, LEONARDO G. COHEN,
AND MARK HALLETT

Transcranial magnetic stimulation (TMS) was introduced by Barker and colleagues in 1985 (1985a, 1985b, 1985c) and rapidly gained popularity as a painless and noninvasive means of brain stimulation, largely replacing transcranial electrical stimulation, which had been developed a few years earlier (Merton et al., 1980) and which, while effective, was painful. Over the years, TMS has gained a place in the armamentarium of electrodiagnostic medicine. However, its chief contribution has been as a tool for clinical and basic neurophysiologists investigating the human motor system in health and disease.

Transcranial magnetic stimulation uses the principle of inductance to get electrical energy across the scalp and skull. A small coil of wire is placed on the scalp, and a powerful current pulse is briefly passed through it. This produces a rapidly changing magnetic field, oriented orthogonally to the plane of the coil, that passes unimpeded through the tissues of the head, causing comparatively little local sensation. The changing magnetic field, in turn, causes a much weaker electrical current to flow in the conductive medium of the brain. This induced current is also in the plane of the coil and is capable of depolarizing neurons. Its strength is, in part, a function of the rate of change of the magnetic field, which, in turn, is a function of the rate of change in the current in the coil. Other factors include the strength of the current and the number of windings in the coil. Therefore, to induce enough current to depolarize neurons in the brain, the current passed through the stimulating coil must be quite powerful and must change very rapidly, starting and stopping within a few hundred microseconds.

The stimulators and coils in production today develop about 1.5 to 2 Tesla at the face of the coil and appear to be able to activate neurons in the cerebral cortex 1.5 to 2 cm from the surface of the coil (Epstein et al., 1990; Rudiak et al., 1994). An important fact about TMS is that, because of the orientation of the magnetic field perpendicular to the surface of the brain, under most conditions it has a strong tendency to activate intracortical axons and interneurons rather than cortical output cells (Amassian et al., 1989; Rothwell et al., 1991). This is probably because these elements lie parallel to the surface of the brain, orthogonal to the magnetic field, and thus in the plane of the induced current.

Mapping with Transcranial Magnetic Stimulation

Mapping requires relatively focal activation of the brain, and an early innovation in the design of stimulating coils made this possible. So-called butterfly or eight-shaped coils consist of two loops of windings that intersect in the middle. The magnetic field is maximal at the intersection and weaker elsewhere (Cohen et al., 1990; Roth et al., 1991).

The method generally employed for mapping the cortical representation of a muscle is to apply a standard stimulus to a grid of points distributed across the scalp and record the resulting motor-evoked potentials (MEPs). Plotting the average MEP amplitude evoked at each site against the site's Cartesian coordinates with respect to the grid generates a map of the motor representation of the target muscle as projected onto the scalp (Fig. 15-1A). The site where the MEPs of maximal amplitude can be evoked in the target muscle has been called the *optimal position*. Plots of the threshold for evoking a standard MEP at different scalp sites have also been made. In our experience, the two techniques are functionally, if not physiologically, equivalent. Motor-evoked potential latencies have also been plotted topographically (Fuhr et al., 1991). We have found that the most reliable measure of the central tendency of TMS amplitude maps is the amplitude-weighted center of gravity (Wassermann et al., 1992), but this rarely differs widely from the optimal position (Wassermann et al., 1992, 1996). We have also found that the center of gravity of the map of a hand muscle lies on the scalp directly over the central sulcus and near the location of the hand representation, as estimated by $H_2{}^{15}O$ positron emission tomography (PET) scanning (Wassermann et al., 1996).

In a detailed study designed to determine the requirements for the spacing of stimulation sites and the number of stimuli required at each site for producing reliable maps (Brasil-Neto et al., 1992a), it was found that the error in locating an optimal position increased with spacings above 0.5 cm. The number of stimuli required to generate an estimate within 30% of the theoretical true MEP amplitude ranged from 2 to over 100. Reliability was related directly to MEP amplitude. Therefore, more stimuli were required with lower stimulus intensity, greater distance

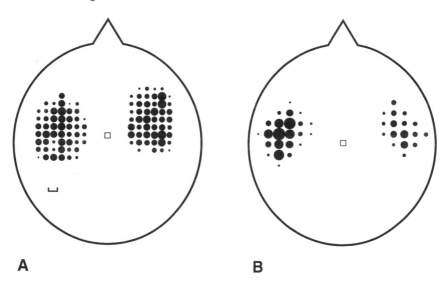

A   **B**

Figure 15-1. (A). Map of the cortical representations of the abductor pollicis brevis (thumb) muscles of a normal subject. Circles indicate the average amplitude of the MEPs evoked with three trials of stimulation at sites 1 cm apart on the scalp. Amplitudes are scaled to the size of the compound muscle action potential (CMAP) evoked in each muscle with supramaximal stimulation of the median nerve. The bar indicates 50% of the CMAP amplitude. (B). Similar map obtained from a patient with a small infarct involving the internal capsule on the right. Ten stimuli were delivered at each scalp site. The map is scaled to the largest average MEP evoked on either side. The squares in the center of each map indicate the vertex. The right muscle is shown on the left and vice versa.

from the optimal position, and in proximal muscles whose representations produce smaller MEPs when stimulated.

In one early study (Wassermann et al., 1992), we used TMS to map the cortical representations of four upper extremity muscles (the abductor pollicis brevis, flexor carpi radialis, biceps, and deltoid) in the contralateral hemispheres of ten normal subjects. Three stimuli were delivered to scalp positions 1 cm apart which were registered with reference to the vertex (top of the head) as defined by the International 10–20 system, which uses scalp landmarks to standardize positions on the head. The amplitude and latency of the resulting MEPs were averaged for each position. Maps were described in terms of the number of excitable scalp positions, the average latencies and amplitudes of the MEPs evoked at all sites, the locations of optimal positions, and the threshold for producing MEPs with stimulation at the optimal position. We compared different muscles across subjects and the same muscles on the left and right sides in individual subjects. Distal muscles had larger representations with higher-amplitude MEPs and lower thresholds. This finding is consistent with classical maps made by electrical stimulation of the cortical surface (Penfield & Boldrey 1937; Woolsey et al., 1952) and reflects the fact that these muscles have stronger corticospinal projections to the spinal cord. However, it is at odds with more modern maps made with intracortical microstimulation in primates (e.g., Donoghue et al., 1992; Waters et al., 1990) in which the area of cortex where stimulation produced movement in distal muscles is sometimes smaller than that of other muscles. This discrepancy may reflect the fact that the size of TMS maps is related to the excitability and density of projecting fibers of the cortical motor representations rather than simply to their areal extent. The MEP amplitude-weighted centers of gravity and the optimal positions of the maps showed a tendency to lie in the predicted somatotopic order, with the proximal muscles represented medially and posteriorly to the distal muscles. Other investigators (Wilson et al., 1993) have produced statistically enhanced maps showing slight but reliable differences in the scalp locations of two intrinsic hand muscles.

Conventional, short-latency, low-threshold MEPs to TMS are believed to be conducted via corticomotoneuronal pathways from the primary motor cortex (M1) (Rothwell et al., 1991). These direct pathways which underlie fine, individuated movements of the distal extremities, are believed to be primarily contralateral in their distribution (Lemon, 1993). This may explain the difficulty of producing MEPs with TMS in muscles ipsilateral to the stimulated hemisphere in normal subjects, although inhibitory phenomena are easily evoked (Wassermann et al., 1991). Nevertheless, in a study of six normal subjects (Wassermann et al., 1994), we found two who had reproducible MEPs in the ipsilateral first dorsal interosseous and deltoid when these muscles were activated voluntarily during stimulation. Both of these subjects (one of whom was the senior author) were neurologically normal and unremarkable in terms of motor skills. We mapped the scalp distributions of these motor representations and found that the ipsilateral hand was represented near the contralateral hand but also, and most robustly, laterally and anteriorly where it overlapped the representation of the contralateral face (Fig. 15-2). This finding has been subsequently confirmed in ten normal subjects (Ziemann et al., 1999).

Changes in Transcranial Magnetic Stimulation Maps after Peripheral Lesions

The dramatic effects of deafferentation (Merzenich et al., 1983a, 1983b; Pons et al., 1991) and amputation (Merzenich et al., 1984) on body representations in primate somatosensory cortex are well known. Less familiar, however, is the fact that amputation and deafferentation affect motor as well as sensory representations in a similar manner, causing increased excitability and possible expansion of the representations of neighboring body parts. Most of the evidence for these effects comes from TMS studies of humans.

Patients with spinal cord transections show increased MEP amplitudes and expanded maps of muscles innervated by spinal segments just above the level of the lesion (Levy et al., 1990; Topka et al., 1991), suggesting a change in the cortical representation of these muscles. In other studies (Cohen et al., 1991a) of subjects with traumatic, surgical, and congenital amputations of the arm near the elbow, TMS

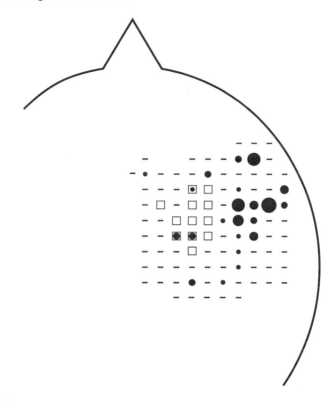

Figure 15-2. Data from a single subject showing the cortical representation of both first dorsal interosseous (index finger) muscles on the right hemisphere. Circles represent sites where statistically significant MEPs were evoked in the ipsilateral (right) muscle with ten trials of stimulation. Their size is proportional to the average amplitude. Squares indicate sites where the largest MEPs (≥50th percentile) were evoked in the contralateral (left) muscle. Dashes represent other stimulated sites.

maps were made of muscles proximal to the stump and their homologs in the other arm. The apparent motor representation areas targeting the muscles immediately proximal to the stump were larger than those for the same muscles in the intact arm. This finding could be interpreted as an expansion of the representation of the muscles proximal to the stump. However, the threshold for activation of the muscles proximal to the amputation was also decreased compared with that of their homologs on the intact side. As in the maps of intact subjects described above, increases in the excitability and in the extent of the excitable area can be difficult to distinguish with TMS. Another feature of this type of change and the analogous effect seen after reversible deafferentation (see below) is that the difference in the excitability of the muscles proximal to the lesion and their contralateral homologs disappears with voluntary activation of the muscles (Ridding & Rothwell, 1995).

This type of reorganization appears to happen very soon after the onset of the deafferenting lesion. In one experiment (Brasil-Neto et al., 1992b), a pneumatic

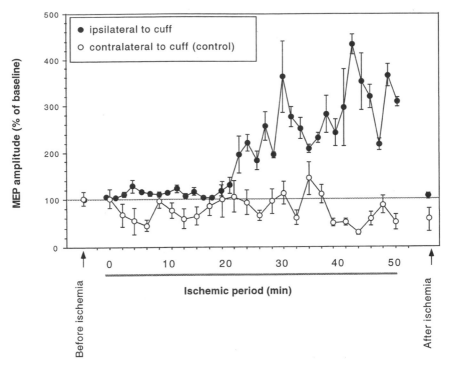

Figure 15-3. Data from a single subject showing the amplitude of MEPs recorded simultaneously from both biceps muscles before, at 2 minute intervals during, and after ischemic paralysis created by a tourniquet applied just below the elbow. Each point is the average of ten trials of stimulation with a large, round coil that produced activation of both hemispheres. Bars show the standard deviation.

tourniquet was placed just below the elbow in normal subjects, and anesthesia was produced both by the ischemia from the cuff and by a regional lidocaine infusion. Transcranial magnetic stimulation was delivered with a round coil that stimulated both hemispheres simultaneously. Anesthesia was demonstrated by the absence of voluntary movement, MEPs, and sensation below the cuff. Within minutes of the onset of anesthesia, the amplitude of MEPs to TMS in the muscles proximal to the anesthetized forearm increased dramatically and then returned to preanesthesia levels soon after the anesthesia wore off (Fig. 15-3). There was no such change in the MEPs evoked by the same stimuli in the muscles of the other arm.

In a follow-up study (Brasil-Neto et al., 1993) designed to determine the location at which this rapid change in excitability occurred, H-reflexes (the electrical equivalent of deep tendon reflexes), MEPs to TMS, and MEPs to transcutaneous electrical stimulation of the spinal cord and motor cortex were recorded before and after application of the tourniquet. The amplitudes of MEPs to TMS, but not to electrical stimulation of the brain or spinal cord, were larger in the biceps on the side with the cuff during ischemia. The H-reflex was unaffected by ischemia, indicating that the excitability of the spinal motoneurons to segmental sensory input remained unchanged. Electrical brain stimulation produces MEPs primarily by direct stimulation of the axons of corticospinal neurons (Rothwell et al., 1994), whereas TMS appears to have much of its effect at a presynaptic level (Amassian et al., 1989; Rothwell et al., 1991). Electrical stimulation of the spinal cord clearly acts below the cortical level as well. The fact that MEPs evoked by TMS, but not by electrical stimulation, changed with reversible denervation strongly suggests an increase in the excitability of cells within the motor cortex. This type of modulation of excitability following deafferentation must be mediated by changes in sensory systems, raising the possibility that the body representation in M1 is maintained dynamically by transcortical inputs from the somatosensory cortex. Strong, topographically specific excitatory projections from somatosensory areas onto output cells in M1 exist (Zarzecki, 1989, 1991) and could mediate this effect.

Other manipulations induce reorganization of motor maps that can be detected with TMS but that occur through different mechanisms. Mano and colleagues (1995) described four patients with complete upper limb paralyses from traumatic injuries of the cervical nerve roots who underwent surgical connection of an intercostal nerve (which normally innervates the rib muscles of a single segment) to the musculocutaneous nerve (which normally supplies the biceps muscle) to restore function in the upper arm. Four to 6 months after the operation, electrical activity could be recorded from the biceps muscle on the operated side during deep breathing, and MEPs were present with TMS. Over 1 to 2 years, the patients gradually acquired the ability to activate the biceps independent of respiration. Transcranial magnetic stimulation mapping of the cortical representation of the reinnervated biceps showed a gradual shift in its location over 4 to 33 months. During this time, it was observed to move from the area of the intercostal muscles to a location more lateral on the scalp near the cortical representations of the other arm muscles. These findings demonstrate a profound reorganization in the output map of the motor cortex, probably resulting from the formation of new connections within and between the motor cortex and the spinal cord.

Transcranial Magnetic Stimulation Studies after Central Lesions

Emergent Ipsilateral Motor Representations

It is a common clinical observation that even devastating unilateral cerebral injuries, such as surgical removal of an entire cerebral hemisphere, can be followed by dramatic recovery of motor function, particularly when the lesion occurs at an early age. To investigate the mechanisms underlying this phenomenon, we studied patients who had undergone surgical hemispherectomy for intractable epilepsy (Cohen et al., 1991b; Pascual-Leone et al., 1992). One patient was a 32-year-old man who had had the left hemisphere removed at 7 years of age. Transcranial magnetic stimulation of the remaining (right) hemisphere caused bilateral activation of the deltoid and biceps muscles. Transcranial magnetic stimulation mapping showed that the muscles on the right were optimally activated by stimulation of scalp positions slightly anterior and lateral to those activating the homologous muscles on the normal left side. Similarly, movements about the right elbow were associated with cerebral blood flow increases on $H_2^{15}O$ PET scanning in an area centered 1.4 cm anterior and lateral to that activated by the same movements on the left. These results indicate that ipsilateral and contralateral representations in the remaining hemisphere are topographically differentiated, with ipsilateral representations having a more anterior and lateral scalp distribution. The location of the representation of the ipsilateral muscles in this and other similar cases bears a suggestive resemblance to the location of the ipsilateral hand representation that we found in the normal subjects (Wassermann et al., 1994). It is possible that this area, anterior and lateral to the representation of the contralateral upper extremity, contains a latent bilateral representation that can become functional under certain circumstances. It may also be relevant that bilateral upper extremity control has been imputed to a similarly located zone of the primary motor cortex in monkeys (Aizawa et al., 1990).

In another study of hemispherectomy patients (Pascual-Leone et al., 1992), we found that those who were operated on at a very early age had a better chance of substantial recovery of motor function that was associated with the development of a distinct representation of the ipsilateral proximal arm muscles, again lying anterolateral to the contralateral representation. Patients who were operated on at an older age had a poorer recovery, and the ipsilateral and contralateral representations in the intact hemisphere could not be distinguished spatially.

Other evidence of the capacity of the intact hemisphere to assume or retain control of the ipsilateral muscles after congenital and childhood cerebral lesions comes from the work of Carr et al. (1993). They found large, short-latency, ipsilateral MEPs to TMS in the hand muscles of 21 of 33 young subjects with hemiplegic cerebral palsy. Eleven of these subjects had intense mirror movements (involuntary mimicking by the opposite limb) of a type rarely, if ever, seen after brain lesions in adults. These subjects also showed evidence of synchronous firing of motor units in the homologous muscles on both sides of the body, implying abnormal or abnormally preserved branching of corticospinal axons to both sides of the spinal cord. Good function of the affected hand was associated with MEPs to stimulation of the contralateral motor cortex, indicating intact normal pathways. Ipsilateral MEPs were found in subjects with both good and poor function of the affected hand. When contralateral MEPs were not present, hand function was poor unless intense mirroring was present. Therefore, ipsilateral MEPs by themselves are not evidence of functionally significant ipsilateral control.

Ipsilateral responses have also been recorded in patients with smaller cerebral lesions acquired in adulthood. However, there these responses may be a marker of poor recovery. Turton et al. (1996) studied 21 patients within 5 weeks of the onset of a stroke and then at regular intervals over the next 12 months. They found that the presence of contralateral MEPs at the start of the study was a good indicator of recovery. In addition, contralateral MEPs appeared at or just before the time of recovery of hand movement in those who recovered it later during the study. However, this relationship between contralateral MEPs and voluntary activation did not hold for more proximal muscles. Turton et al. also found nine subjects with ipsilateral MEPs in affected hand muscles evoked by stimulation of the intact hemisphere, most of whom had poor recovery of hand function. These ipsilateral MEPs had low amplitude and resembled the ipsilateral MEPs that we found in normal subjects more closely than those seen in the proximal muscles of hemispherectomy patients and patients with cerebral palsy. They concluded that the underlying mechanism of such responses was not necessarily beneficial in terms of recovery.

In a study of five patients with infarcts of the internal capsule involving the corticospinal tract, Fries et al. (1991) recorded bilateral MEPs to transcranial electrical and magnetic stimulation of the lesioned hemisphere alone. The authors suggested that these responses may have been conducted by corticoreticulospinal pathways unmasked by the lesion. To our knowledge, this observation has not been reproduced elsewhere.

We have searched for ipsilateral MEPs in more than ten stroke patients with various types of lesions and courses of recovery. All were studied at least 2 months following their strokes. We stimulated repeatedly at maximal intensity over both hemispheres in the optimal location for activating the contralateral hand, and also in the anterolateral area, where we produced ipsilateral responses in the normal subjects and in those with early hemispherectomy. Electromyographic (EMG) signals from the ipsilateral muscles were rectified and averaged while the subject maintained a moderate degree of voluntary muscle contraction. We found ipsilateral MEPs in only one patient with a lesion of the internal capsule, but these MEPs could be evoked with stimulation of either hemisphere and therefore appeared to be a normal finding. Most of these patients had some degree of mirroring with the unaffected hand when making movements with the recovered hand.

Changes in Contralateral Motor Representations

Soon after its development, TMS was used to investigate the pathophysiology of hemiparesis after cerebral lesions (Bridgers, 1989). The presence of MEPs to TMS early after the onset of hemiparesis has been associated with eventual recovery in most studies (Catano et al., 1995, 1996; Rapisarda et al., 1996; Turton et al., 1996). However, other investigators have not found this to be true (Arac et al., 1994). These clinically oriented studies have not generally examined the specific effects of lesions in different brain areas on MEP thresholds or other electrophysiological parameters.

The only consistent findings that we have discovered after stroke in adults have been decreased cortical excitability and constricted TMS maps in the lesioned hemisphere following recovery from even relatively small subcortical infarcts that produce only transient weakness (Fig. 15-1B). This is not surprising if one assumes that these lesions disrupt the descending motor pathways that conduct the MEP. Analyses of neuroimaging studies to determine the exact fiber groups affected by these lesions are underway. It is also of interest that subjects with similar lesions have abnormally high increases in regional cerebral blood flow during movements of the affected hand on $H_2{}^{15}O$ PET scans in other laboratories (Chollet et al., 1991; Di Piero et al., 1992; Weiller et al., 1992, 1993) as well as our own. This suggests that in cases where a lesion in the output pathways raises the threshold for muscle activation by TMS, the threshold for natural corticospinal activation is elevated as well.

Conclusions

Transcranial magnetic stimulation has proven to be a convenient and valid tool for the investigation of the human motor system in normal subjects and patients with lesions. While motor maps made with TMS are perhaps not an accurate representation of the detailed functional topography of the motor cortex, they are generally consistent within and across individuals, and show reproducible changes after central and peripheral lesions and manipulations. Using TMS, we and other investigators have discovered selective excitability increases in the representations of body parts proximal to deafferenting lesions in the arm or the spinal cord. These changes after a reversible nerve lesion become detectable within minutes. More gradual and profound reorganization in the somatotopic map in M1 follows a peripheral nerve cross.

After large hemispheric lesions early in life, TMS has revealed functioning representations of both sides of the body in the remaining healthy motor cortex. There is some resemblance between the representation of the ipsilateral upper extremity in these cases and that detected with TMS in some normal individuals. This finding suggests the existence of a latent ipsilateral motor representation that can be potentiated and made to function under some circumstances. We have not encountered this type of reorganization after lesions acquired in adulthood. There, TMS has been helpful primarily in clarifying the pathophysiology of the lesions themselves.

References

Aizawa, H., Mushiake, M., and Tanji, J. (1990) An output zone of the monkey primary motor cortex specialized for bilateral hand movement. *Experimental Brain Research,* 82: 219–221.

Amassian, V.E., Cracco, R.Q., Maccabee, P.J., Cracco, J.B., Rudell, A., and Eberle, L. (1989) Suppression of visual perception by magnetic coil stimulation of human occipital cortex. *Electroencephalography and Clinical Neurophysiology,* 74:458–462.

Arac, N., Sagduyu, A., Binai, S., and Ertekin, C. (1994) Prognostic value of transcranial magnetic stimulation in acute stroke. *Stroke,* 25:2183–2186.

Barker, A.T., Freeston, I.L., Jalinous, R., Merton, P.A., and Morton, H.B. (1985a) Magnetic stimulation of the human brain. *Journal of Physiology (London),* 369:3P (Abstract).

Barker, A.T., Jalinous, R., and Freeston, I.L. (1985b) Noninvasive magnetic stimulation of the human motor cortex. *Lancet,* 1:1106–1107.

Barker, A.T., Jalinous, R., Freeston, I.L., and Jarratt, J.A. (1985c) Motor responses to noninvasive brain stimulation in clinical practice. *Electroencephalography and Clinical Neurophysiology,* 61:570.

Brasil-Neto, J., Cohen, L.G., Panizza, M., Fuhr, P., and Hallett, M. (1992a) Optimal focal transcranial magnetic activation of the human motor cortex: Effects of coil orientation, shape of induced current pulse, and stimulus intensity. *Journal of Clinical Neurophysiology,* 9:132–136.

Brasil-Neto, J.P., Cohen, L.G., Pascual-Leone, A., Jabir, F.K., Wall, R.T., and Hallett, M. (1992b) Rapid reversible reorganization in human motor system following transient deafferentation. *Neurology,* 42:1302–1306.

Brasil-Neto, J.P., Valls-Solé, J., Pascual-Leone, A., Cammarota, A., Amassian, V.E., Cracco, R., Maccabee, P., Cracco, J., Hallett, M., and Cohen, L.G. (1993) Rapid modulation of human cortical motor outputs following ischemic nerve block. *Brain,* 116: 511–525.

Bridgers, S.L. (1989) Magnetic cortical stimulation in patients with hemiparesis. In: *Magnetic Stimulation in Clinical Neurophysiology,* S. Chokroverty Ed. Boston: Butterworth's. 233–247.

Carr, L.J., Harrison, L.M., Evans, A.L., and Stephens, J.A. (1993) Patterns of central motor reorganization in hemiplegic cerebral palsy. *Brain,* 116:1223–1247.

Catano, A., Houa, M., Caroyer, J.M., Ducarne, H., and Nocl, P. (1995) Magnetic transcranial stimulation in non-haemorrhagic sylvian strokes: Interest of facilitation for early functional prognosis. *Electroencephalography and Clinical Neurophysiology,* 97:349–354.

Catano, A., Houa, M., Caroyer, J.M., Ducarne, H., and Noel, P. (1996) Magnetic transcranial stimulation in acute stroke: Early excitation threshold and functional prognosis. *Electroencephalography and Clinical Neurophysiology,* 101:233–239.

Chollet, F., Di Piero, V., Wise, R.J., Brooks, D.J., Dolan, R.J., and Frackowiak, R.S. (1991) The functional anatomy of motor recovery after stroke in humans: A study with positron emission tomography. *Annals of Neurology,* 29:63–71.

Cohen, L.G., Bandinelli, S., Findlay, T.W., and Hallett, M. (1991a) Motor reorganization after upper limb amputation in man. *Brain,* 114:615 627.

Cohen, L.G., Roth, B.J., Nilsson, J., Dang, N., Panizza, M., Bandinelli, S., Friauf, W., and Hallett, M. (1990) Effects of coil design on delivery of focal magnetic stimulation. Technical considerations. *Electroencephalography and Clinical Neurophysiology,* 73:350–357.

Cohen, L.G., Roth, B., Wassermann, E.M., Fuhr, P., Topka, H.R., and Schultz, J. (1991b) Magnetic stimulation of the human cerebral cortex, an indicator of reorganization in motor pathways in certain pathological conditions. *Journal of Clinical Neurophysiology,* 8:56–65.

Di Piero, V., Chollet, F.M., MacCarthy, P., Lenzi, G.L., and Frackowiak, R.S.J. (1992) Motor recovery after acute ischaemic stroke: A metabolic study. *Journal of Neurology, Neurosurgery and Psychiatry,* 55:990–966.

Donoghue, J.P., Leibovic, S., and Sanes, J.N. (1992) Organization of the forelimb area in squirrel monkey motor cortex: Representation of digit, wrist and elbow muscles. *Experimental Brain Research,* 89:1–19.

Epstein, C.M., Schwartzenberg, D.G., Davey, K.R., and Sudderth, D.B. (1990) Localizing the site of magnetic brain stimulation in humans. *Neurology,* 40:666–670.

Fries, W., Danek, A., and Witt, T.N. (1991) Motor responses after transcranial electrical stimulation of cerebral hemispheres with a degenerated corticospinal tract. *Annals of Neurology,* 29:646–650.

Fuhr, P., Cohen, L.G., Roth, B., and Hallett, M. (1991) Latency of motor evoked potentials to focal transcranial stimulation varies as a function of scalp positions stimulated. *Electroencephalography and Clinical Neurophysiology,* 81:81–89.

Lemon, R.N. (1993) The G.L. Brown Prize Lecture. Cortical control of the primate hand. *Experimental Physiology,* 78:263–301.

Levy, W.J., Amassian, V.E., Traad, M., and Cadwell, J. (1990) Focal magnetic coil stimulation reveals motor cortical system reorganized in humans after traumatic quadriplegia. *Brain Research,* 510:130–134.

Mano, Y., Nakamuro, T., Tamura, R., Takayanagi, T., Kawanishi, K., Tamai, S., and Mayer, R.F. (1995) Central motor reorganization after anastomosis of the musculocutaneous and intercostal nerves following cervical root avulsion [see comments]. *Annals of Neurology,* 38:15–20.

Merton, P.A., and Morton, H.B. (1980) Stimulation of the cerebral cortex in the intact human subject. *Nature,* 285:227 (Letter).

Merzenich, M.M., Kaas, J.H., Wall, J.T., Nelson, R.J., Sur, M., and Felleman, D.J. (1983a) Topographic reorganization of somatosensory cortical areas 3b and 1 in adult monkeys following restricted deafferentation. *Neuroscience,* 258:33–55.

Merzenich, M.M., Kaas, J.H., Wall, J.T., Sur, M., Nelson, R.J., and Felleman, D.J. (1983b) Progression of change following median nerve section in the cortical representation of the hand in areas 3b and 1 in adult owl and squirrel monkeys. *Neuroscience,* 10:639–665.

Merzenich, M.M., Nelson, R.J., Stryker, M.P., Cynder, M.S., Shoppmann, A., and Zook, J.M. (1984) Somatosensory cortical map changes following digit amputation in adult monkeys. *Journal of Comparative Neurology,* 224:591–605.

Pascual-Leone, A., Chugani, H.T., Cohen, L.G., Brasil-Neto, J.P., Valls-Solé, J., Wassermann, E.M., Fuhr, P., and Hallett, M. (1992) Reorganization of human motor pathways following hemispherectomy. *Annals of Neurology,* 32:261.

Penfield, W., and Boldrey, E. (1937) Somatic motor and sensory representation in the cerebral cortex of man as studied by electrical stimulation. *Brain,* 60:389–443.

Pons, T.P., Garraghty, P.E., Ommaya, A.K., Kaas, J.H., Taub, E., and Mishkin, M. (1991) Massive cortical reorganization after sensory deafferentation in adult macaques [see comments]. *Science,* 252:1857–1860.

Rapisarda, G., Bastings, E., Maertens de Noordhout, A., Pennisi, G., and Delwaide, P.J. (1996) Can motor recovery in stroke patients be predicted by early transcranial magnetic stimulation? *Stroke,* 27:2191–2196.

Ridding, M.C., and Rothwell, J.C. (1995) Reorganisation in human motor cortex. *Canadian Journal of Physiology and Pharmacology,* 73:218–222.

Roth, B.J., Saypol, J.M., Hallett, M., and Cohen, L.G. (1991) A theoretical calculation of the electric field induced in the cortex during magnetic stimulation. *Electroencephalography and Clinical Neurophysiology,* 81:47–56.

Rothwell, J., Burke, D., Hicks, R., Stephen, J., Woodforth, I., and Crawford, M. (1994) Transcranial electrical-stimulation of the motor cortex in man—further evidence for the site of activation. *Journal of Physiology (London),* 481:243–250.

Rothwell, J.C., Thompson, P.D., Day, B.L., Boyd, S., and Marsden, C.D. (1991) Stimulation of the human motor cortex through the scalp. *Experimental Physiology,* 76:159–200.

Rudiak, D., and Marg, E. (1994) Finding the depth of magnetic brain stimulation: A reevaluation. *Electroencephalography and Clinical Neurophysiology,* 93:358–371.

Topka, H., Cohen, L.G., Cole, R., and Hallett, M. (1991) Reorganization of corticospinal pathways following spinal cord injury. *Neurology,* 41:1276–1283.

Turton, A., Wroe, S., Trepte, N., Fraser, C., and Lemon, R.N. (1996) Contralateral and ipsilateral EMG responses to transcranial magnetic stimulation during recovery of arm and hand function after stroke. *Electroencephalography and Clinical Neurophysiology,* 101:316–328.

Wassermann, E.M., Fuhr, P., Cohen, L.G., and Hallett, M. (1991) Effects of transcranial magnetic stimulation on ipsilateral muscles. *Neurology,* 41:1795–1799.

Wassermann, E.M., McShane, L.M., Hallett, M., and Cohen, L.G. (1992). Noninvasive mapping of muscle representations in human motor cortex. *Electroencphalography and Clinical Neurophysiology,* 85:1–8.

Wassermann, E.M., Pascual Leone, A., and Hallett, M. (1994) Cortical motor representation of the ipsilateral arm. *Experimental Brain Research,* 100:121–132.

Wassermann, E.M., Wang, B., Zeffiro, T.A., Sadato, N., Pascual-Leone, A., Toro, C., and Hallett, M. (1996) Locating the motor cortex on the MRI with transcranial magnetic stimulation. *NeuroImage,* 3:1–9.

Waters, R.S., Samulack, D.D., Dykes, R.W., and McKinley, P.A. (1990) Topographic organization of baboon primary motor cortex: Face, hand, forelimb, and shoulder representation. *Somatosensory and Motor Research,* 7:485–514.

Weiller, C., Chollet, F., Friston, K.J., Wise, R.J., and Frackowiak, R.S. (1992) Functional reorganization of the brain in recovery from striatocapsular infarction in man. *Annals of Neurology,* 31:463–472.

Weiller, C., Ramsay, S.C., Wise, R.J.S., Friston, K.J., and Frackowiack, R.S.J. (1993) Individual patterns of functional reorganization in the human cerebral cortex after capsular infarction. *Annals of Neurology,* 33:181–189.

Wilson, S.A., Thickbroom, G.W., and Mastaglia, F.L. (1993) Transcranial magnetic stimulation mapping of the motor cortex in normal subjects. The representation of two intrinsic hand muscles. *Journal of Neurological Science,* 118:134–144.

Woolsey, C.N., Settlage, P.H., Meyer, D.R., Sencer, W., Hamuy, T.P., and Travis, A.M. (1952) Patterns of localization in precentral and supplementary motor areas and their relation to the concept of a premotor area. *Research Publications of the Association for Research in Nervous and Mental Disorders,* 30:238–264.

Zarzecki, P. (1989) Influence of somatosensory cortex on different classes of cat motor neuron. *Journal of Neurophysiology,* 62:487–494.

Zarzecki, P. (1991) The distribution of corticocortical, thalamocortical, and callosal inputs on identified motor cortex output neurons: Mechanisms for their selective recruitment. *Somatosensory and Motor Research,* 8:313–325.

Ziemann, U., Ishii, K., Borgheresi, A., Yaseen, Z., Battaglia, F., Hallett, M., Cincotta, M., and Wassermann, E.M. (1999) Dissociation of the pathways mediating ipsilateral and contralateral motor-evoked potentials in human hand and arm muscles *Journal of Physiology (London),* 518:895–906.

16

Methodological Issues in Functional Magnetic Resonance Imaging Studies of Plasticity Following Brain Injury

TIMOTHY C. RICKARD

Functional magnetic resonance imaging (fMRI) holds great promise of providing fundamental new insights into the plasticity of neural organization that may accompany recovery of function after brain damage. In principle, comparison of the activation patterns of patients and normal subjects can provide direct information not only about whether neural plasticity has occurred, but also about its location and extent. However, there are a number of factors that can lead to activation differences between patients and controls that are completely unrelated to any plasticity effect that may be present. Taken as a group, these factors present a significant challenge to researchers in this area. This chapter provides a brief tour of some of the more important of these challenges from the perspectives of both methodology and data interpretation.

The focus is on delineation of some critical conditions necessary to infer *neural plasticity,* that is, the emergence of unique patterns in the connectivity and functioning of one or more neural networks following brain injury that are not usually observed in the normal brain. These neural-level changes may reflect the operation of a specialized plasticity mechanism that induces reorganization after injury, or they may reflect the operation of the same learning mechanisms operating in the normal, uninjured brain (Stiles, 1995). In either case, this broad definition assumes genuine reorganization of neural networks such that new tissue comes to perform a cognitive function similar to that previously performed by the damaged tissue (contrast this to patients' use of compensatory strategies that are also available to normals, as discussed in the section "Strategy Differences").

It is important to recognize at the outset that fMRI currently has spatial resolution on the order of about 0.50 cc^3. Effective resolution for inferring neural plasticity in a patient is often limited further by differences in anatomical structure and functional localization that are present even among normal brains. Thus, investigation of plasticity using fMRI implicitly assumes that at least some varieties of neural plasticity can be observed on a rather large spatial scale (as would be the case, for example, for left-to-right hemisphere transfer of function). Finally, this chapter assumes that the reader has a working knowledge of some of the basic aspects of fMRI task design and data analysis. For general discussions of fMRI methodology, see Aine (1995) and Kim and Ugurbil (1997).

The Ideal Functional Magnetic Resonance Imaging Plasticity Study

This chapter is organized around what appear to be the ideal conditions for allowing inferences about neural plasticity using fMRI. My argument is not that all such conditions need to be met for a study to be informative. Rather, discussion of a set of ideal conditions focuses attention on a number of the major potential sources of methodological and interpretational difficulty. This chapter also focuses on issues related to the study of plasticity for relatively high-level cognitive processes (e.g., language or numerical cognition). This focus in part reflects my own background and in part is motivated by the fact that studies of relatively high-level cognitive processes are the most problematic with respect to controlling for various potentially confounding factors. Studies of basic perceptual and motor tasks are also susceptible to at least a subset of these factors.

Three broad criteria for an *ideal* fMRI study of plasticity are as follows: (*1*) there must be clear evidence of significant (ideally, complete) behavioral recovery of function in the patient; (*2*) the cognitive or information-processing steps executed by the patient and controls in the service of the task should be equivalent (or, if they are not equivalent, the differences should be specifically identified); and (*3*) there must be statistically significant activation in the candidate plasticity area for the patient but not for the controls. On close inspection, achieving each of these criteria (especially the latter two) requires attention to often complex issues in design, analysis, and interpretation.

Clear Evidence of Recovery of Behavioral Function in the Task Domain of Interest

Behavioral evidence of significantly recovered cognitive function after injury is an important precondition for studying cognitive-neural plasticity with fMRI. Two major factors regarding recovery of behavioral function should be considered in single-case patient designs. First, ideally, at least two behavioral measures should be taken: one after the acute postinjury stage and the other at a later point (perhaps after remedial training in the task domain of interest). The first measure demonstrates initial impairment, and the second demonstrates recovery of function. The demonstration of initial impairment *after* the acute stage of recovery is crucial. If the initial measure documenting impairment occurs during the acute stage, then an inference of neural plasticity as the underlying cause of recovered function is dubious because recovery may have reflected only a return to normal operation of undamaged tissue that was only temporarily compromised by the injury (e.g., due to temporary swelling or pressure).

Researchers may often be tempted to infer that neural plasticity has occurred even without direct evidence that there was any deficit after the acute phase. This temptation may be particularly great if the nature and locus of an injury suggest that a particular deficit should be present but is not observed. Although there may be individual cases in which this approach is reasonable (e.g., when the injury is located in well-understood perceptual or motor regions of the brain), in general it should be used with caution. For example, language production is generally believed to have dominantly left temporofrontal localization in normal right-handers. It may thus appear natural to infer recovery of function automatically (even in the absence of direct evidence of a deficit after the acute stage) if a right-hander who previously suffered left temporofrontal damage appears to have relatively preserved language production. However, this approach has a potentially serious pitfall: unless the statistical distribution of localization of these functions in the normal population is extremely well documented, it may be difficult to distinguish a true plasticity effect from the possibility that the patient had a naturally atypical pattern of functional localization prior to the injury. For this reason, it is always preferable to have direct evidence of an initial deficit after the acute stage of injury, followed by recovery of function over time.

A second factor to consider carefully is the precision of the mapping between the neuropsychological evidence documenting recovery of function and the actual task to be used in the fMRI experiment. Most standard neuropsychological testing is relatively broad in scope, covering general domain functions such as language comprehension, visual attention, and long-term memory. However, due to technical and practical limitations, fMRI tasks are typically hyperspecific, focusing on only a small subset of the stimuli and task situations that constitute a more general domain of interest. Even if clear recovery of cognitive function is indicated by neuropsychological tasks, one must consider whether the specific fMRI task employed captures the same set of mental processes. Ideally, the fMRI task should be almost identical to the neuropsychological tests on which the inference of behavioral recovery of function was based. One powerful approach to dealing with this issue involves testing the patient repeatedly over time on both the general neuropsychological battery and the specific tasks to be used in the fMRI study. Performance improvements should be observable on both.

Cognitive Equivalence for Patients and Controls

Valid interpretation of any differences obtained in fMRI activation for controls and patients also requires careful evaluation of whether or not cognitive equivalence exists between normal and patient populations in the task domain of interest. *Cognitive equivalence* refers to equivalence of the underlying information-processing stages and processes, as well as the efficiency and nature of the execution of those processes. It may be very difficult to demonstrate conclusively a null hypothesis of pure cognitive equivalence in most cases. Nevertheless, it is imperative to explore this issue to the extent possible, since interpretation of any obtained differences in activation patterns would be profoundly different under conditions of cognitive equivalence than under conditions of clear cognitive nonequivalence. The discussions in the sections "Strategy Differences," "Performance Differences," and "Skill Level Differences" elaborate on this point.

Strategy Differences. The most obvious violation of the principle of cognitive equivalence is the use of different strategies by patients and controls to solve a given task. If a patient has recovered a function by applying an alternative compensatory strategy that is also available to normals, but that normals do not typically use (perhaps because it is less obvious or requires more effort), then neural plasticity as defined previously has not necessarily occurred. The point here is not that use of compensatory strategies by patients is uninteresting. Rather, it is that a fundamentally different type of plasticity would be indicated under such conditions.

There are several ways to evaluate possible strategy differences. For example, carefully employed concurrent or retrospective protocols can often provide veridical characterizations of subjects' strategies (e.g., Ericsson & Simon, 1994). Also, different strategies for performing a task often imply specific and unique patterns in error and reaction time (RT) data (Siegler, 1988). Converging evidence from verbal protocols, errors, and RT patterns can often provide definitive evidence regarding strategy use, although protocols can also distort performance under some conditions (Ericsson & Simon, 1994; Kirk & Ashcraft, 1997).

Performance Differences. *Performance differences* refer to differences in observable measures of behavioral performance, such as RT and error rate. In general, patients can be expected to be slower and more error prone than normal control subjects, even if they have exhibited substantial recovery of function and even if identical strategies are used by patients and by normals. Performance differences create a potentially serious obstacle to interpretation because fMRI brain activity patterns may be highly sensitive to such effects (Carpenter et al., 1997). Various factors, including differences in the duration of one or more stages of information processing, cognitive processes uniquely induced by high error rates, speed–accuracy trade-offs, and possible nonlinear relations between patterns of brain activity and the degree of mental effort required, might all provide accounts of obtained activation differences between patients and normal controls independent of any hypothesized neural plasticity effect.

It is also important to keep in mind that in some cases neural plasticity in the patient may occur within the same brain areas that are also activated by a particular task in the normal population. That is, it is possible that some types of plasticity will alter neither the extent nor the magnitude of fMRI activation observed for a patient (in comparison to controls). Thus, even if there is clear evidence of behavioral recovery of function for the patient, it does not necessarily follow that neural plasticity is the cause of any abnormal pattern of activity observed in that patient. In the realistic case in which the patient has a residual performance deficit relative to normals, an atypical pattern of activation for the patient might reflect nothing more than differences in information processing caused by the greater level of task difficulty posed for the patient.

One possible approach to evaluating the role of performance differences in obtained activation patterns is to incorporate at least two levels of task difficulty in the fMRI study for both patients and normal controls while also ensuring performance overlap, such that normal control performance in the difficult condition is worse (as measured by RT and error rate) than patient performance in the easy condition. If normals show one pattern of activity over each of the two overlapping difficulty levels and patients show a second stable pattern over each of the two overlapping levels, then performance differences as the sole cause of these findings can probably be rejected with reasonable confidence.

An alternative approach involves performing fMRI scans at multiple points during remedial training. If behavioral performance improves monotonically, and if fMRI activation in the patient also increases monotonically in an area not activated in normals, then a strong inference that that area is the site of new learning in the patient is warranted. This method may prove quite powerful, since in this case the performance artifact hypothesis and the true plasticity hypothesis make opposing predictions.

Skill Level Differences. Another way in which the principle of cognitive equivalence can be violated is if patients and controls perform a task using the same strategy but at different skill levels. Recent neuroimaging work has shown that as skill improves with practice on a task, the neural networks involved in performance can also change. For example, Raichle and colleagues (1994) showed that before practice, one neural network may be involved in naming a verb appropriate to a noun given as a cue. After practice in retrieving particular verbs appropriate to the same set of nouns, however, another network may be involved. Raichle et al. believed the former network to be involved in controlled search for an appropriate verb and the later network to reflect automatic learned retrieval of particular verbs for each noun.

In principle, it is possible that the strategy employed (at a consciously interpretable level), as well as the measurable behavioral performance, can be roughly equivalent in patients and normals, but that the skill level, and thus the underlying neural networks involved in performance, are different. Consider the controlled versus automatic word generation pathways of Raichle et al. (1994). Assume that a patient has selective damage to the automatic pathway, and assume an experimental design in which the same nouns are used as cues several times over the course of the experiment. The activation pattern obtained for the normal controls in this design would reflect primarily activity in the automatic pathway. In contrast, activation in the patient would reflect exclusively activity in the nonautomatic, or controlled, pathway. Under these conditions, activation in the controlled pathway for the patient would probably be greater than that for normals (note that, in this example, behavioral performance differences would also be expected). However, it would clearly not be appropriate to interpret this finding as evidence of neural plasticity in the patient.

Clear Evidence of Activation in the Candidate Area for Patients But Not for Normals

There are additional complications involved in inferring whether or not brain areas activated in patients who have already recovered function can be considered different from the brain areas activated in normal control subjects. First, there is substantial individual variability in the anatomical structure of different brains. Major anatomical landmarks (such as the central sulcus) may differ between brains by as much as 1 cm or more, even after both brains have been normalized using the best existing methods. Second, there are individual differences in localization of function above and beyond the anatomical differences (although the magnitude of these effects is currently unknown). In combination, these two factors probably produce a great degree of variability in the neural locus of function in two randomly selected normal brains even after precise normalization. These facts make the effective resolution of fMRI, when applied to intersubject analyses, substantially lower than the current technical limit of around 0.50 cc^3.

There are two major approaches to comparing activation across brains. The first is to use recognizable anatomical structures (such as the central sulcus) as a standard of reference for each brain. This approach may be appropriate if the activations of interest are proximal to major landmarks. However, for many brain areas (such as the parietal cortex) there may be substantial individual differences in the patterns of cortical folding that preclude a standard landmark approach. An alternative approach, which is less precise but perhaps more generally applicable, involves normalizing all brains to a standard atlas, such as that of Talairach and Tournoux (1988). Comparison of areas across subjects in a normalized brain space has the disadvantage of reducing effective spatial resolution. However, it has the advantage of providing an objective and unbiased transformation into a standardized space that can greatly facilitate quantitative approaches to analysis (for a recent discussion, see Zeffiro et al., 1997). The discussion below presumes that this second method has been applied; that is, it assumes that the brains of patients and normal control subjects have all been normalized to the same standard space.

If the statistical properties of the combined anatomical and functional variability of localization of specific cognitive processes were known and tabulated in some sort of atlas, then determination of whether activation is or is not located where it is expected to be in the normalized brain of the patient might be relatively straightforward. Barring that, researchers must collect data from a large enough sample of normals such that the patient's activation can be demonstrated to be outside of the expected range for normals. One possible method might involve (*1*) determining some measure of centrality of each cluster of activated voxels, perhaps by calculating the center of mass, and (*2*) performing an appropriate statistical test

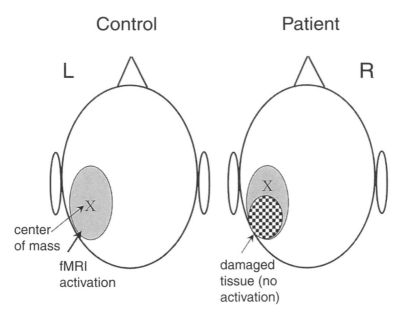

Figure 16-1. Simplified hypothetical results of a center of mass analysis (shown by the **X**) for a patient with left parietal damage and for a normal control subject. In this case, there is no evidence of plasticity. Results of the center-of-mass analysis, however, incorrectly suggest that there is adjacent tissue plasticity.

to evaluate whether the center of mass of the patient's cluster is reliably different from that the corresponding cluster or clusters in the normal control group. This approach is intuitively reasonable. However, it is problematic because the lack of activity in the damaged area in the patient can itself result in a shifted center of mass for a cluster relative to normals even if no plasticity detectable using fMRI is present. The highly simplified picture in Figure 16-1 depicts this scenario. On the left, an activation cluster for a normal subject is portrayed. On the right, the same cluster is shown for a patient who has sustained injury and has no neural function in an area that overlaps with the cluster. In this example, the perimeters of the activation cluster are identical for the normal subject and the patient (aside from the damaged portion itself). Thus, there is really no evidence of plasticity in this hypothetical result. However, a center of mass analysis would generate a different center coordinate for the patient than for the control simply because the centroid of the activation has shifted for the patient (see the loci of the **X**'s in Fig. 16-1). Thus, a pure center-of-mass analysis would lead the researcher to conclude that plasticity has been observed when in fact it has not.

A more appropriate approach would involve conducting a center-of-mass analysis, but only after first adjusting the activation in the normalized brain of the control subject to be zero in the area corresponding to the area damaged in the normalized brain of the patient. After this adjustment, the center-of-mass coordinates

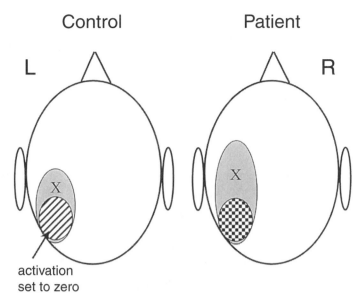

Figure 16-2. Simplified hypothetical results of a modified center-of-mass analysis (shown by the X) for a patient with left parietal damage and for a normal control subject. In this analysis, activation for the normal subject has been set to zero in the area corresponding to the damage in the patient. The result suggests adjacent tissue plasticity.

for the normal subject and the patient would be identical for the example depicted in Figure 16-1. If, however, there is plasticity in the patient on a scale detectable using fMRI, the center of mass would be shifted for the patient, as depicted in Figure 16-2.

A modified center-of-mass result such as that depicted in Figure 16-2 might tempt a researcher to conclude that there is an area activated in the patient that is not activated in the control subject. However, it is important to keep in mind the fact that all neuroimaging analysis techniques artificially dichotomize each measured brain area (or voxel cluster) into active and inactive categories to allow data to be synthesized and condensed into a comprehensible form. Thus, failure of an area to reach a statistical significance threshold in a given subject, regardless of the technique employed, does not imply that such areas are not activated at all by the task. Rather, the magnitude of activation in that area may simply be too small to be detected reliably given the available statistical power. This possibility is demonstrated by the results of a recent fMRI investigation of basic arithmetic in normal subjects (Rickard et al., 1997). In this study, a simple arithmetic verification task (e.g., $4 \times 7 = 32$; true of false?) was alternated with a perceptual-motor control condition. An axial anatomical slide with overlayed functional results is depicted for an example subject in Figure 16-3. On the top, a strict voxel-level activation threshold was used in the statistical analysis. On the bottom, a much more liberal voxel-level threshold was used. The liberal threshold analysis clearly shows acti-

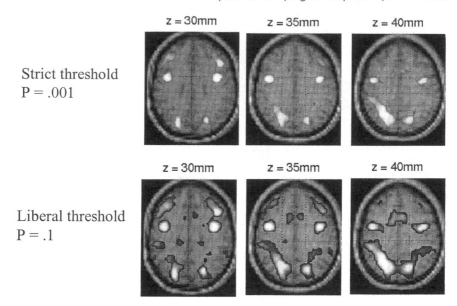

Figure 16-3. Functional magnetic resonance imaging results for a normal subject performing a multiplication verification task (e.g., $4 \times 7 = 32$; true or false?). The top panel shows the results for a high-voxel-level significance threshold, and the bottom panel shows the results for a low-voxel-level significance threshold.

vations not present in the strict threshold analysis. Particularly interesting is the anterior extension of the right parietal activation cluster, which is evident only in the liberal threshold analysis.

In applying fMRI to plasticity research, it is critical to keep in mind this contrast between the *all-or-none* activation differences between patients and controls and the *relative-intensity* activation differences. A conclusion of all-or-none activation differences requires an area to be reliably active in a patient but the corresponding area in normals to show no activity even under conditions in which statistical power to detect a small effect size is substantial. To date, there appear to be no plasticity studies using any neuroimaging technique that have clearly demonstrated all-or-none activation differences using this criterion. Indeed, it is possible that this strong form of plasticity does not exist in nature, or that it exists only in circumscribed brain regions, such as plasticity within the motor system or plasticity exhibited in adults who sustained injury during early childhood. From a neurophysiological perspective, relative intensity differences appear to be more likely to occur than all-or-none differences. It seems more natural that already existing connectivity in an area would be modified to facilitate lost function than that an entirely new area previously unrelated to the impaired function in the patient would come into play.

Approaches to Testing for Plasticity in Three Special Cases

In this section, I will outline what appear to be some unique challenges and opportunities posed by three different candidate types of plasticity observable through fMRI. First, however, it is worthwhile to discuss a potentially important pattern in brain activation that appears to be emerging in the recent literature. Specifically, for many types of tasks, there appears to be a substantial hemispheric symmetry in activation. As an example, in the Rickard et al. (1997) arithmetic study described previously, there was statistically significant and symmetrical activation in prefrontal, Broca's, parietal, and fusiform/lingual areas in each of eight subjects (an example of this symmetry can be seen in Fig. 16-3). In that study, the intensity level of activity was often asymmetric (e.g., greater activation in the left hemisphere in some case; see Fig. 16-3), but bilateral activation clusters were still detectable above the threshold in nearly every case. Note that nothing about a finding of hemispherically symmetric activation requires an inference of hemispherically symmetric function. It could be that different (but perhaps complementary) functions are performed in the two hemispheres. The point, for our purposes, is simply that, empirically speaking, symmetric patterns of activation appear to be the rule for at least some types of tasks (see Smith et al., 1995, for a related discussion). Interestingly, this hypothesis also raises the possibility that some positron emission tomography (PET) and fMRI results in the literature that have been interpreted as showing purely uni-hemispheric activity in fact represent cases in which only one of the two hemispheres obtained an activation level above the statistical reliability threshold employed.

Now consider the first candidate type of plasticity observable with fMRI, which I will call *homologous tissue plasticity* (e.g., see Weiller et al., 1994). The prospect that activation occurs symmetrically in the normal brain has important, albeit not necessarily encouraging, implications for investigation of homologous tissue plasticity using fMRI. Assume, for example, that a patient with extensive left inferior parietal damage shows relatively preserved arithmetic skills. The neuropsychological literature suggests that arithmetic is a dominantly left parietal process in the normal brain. Thus, one reasonable hypothesis would be that the preserved arithmetic skills in this patient reflect homologous plasticity of function in the right inferior parietal areas. Assume that fMRI activation in this patient during performance of arithmetic tasks indeed reveals right-sided inferior parietal activation. This finding might be taken as direct evidence of the hypothesized plasticity effect. However, assume also that results for normals show the symmetric left-right hemisphere inferior parietal activity pattern, as observed by Rickard et al. (1997; see Fig. 16-3). Clearly, based on this set of results alone, it would not be possible to make the strong inference that the right-sided activation in the patient necessarily reflects plasticity of function.

Greater confidence in that conclusion might be possible if, in addition, the patient shows relatively greater activation in the right hemisphere than do the controls. However, if the patient performs more poorly than the controls, even this result might be solely an artifact of performance differences, as outlined previously.

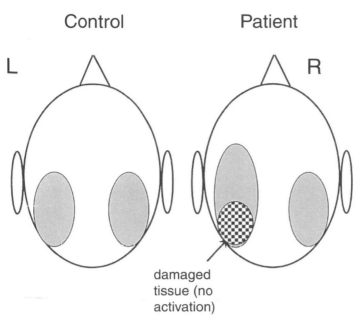

Figure 16-4. Hypothetical fMRI result suggestive of adjacent tissue plasticity in a patient with left parietal injury.

Converging evidence for a plasticity interpretation might be found by using alternative methods, such as transcranial magnetic stimulation, to confirm that the right-sided activity is more critical to task performance for the patient than it is for the controls. An alternative approach would be to conduct fMRI at multiple stages during remedial training, as outlined in the section "Performance Differences." If patient performance improves with training and activation in the homologous (right side) area also increases, then performance differences can be eliminated as a potential artifact.

In the second candidate case, plasticity occurs in the brain tissue adjacent to the cite of injury (i.e., *adjacent tissue plasticity*). Hemispheric symmetry of activation in the normal brain may have more encouraging implications for making inferences about adjacent plasticity. In the example shown in Figure 16-4, left parietal activation has been extended forward due a hypothetical plasticity effect after posterior left-side damage. The result is a left-right activation asymmetry in this patient. Assuming a high degree of symmetry in the normal population, one can, in principle, test an adjacent plasticity hypothesis by quantifying the asymmetry in the patient and showing that it would be rare given the statistical distribution of asymmetry observed for normals. One approach might be to demonstrate that there are brain regions in the patient that show a greater differential between left-sided and right-sided activation than would be expected in normal subjects. Regardless of the method employed, however, this approach in essence turns a between-subjects

Control   Patient

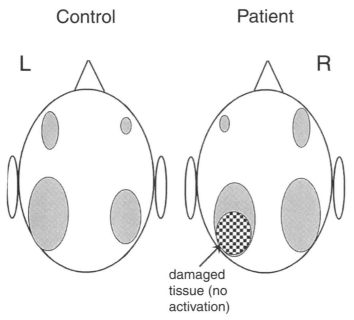

damaged
tissue (no
activation)

Figure 16-5. Example of a possible systems-level plasticity effect.

design, as presumed in earlier discussions, into a within-subjects (left versus right) design. This approach *may* provide statistical leverage if there is highly consistent hemispheric symmetry for normals in the task domain of interest.

A third general type of plasticity to be considered briefly will be termed *systems level plasticity.* This term is used to refer to distal changes in activity patterns accompanying recovery of function after brain injury. For example, consider Figure 16-5. On the left side of the figure, a hypothetical task in normals activates bilateral parietal and prefrontal areas (similar to the study of Rickard, et al., 1997; see Fig. 16-3), with stronger left-sided than right-sided activation in both locations. The right side of Figure 16-5 shows a candidate systems-level plasticity effect for the same task for a patient in whom the left parietal area is damaged and the right parietal area, as well as the right pre-frontal area, shows greater activation than in normals. Such a systems-level effect may prove to be fairly common and could reasonably be used to buttress a claim of plasticity in this example. However, note that the increase in right prefrontal activity in this example might just as reasonably reflect only a correlated increase in activation resulting from the increased right parietal activation. That is, any factor that increases posterior activity might increase anterior activity within the same hemisphere, quite independently of any neural plasticity per se. So, even if true neural plasticity is exhibited in the right posterior area (an inference that is subject to the complications outlined previously), the increase in right anterior activity might not reflect neural plasticity.

There are likely to be many different systems-level plasticity patterns, and detailed treatment of each of these is beyond the scope of this chapter. The important point, for our purposes, is that the issues that complicate inferences regarding neural plasticity in the preceding examples are at least as problematic in the case of systems-level plasticity.

Plasticity Effects Following Injury in Childhood Versus Adulthood

An especially promising application of fMRI to plasticity research involves comparison of activation patterns in a patient group that sustained an injury in early childhood to activation patterns in a patient group that sustained roughly equivalent injury in adulthood. Assume that both groups exhibit at least minimal performance on the task of interest but that the childhood injury group exhibits better, possibly near-normal, performance (as is often observed to be the case; see Stiles, 1995, for a review in the domain of visuospatial skills). Assume also that the task domain of interest is language and that the locus of injury is in the left temporofrontal language areas. Now consider an fMRI task that is within the capability of both groups and that taps language skills. One reasonable outcome would be that, relative to normal controls, the adult-injured patients would show only minimal right homologous activation (in the range of that observed for normals) but that the childhood-injured patients would show right homologous activation of much greater magnitude. Indeed, right hemisphere activation in the childhood-injured patients may match or even exceed left hemisphere activation in a normal control group. This hypothetical but plausible finding would allow strong inferences about relative plasticity effects following injury in childhood versus adulthood because it would place level of performance in opposition to the obtained differences in activation intensity. That is, the adult-injured group would exhibit poorer performance but would not exhibit unusual right hemisphere activation patterns. In contrast, the childhood-injured group would show nearly normal performance and would exhibit unusually strong right hemisphere activity patterns consistent with plasticity. The fact that fMRI activation generally appears to increase with increasing task difficulty (as indexed by decreased performance; see Carpenter et al., 1997) would thus be unable to explain the activation pattern of the childhood-injured group.

Conclusion

Functional magnetic resonance imaging appears to be well suited to the exploration of plasticity in the human brain following injury. In principle, this approach should be able to help answer at least two fundamental questions simultaneously: (*1*) what areas of the brain exhibit plasticity in response to a particular type and locus of injury? and (*2*) how does the degree of plasticity depend on the age at the time of injury? Although the obstacles to valid interpretation summarized in this chapter are indeed challenging, they do not appear to be insurmountable, at least for some types of research questions. In addition, inevitable improvements in the resolution and precision of fMRI, advances in complementary fields such as functional neuroanatomy and computational neuroscience, and the use of other emerging tools (such as magnetoencephalography and transcranial magnetic stimulation) as sources of converging evidence should ensure a central and productive role for neuroimaging techniques like fMRI in future studies of neuroplasticity following brain injury.

ACKNOWLEDGMENTS

I am grateful to Jordan Grafman for many productive conversations regarding neuroplasticity and to Gianpaolo Basso for assistance preparing figures.

References

Aine, C.J. (1995) A conceptual overview and critique of functional neuroimaging techniques in humans: I MRI/FMRI and PET. *Critical Reviews in Neurobiology,* 9:229–309.

Carpenter, M.P., Just, M.A., and Keller, T.A. (1997, March) Computational and fMRI studies of working memory in language comprehension. Paper presented at the 4th annual meeting of the Cognitive Neuroscience Society, Boston.

Ericsson, K.A., and Simon, H.A. (1984) *Protocol Analysis: Verbal Reports as Data.* Cambridge, MA: MIT Press.

Kim, S.G., and Ugurbil, K. (1997) Functional magnetic resonance imaging of the human brain. *Journal of Neuroscience Methods,* 74:229–43.

Kirk, E.P., and Ashcraft, M.H. (1997, November) Verbal Reports on Simple Addition: A demanding Task. Poster presented at the 38th annual meeting of the Psychonomics Society, Philadelphia.

Raichle, M.E., Fiez, J.A., Videen, T.O., Pardo, J.V., Fox, P.T., and Peterson, S.E. (1994) Practice-related changes in human brain functional anatomy during nonmotor learning. *Cerebral Cortex,* 4:8–29.

Rickard, T.C., Romero, S., Bassa, G., Wharton, C., Flitman, S., and Grafman, J. (1997) The calculating brain: An fMRI study. Submitted.

Siegler, R.S. (1988) Strategy choice procedures and the development of multiplication skill. *Journal of Experimental Psychology: General,* 117:258–275.

Stiles, J. (1995) Plasticity and development: Evidence from children with early focal brain injury. In B. Julesz and I. Kovacs (eds.), *Maturational Windows and Adult Cortical Plasticity.* Reading, MA: Addison-Wesley.

Talairach, J., and Tournoux, P. (1988) *Co-Planar Stereotaxic Atlas of the Human Brain.* New York: Thieme.

Weiller, C., Isenee, C., Rijntjes, M., Huber, W., Muller, S., Bier, D., Dutschka, K., Woods, R.P., Noth, J., and Diener, H.C. (1994) Recovery from Wernicke's aphasia: A positron emission tomographic study. *Annals of Neurology,* 37:723–732.

Zeffiro, T.A., Eden, G.F., Woods, R.P., and VanMeter, J.W. (1997) Intersubject analysis of fMRI data using spatial normalization. *Advances in Experimental Medicine and Biology,* 413:235–240.

17

Neuroimaging of Functional Recovery

RANDY L. BUCKNER AND STEVEN E. PETERSEN

A fundamental issue in studying recovery after brain damage is trying to understand how remaining (intact) brain regions support compensated capabilities. This broad issue directly prompts exploration of two related questions: (*1*) What are the brain pathways that support functioning in a given domain in the intact brain and (*2*) How are these pathways changed in the damaged brain? To answer these questions it is essential to have methods that allow observation of neural activity in the intact and damaged brain. For these methods to be truly useful they must be robust enough to identify brain areas active in different patient groups and individual subjects.

Functional neuroimaging provides one set of methods that might fulfill these requirements (Frackowiak & Friston, 1995; Posner & Raichle, 1994; Roland, 1993). In about an hour or two, a patient can be led through a noninvasive battery of imaging procedures that yields a picture of active brain areas across a number of conditions. Imaging can be done on normal as well as compromised brains.

However, current neuroimaging methods have various limitations and challenges. For example, these methods depend on indirect measurements of brain activity (hemodynamics) that are both sluggish in timing and poorly understood. Nonetheless, careful application of neuroimaging techniques can provide a window through which to view the neural basis of mental functions, including recovery following brain damage.

In this context, this chapter describes how functional neuroimaging techniques are being applied to elucidate human brain function. The basis of commonly used techniques focusing on positron emission tomography (PET) and functional MRI (fMRI) will be discussed, and then we will give some recent examples of how imaging has informed the understanding of the recovery of language function following left hemisphere damage.

318

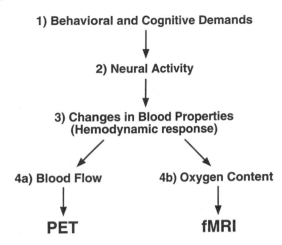

Figure 17-1. The logic and assumptions underlying PET and fMRI brain imaging are illustrated. Both methods rely on the observation that changes in (1) behavioral and cognitive task demands lead to changes in (2) neural activity. Through poorly understood mechanisms, changes in neural activity correlate closely with changes in (3) blood properties. It is these indirect measurements of neural activity on which both PET and fMRI base their measurements. Positron emission tomography measures brain activity through blood property change relating to (4a) blood flow, while fMRI measures a related property involving change in (4b) oxygen content (often referred to as the *BOLD-contrast mechanism*).

Methodological Considerations

Positron emission tomography and fMRI both take advantage of a fortuitous physiologic property: When a region of the brain increases its activity, both blood flow and the oxygen content of the blood in that region increase (Fig. 17-1). Positron emission tomography employs radiolabeled tracers to visualize blood flow changes related to neural activity (Raichle, 1987). Functional magnetic resonance imaging, which has been widely applied only in the past 5 years, most commonly visualizes neural activity indirectly through changes in oxygen content in the blood (Kwong et al., 1992; Ogawa et al., 1990, 1992). Other metabolic and hemodynamic contrast signals appropriate for both PET and fMRI also exist but are much less commonly used.

Several observations further suggest that the signals detected by PET and fMRI are valid measurements of local changes in neuronal activity. First, studies of primary visual cortex activation in relation to its well-understood retinotopic organization have demonstrated predictable activation patterns (e.g., DeYoe et al., 1996; Engel et al., 1997; Fox et al., 1987; Sereno et al., 1995) and suggest a current practical resolution of about 3 to 6 mm (e.g., Engel et al., 1997; Raichle, 1987). Resolution at this level can be used to map within large cortical areas (e.g., V1) and to identify smaller cortical areas (e.g., lateral intraparietal area (LIP)). This resolution also can distinguish between separate subcortical structures such as the amyg-

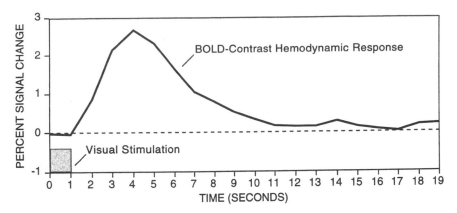

Figure 17-2. The temporal evolution of the hemodynamic signal on which both PET and fMRI base their measurements is illustrated for a 1 second visual stimulation (shown as a shaded rectangle). The response labeled "BOLD-Contrast Hemodynamic Response" shows the time course of the signal change in a visual cortex region. While tightly locked to the stimulation event, the sluggish hemodynamic response does not begin for about 2 seconds, peaks at about 4 to 6 seconds, and takes 10 to 12 seconds to evolve. This temporal blurring presents a challenge to brain imaging using PET and fMRI, but the problem can be overcome in certain instances (see text).

dala and the hippocampus. Imaging at this resolution, however, cannot resolve the columnar organization within a functional area. Second, neuroimaging tracks neuronal activity temporally. When prolonged or multiple visual stimuli are presented to subjects, the signal summates across the separate (Dale & Buckner, 1997; Fox & Raichle, 1985) and continuous (Boynton et al., 1996; Konishi et al., 1996) evoked neuronal events, as would be predicted for a measurement linked to neuronal activity (although modest deviations from this pattern can be found; Friston et al., 1997; Vazquez & Noll, 1998).

Neuroimaging methods have also demonstrated reliability across independent subject groups and even across imaging modalities (e.g., PET compared to fMRI; Clark et al., 1996; Ojemann et al., 1998). Critically important to patient studies, both techniques can measure brain pathways active in individual subjects, and do so quite reliably. This is illustrated in Plate 3 for a memory task.

However, both techniques have several important limitations that must be considered. It is unlikely that PET or currently applied fMRI will provide much information about local physiologic properties (e.g., whether a net activity change relies on inhibitory or excitatory synapses or on relative combinations of the two). In this regard, studies with current functional neuroimaging methods yield information about net changes in activity (both excitatory and inhibitory) within brain regions spanning several millimeters. Furthermore, hemodynamics in response to neuronal activity are revealed on a temporal scale far longer than that of the neuronal activity itself. For a sensory event lasting for only a fraction of a second, hemodynamic changes will take place over a 10 to 12 second period (Bandettini, Blamire 1993; et al., 1992; see Fig. 17-2).

While this limitation is less apparent for PET methods that average data over time periods of about 1 minute, this temporal "blurring" of the signal is a true limitation for fMRI studies that extend to measurements of a second or less (Cohen & Weisskoff, 1991). However, the restrictions on measurements are perhaps not as severe as one might imagine. For example, various fMRI methods have taken advantage of the reliable timing of the evoked blood flow signal to demonstrate temporal resolution at the subsecond level (Burock et al., 1998; Luknowsky et al., 1998; Rosen et al., 1998a). Changes in neural activity associated with individual trials or components of a trial of a task can be observed (Cohen et al., 1997; Courtney et al., 1997; Shulman et al., 1998). Richter et al. (1997), in a dramatic example of the temporal resolution and sensitivity of fMRI, captured brain activity associated with a *single* momentary cognitive act of mentally rotating a stimulus without recourse to averaging over events. However, examination of the temporal cascade of brain activity across areas on the order of tens to hundreds of milliseconds will probably remain the domain of techniques more directly coupled to neuronal activity, such as electroencephalography (EEG), magnetoencephalography (MEG) and perhaps human optical imaging.

Several differences beyond temporal precision exist between PET and fMRI that are worth mentioning. In contrast to PET, fMRI is completely noninvasive, requiring only that the subject lay still within the MRI scanner and comply with the behavioral procedures (DeYoe et al., 1994). In addition, fMRI is relatively inexpensive and can be performed on scanners available in most major hospitals, making it available for widespread clinical use. However, fMRI is extremely sensitive to brain motion and a number of other artifacts that can impede examination of brain function. The most severe challenge is motion.

Brain motion on the order of millimeters disrupts the ability to interpret fMRI data. Even motion associated with the respiratory and cardiac cycles can affect functional imaging of the brain. Motion correction algorithms (e.g., Woods et al., 1998) and head immobilization techniques are routinely used to reduce these difficulties, but motion remains a serious challenge to fMRI studies, especially studies of patients. In particular, it is difficult (but not impossible) to image overt speech production during fMRI studies because of the head motion and the changes in air volume associated with overt speech (e.g., see Birn et al., 1999; Phelps et al., 1997).

While PET has the disadvantages of invasiveness and temporal sampling, there is one area in which it has a clear current advantage: quantitation. Positron emission tomography can provide relatively accurate measurements of absolute blood flow (and some other metabolic measures). For this reason, images of functional as well as structural lesions can be obtained, including images of areas distant from structural lesions that show metabolic abnormalities. Images of functional lesions can potentially be correlated with behavioral measures, much as structural lesions can.

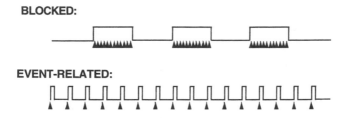

Figure 17-3. Two separate paradigms are illustrated: blocked and event-related. In the blocked paradigm, many task trials (arrowheads) of the same kind are presented sequentially, and the entire epoch is averaged together. Brain activation changes are measured by contrasting extended epochs in which subjects perform a target task to other extended epochs (shown as the intervening time periods between sequential trials in the blocked paradigm) in which a reference control task is performed. By contrast, in the event-related paradigm, individual trials are isolated and there are no separate task trial blocks. Recent methods have demonstrated that event-related paradigms can isolate individual trials spaced just a few seconds apart (see text).

Applications of Neuroimaging Techniques

Beyond basic technical considerations, one must consider issues of the practical application of neuroimaging techniques to questions about human higher brain function and recovery. Namely, how can tasks and trials within a task be constructed to disentangle brain-based cognitive operations? This topic presents a number of challenges, and no single answer exists. The basic paradigm construct most commonly used is to have subjects engage in a target task for a period of time (perhaps multiple trials of a word generation task) and then contrast that task period to periods in which subjects perform a reference task (perhaps a matched task involving viewing of words with no production or something as simple as having a subject fixate a small plus sign).

The logic of this paradigm construct is that brain activity will change between the two task states and correlate selectively with the manipulated task demands. When fMRI is used, images are taken of the brain repeatedly in sequence (as rapidly as one set of whole-brain images every 2 seconds). Brain areas of activation are identified by examining which specific regions change signal intensity as the task state changes from the reference condition (word viewing or fixation) to the target task (word generation). One example of such a paradigm construct is illustrated in Figure 17-3A.

Statistical procedures ranging from simple, direct comparisons between task states to complex assessments of interactions and correlation among task states can then be employed to identify those regions whose activity change is unlikely to occur by chance (Frackowiak & Friston, 1995). Correlation of activity with subject performance is also possible.

More recently, paradigms that isolate individual trials of tasks have been developed—so-called event-related procedures (Buckner et al., 1996a; Dale & Buckner, 1997; Josephs et al., 1997; Rosen et al., 1998a; Zarahn et al., 1997). An example of an event-related paradigm is illustrated in Figure 17-3B. These procedures allow experimenters to contrast activity associated with different types of trials and even to disentangle the activity associated with subcomponents of a trial. For example, trials of one type (e.g., trials performed correctly) can be contrasted to separate trials of another type (e.g., trials performed incorrectly). Important to patient explorations, event-related procedures can allow removal of individual trials (or MRI images) associated with gross head movement or bad performance.

As an example of how such paradigms can be used to study language, let us consider a target language task referred to as the *word-stem completion task,* which has an extensive history in both PET and fMRI studies. This task involves presenting subjects with visual word-stem cues (e.g., "cou____", "str____") and asking them to generate complete words (e.g., "courage," "string"). This task requires visual processing and motor production (when overt speech is required), and also places demands on lexical access and word selection. A number of studies using both PET (Buckner et al., 1995a, 1995b; Schacter et al., 1996a; Squire et al., 1992) and fMRI (Buckner et al., 1996a; Ojemann et al., 1998) have explored this task. Older adults (Backman et al., 1997; Schacter et al., 1996b) and patients (Buckner et al., 1996b) have been studied as well, making the task particularly useful for illustrating how neuroimaging can be applied to questions of clinical interest.

Examination of either blood flow changes with PET or related changes with fMRI demonstrate robust activity within a network of brain areas when word-stem completion is contrasted to a low-level reference task in which subjects simply fixate a cross-hair. These areas include visual and motor regions, medial and lateral cerebellum, and frontal regions near classically defined Broca's area. The areas of frontal activation, particularly those localized inferiorly near the ventral portion of the inferior frontal gyrus and operculum, are most often strongly left lateralized.

By relying on convergent data across tasks and laboratories, it is possible to begin to define the processing contributions of specific brain areas to word-stem completion task performance. For example, the left frontal region that is activated near the operculum during word-stem completion can be shown to be active across a wide range of tasks requiring manipulation of verbal materials, regardless of whether speech is required. This finding suggests that this area plays a role in lexical access or representation of verbal materials (Buckner & Petersen, 1996; Gabrieli et al., 1998). Verbal fluency tasks, elaborate speech production tasks, and verbal working memory tasks all rely on this process and depend on left frontal participation in the normal intact brain.

Given the ability to make such observations, it is not surprising that these techniques can be applied to the study of recovery. The following section describes neuroimaging data suggesting that the right frontal cortex may compensate, in certain instances, for damaged left frontal regions.

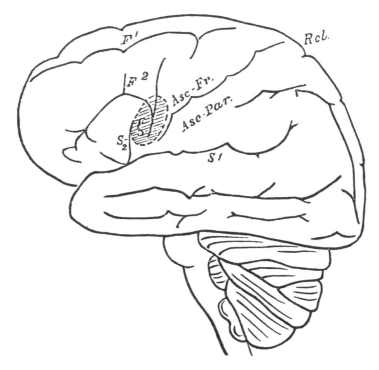

Figure 17-4. The original illustration of Barlow's famous patient is presented (Barlow, 1877). The hatched portion of the brain shows the location of the area on the right side that was believed to participate in recovery of speech function. This illustration represents some of the earliest data suggesting that functional recovery following left hemisphere injury may be supported by atypical right hemisphere involvement.

Example: Is Right Frontal Cortex Used During Language Recovery Following Left Hemisphere Stroke?

The idea that right frontal regions compensate for functional damage to the left frontal cortex was suggested on the basis of a case study of a 10-year-old boy who suffered serial lesions to the left and then the right hemispheres (Barlow, 1877). The patient largely recovered from an initial aphasia associated with right hemiplegia. Four months later, a second lesion reintroduced aphasia, but this time associated with left hemiplegia. Examination of the postmortem brain localized the earlier infarct to an area the size of "a shilling" within the left inferior frontal cortex (near the region now defined as Broca's area) and the later infarct to a region of tissue softening in the right homolog (Fig. 17-4). The implication of this extraordinary case was that the right hemisphere played a role in functional recovery after the initial insult—specifically, the homologous region in the right frontal cortex near the inferior frontal gyrus.

The findings in a number of more modern studies have been consistent with Barlow's observation, including several further cases of serial left and then right lesions producing aphasia (Vallar, 1990). Additional evidence comes from sodium amytal injections, which can pharmacologically inactivate the spared right hemisphere in left hemisphere stroke patients and sometimes produce language impairments in recovered aphasics (Kinsbourne, 1971). Thus, a number of sources indicate that right hemisphere compensation appears to contribute to recovery from aphasia. However, as has been noted, the complex process of recovery in any given individual is unique and may involve multiple mechanisms, such as the use of preserved left hemisphere regions (Cappa & Vallar, 1992). Functional brain imaging is able to bring a new perspective to this work by characterization, on a patient-by-patient basis, of the brain areas used during recovered language function. To illustrate the potential of using functional brain imaging to understand recovery, we turn to a case study of patient LF1 and several recent extensions of this study.

Patient LF1 was our first exploration of functional recovery after stroke (Buckner et al., 1996b); similar investigations have been conducted in many other laboratories (e.g., Ohyama et al., 1995). LF1 (named for "Left Frontal" patient 1) was a 72-year-old retired professional who presented with speech difficulties on waking one morning. He was familially right-handed. Clinical evaluation, including computed tomography (CT) and MRI, revealed a left frontal infarct consistent with stroke. The extent of the infarct included the inferior portion of the frontal gyrus and the frontal operculum, sparing the anterior portion of the temporal lobe. Neuropsychological evaluation 1 month after the stroke showed that LF1 was extremely intelligent, with a premorbid IQ probably above 120. As an example of his high intelligence, he performed in the top 1st percentile on nonverbal tests of block design and visual reproduction. Consistent with the location of his stroke and the nature of his initial presentation, he was severely impaired on many verbal fluency tests but not on tests of nonverbal design fluency. At 6 months, LF1 still had significant speech impairments and was classified as a mildly nonfluent aphasic.

LF1 was also tested on a number of tasks motivated by the neuroimaging literature. Predictably, he was found to be impaired on several tests tapping verbal fluency, such as verb generation to nouns and synonym generation. However, to our surprise, there was a class of word generation tasks that LF1 could perform at near-normal levels. One task within this preserved group was the word-stem completion task described above. LF1 performed 85% to 90% percent correctly over several testing sessions, including a session 1 month after his stroke. The overlap between LF1's lesion and normal subjects' frontal activation during this task can be seen in Plate 4 (Buckner et al., 1995a, 1995b, for a discussion of the normal functional anatomy used during this task).

The finding that LF1 performed well on a task that normally activated his missing left frontal cortex positioned him as a patient likely to be using compensatory anatomy. Positron emission tomography functional brain imaging was used to determine the nature of his compensatory pathway. LF1 was imaged while he performed the word-stem completion task; the results can be seen in Plate 4. Whereas normal subjects show robust activation of left frontal cortex during word-stem completion, LF1 showed significant activation on the right. Comparison to a group of control subjects (not age-matched) revealed that none of them exhibited right frontal activation to the same degree as LF1; however, certain subjects exhibited modest, but still significant, right frontal activation—a finding subsequently confirmed with fMRI (Ojemann et al., 1998). The data support the hypothesis that LF1 was using a right prefrontal region to compensate after his left frontal stroke. His compensation was incomplete, as he was able to perform only certain word production tasks.

The presence of weak right frontal activation in normal subjects (combined with the finding that LF1 showed good performance on word-stem completion 1 month after his stroke) suggests that the recovery mechanism observed was compensatory rather than due to a process of new growth. It can be speculated that LF1, having lost the use of the normal left dominant pathway for speech production, was able to recruit the participation of a less used right frontal region.

Two recent follow-up studies have been conducted by Maurizio Corbetta and colleagues that expand on the initial observation concerning patient LF1 (Rosen et al., 1998b, 1998c). First and most important, a group of new chronic patients ($n = 3$) and age-matched control subjects ($n = 6$) were examined to determine if the observation in LF1 was an oddity or if it would generalize to additional patients. This issue is important because there has been at least one observation (since that of LF1) of strong right frontal activation in a normal, familial right-handed subject performing the same word-stem completion task eliciting LF1's right frontal activation (Chee et al., 1998).

The new patients had all suffered strokes that included the left frontal operculum and, on initial presentation, exhibited nonfluent aphasia. These patients were imaged in their chronic phase 6 months to 1 year after the onset of aphasia. Relevant to the question of generalization, the three patients (when averaged together) showed significant activation in the right frontal operculum in a region nearly homologous to the region activated by the control subjects on the left side. Both the patients and the control subjects performed the word-stem completion task at moderate to good levels (67% correct for patients, 84% correct for controls). Rosen et al. (1998b) extended this finding to fMRI and demonstrated, using a covert word-stem completion paradigm, that right frontal activation could be detected in one of the patients. Thus, the finding in LF1 generalizes both to additional subjects and to fMRI studies using covert procedures.

The second study, however, provides data that must be considered when interpreting the presence of activation in the right frontal cortex as being directly related to recovery. Rosen et al. (1998c) examined a patient 1 month after a large frontotemporoparietal infarction. This patient could not perform the word-stem completion task and made stereotyped, unrelated utterances to each word stem. The finding that the patient made utterances to each word stem suggests that effort was being exerted to perform the task but that appropriate completion of the task was impossible at that time. Despite this poor performance, when the patient was imaged using PET, a robust increase in activation was noted in the right frontal operculum similar to that found in LF1 and in the three patients of Rosen et al.

(1998b), who all performed at near-normal levels. Two unanswered questions follow from this recent and still tentative finding. First, why was the region active if it could not support functional compensation at the acute stage? And second, is the right prefrontal activation *responsible* for the recovery in patients like LF1?

While it is too early to draw firm conclusions, the combination of findings across multiple methods (PET, fMRI, serial lesion studies, and Wada tests) suggest the possibility that right hemisphere activation plays a role in a recovery from aphasia. Nonetheless, the problem of early activation in the recovery process has yet to be solved and may provide insights into how rehabilitation may be influenced by observations from neuroimaging. It seems possible that right frontal regions are engaged rapidly after a stroke but that they initially support only minimal linguistic functions; this level may vary from patient to patient. Through some unknown self-organizing process, in certain patients participation of the right-lateralized regions may come to support limited speech function. From a historical perspective, it is worth noting that Barlow's patient (1877) exhibited severe aphasia initially (he could only say "Haw-haw"). Yet within 10 days the patient came to use (apparently) the right frontal cortex, which correlated with recovered speech (this, of course, is just one possible interpretation of Barlow's data). The patient still "occasionally made a mistake, gave the wrong name for a boy, and did not seem always quite to understand what was said to him" (Barlow, 1877 p. 103), suggesting that his recovery was incomplete, much like that of patient LF1.

We conceptualize this process in a simplified way as a *broken-hand* model of recovery. When people break their dominant writing hand, they often gradually begin to write with their already functional nondominant hand, clumsily at first and then better with effort and practice. Right frontal compensation may progress in a similar fashion. A task for the future will be to characterize the progression of activation in the right frontal cortex; to determine whether it correlates with recovery from chronic aphasia; and, in instances where function has not significantly recovered, to determine whether activation predicts later recovery. Functional magnetic resonance imaging methods are readily able to image patients repeatedly over time at different points in their recovery process without notable side effects. Hypotheses such as whether right lateralized brain regions come to compensate for recovered function can be supported and further expanded. Other routes to recovery can also be explored. Perhaps most critically, the characterization of these various activation patterns may have clinical worth by contributing a variable that will help predict which patients can benefit from specific rehabilitative strategies.

References

Backman, L., Almkvist, O., Andersson, J., Nordberg, A., Winbald, B., Reineck, R., and Langstrom, B. (1997) Brain activation in young and older adults during implicit and explicit retrieval. *Journal of Cognitive Neuroscience,* 9:378–391.

Bandettini, P.A. (1993) MRI studies of brain activation: Dynamic characteristics. In *Functional MRI of the Brain.* Berkeley: Society of Magnetic Resonance in Medicine, pp. 144–151.

Barlow, T. (1877) On a case of double hemiplegia, with cerebral symmetrical lesions. *British Medical Journal,* 2:103–104.

Birn, R.M., Bandettini, P.A., Cox, R.W., and Shaker, R. (1999) Event-related fMRI of tasks involving brief motion. *Human Brain Mapping.* 7:106–114.

Blamire, A.M., Ogawa, S., Ugurbil, K., Rothman, D., McCarthy, G., Ellerman, J.M., Hyder, F., Rattner, Z., and Shulman, R.G. (1992) Dynamic mapping of the human visual cortex by high-speed magnetic resonance imaging. *Proceedings of the National Academy of Sciences of the USA,* 89:11069–11073.

Boynton, G.M., Engel, S.A., Glover, G.H., and Heeger, D.J. (1996) Linear systems analysis of functional magnetic resonance imaging in human V1. *Journal of Neuroscience,* 16:4207–4221.

Buckner, R.L., Bandettini, P.A., O'Craven, K.M., Savoy, R.L., Petersen, S.E., Raichle, M.E., and Rosen, B.R. (1996a) Detection of cortical activation during averaged single trials of a cognitive task using functional magnetic resonance imaging. *Proceedings of the National Academy of Sciences of the USA,* 93:14878–14883.

Buckner, R.L., Corbetta, M., Schatz, J., Raichle, M.E., and Petersen, S.E. (1996b) Preserved speech abilities and compensation following prefrontal damage. *Proceedings of the National Academy of Sciences of the USA,* 93:1249–1253.

Buckner, R.L., and Petersen, S.E. (1996) What does neuroimaging tell us about the role of prefrontal cortex in memory retrieval? *Seminars in Neuroscience,* 8:47–55.

Buckner, R.L., Petersen, S.E., Ojemann, J.G., Miezin, F.M., Squire, L.R., and Raichle, M.E. (1995a) Functional anatomical studies of explicit and implicit memory retrieval tasks. *Journal of Neuroscience,* 15:12–29.

Buckner, R.L., Raichle, M.E., and Petersen, S.E. (1995b) Dissociation of human prefrontal cortical areas across different speech production tasks and gender groups. *Journal of Neurophysiology,* 74:2163–2173.

Buckner, R.L., Koutstaal, W., Schacter, D.L., Dale, A.M., Rotte M., and Rosen, B.R. (1998) Functional-anatomic study of episodic retrieval. II. Selective averaging of event-related fMRI trials to test the retrieval success hypothesis. NeuroImage 7:163–175.

Burock, M.A., Buckner, R.L., Woldorff, M.G., Rosen, B.R., and Dale, A.M. (1998) Randomized event-related experimental designs allow for extremely rapid presentation rates using functional MRI. *NeuroReport,* 9:3735–3739.

Cappa, S.F., and Vallar, G. (1992) The role of the left and right hemispheres in recovery from aphasia. *Aphasiology,* 6:359–372.

Chee, M.L., Buckner, R.L., and Savoy, R.L. (1998) Right hemisphere language in a neurologically normal dextral: A fMRI study. *NeuroReport,* 9:3499–3502.

Clark, V.P., Keil, K., Maisog, M., Courney, S., Ungerleider, L.G., and Haxby, J.V. (1996) Functional magnetic resonance imaging of human visual cortex during face matching: A comparison with postiron emission tomography. *NeuroImage,* 4:1–15.

Cohen, J.D., Perlstein, W.M., Braver, T.S., Nystrom, L.E., Noll, D.C., Jonides, J., and Smith, E.E. (1997) Temporal dynamics of brain activation during a working memory task. *Nature,* 386:604–607.

Cohen, M.S., and Weisskoff, R.M. (1991) Ultra-fast imaging. *Magnetic Resonance Imaging,* 9:1–37.

Courtney, S.M., Ungerleider, L.G., Keil, K., and Haxby, J.V. (1997) Transient and sustained activity in a distributed neural system for human working memory. *Nature,* 386:608–611.

Dale, A.M., and Buckner, R.L. (1997) Selective averaging of rapidly presented individual trials using fMRI. *Human Brain Mapping,* 5:329–340.

DeYoe, E.A., Bandettini, P., Neitz, J., Miller, D., and Winans, P. (1994) Functional magnetic resonance imaging (fMRI) of the human brain. *Journal of Neuroscience Methods,* 54:171–187.

DeYoe, E.A., Carman, G.J., Bandettini, P., Glickman, S., Wieser, J., Cox, R., Miller, D., and Neitz, J. (1996) Mapping striate and extrastriate visual areas in human cerebral cortex. *Proceedings of the National Academy of Sciences of the USA,* 93:2382–2386.

Engel, S.A., Glover, G.H., and Wandell, B.A. (1997) Retinotopic organization in human visual cortex and the spatial precision of functional MRI. *Cerebral Cortex,* 7:181–192.

Fox, P.T., Miezin, F.M., Allman, J.M., Van Essen, D.C., and Raichle, M.E. (1987) Retinotopic organization of human visual cortex mapped with positron emission tomography. *Journal of Neuroscience,* 7:913–922.

Fox, P.T., and Raichle, M.E. (1985) Stimulus rate determines regional brain blood flow in striate cortex. *Annals of Neurology,* 17:303–305.

Frackowiak, R.S.J., and Friston, K.J. (1995) Methodology of activation paradigms. In F. Boller and J. Grafman (eds.), *Handbook of Neuropsychology.* Amsterdam: Elsevier, pp. 369–282.

Friston, K.J., Josephs, O., Rees, G., and Turner, R. (1997) Nonlinear event-related responses in fMRI. *Magnetic Resonance Medicine,* 39:41–52.

Gabrieli, J.D.E., Poldrack, R.A., and Desmond, D.E. (1998) The role of left prefrontal cortex in language and memory. *Proceedings of the National Academy of Sciences of the USA,* 95:906–913.

Josephs, O., Turner, R., and Friston, K. (1997) Event-related fMRI. *Human Brain Mapping,* 5:243–248.

Kinsbourne, M. (1971) The minor hemisphere as a source of aphasic speech. *Archives of Neurology,* 25:302–306.

Konishi, S., Yoneyama, R., Itagaki, H., Uchida, I., Nakajima, K., Kato, H., Okajima, K., Koizumi, H., and Miyashita, Y. (1996) Transient brain activity used in magnetic resonance imaging to detect functional areas. *NeuroReport,* 8:19–23.

Kwong, K.K., Belliveau, J.W., Chesler, D.A., Goldberg, I.E., Weisskoff, R.M., Poncelet, B.P., Kennedy, D.N., Hoppel, B.E., Cohen, M.S., and Turner, R. (1992) Dynamic magnetic resonance imaging of human brain activity during primary sensory stimulation. *Proceedings of the National Academy of Sciences of the USA,* 89:5675–5679.

Luknowsky, D.C., Gati, J.S., and Menon, R.S. (1998) Mental chronometry using single trials and EPI at 4 T. *Proceedings of the International Society for Magnetic Resonance in Medicine: 6th Meeting,* 1:167.

Ogawa, S., Lee, T., Nayak, A., and Glynn, P. (1990) Oxygenation-sensitive contrast in magnetic resonance image of rodent brain at high magnetic fields. *Magnetic Resonance Medicine,* 14:68–78.

Ogawa, S., Tank, D.W., Menon, R., Ellerman, J.M., Kim, S.G., Merkle, H., and Ugurbil, K. (1992) Intrinsic signal changes accompanying sensory stimulation: Functional brain mapping with magnetic resonance imaging. *Proceedings of the National Academy of Sciences of the USA,* 89:5951–5955.

Ohyama, M., Senda, M., Kitamura, S., Ishii, K., Mishina, M., and Terashi, A. (1995) Role of the nondominant hemisphere and undamaged area during word repetition in poststroke aphasics. *Stroke,* 27:897–903.

Ojemann, J.G., Buckner, R.L., Akbudak, E., Snyder, A.Z., Ollinger, J.M., McKinstry, R.C., Rosen, B.R., Petersen, S.E., Raichle, M.E., and Conturo, T.E. (1998) Functional MRI studies of word stem completion: Reliability across laboratories and comparison to blood flow imaging with PET. *Human Brain Mapping,* 6:203–215.

Phelps, E.A., Hyder, F., Blamire, A.M., and Shulman, R.G. (1997) FMRI of the prefrontal cortex during overt verbal fluency. *NeuroReport,* 8:561–565.

Posner, M.I., and Raichle, M.E. (1994) *Images of Mind.* New York: Scientific American Books.

Raichle, M.E. (1987) Circulatory and metabolic correlates of brain function in normal humans. In F. Plum and V. Mountcastle (eds.), *The Handbook of Physiology: Section 1. The Nervous System: Vol. V: Higher Functions of the Brain: Part 1.* Bethesda, MD: American Physiological Association, pp. 643–674.

Richter, W., Georgopoulos, A.P., Ugurbil, K., and Kim, S.-G. (1997) Detection of brain activity during mental rotation in a single trial by fMRI. *NeuroImage,* 5:S49.

Roland, P.E. (1993) *Brain Activation.* New York: Wiley-Liss.

Rosen, B.R., Buckner, R.L., and Dale, A.M. (1998a). Event related fMRI: Past, present, and future. *Proceedings of the National Academy of Sciences of the USA,* 95:773–780.

Rosen, H., Fiez, J.A., Hanlon, R., Dromerick, A.W., Linenweber, M., Petersen, S.E., Raichle, M.E., and Corbetta, M. (1998b) Functional imaging of recovery in patients with Broca's aphasia and left frontal opercular damage. *NeuroImage,* 7:S23.

Rosen, H., Petersen, S.E., Linenweber, M., Fiez, J.A., White, D., Chapman, L., and Corbetta, M. (1998c) Right frontal activation speech production in a patient with subacute aphasia. *Society for Neuroscience Abstracts,* 24:20.

Schacter, D.L., Alpert, N.M., Savage, C.R., Rauch, S.L., and Albert, M.S. (1996a) Conscious recollection and the human hippocampal formation: Evidence from positron emission tomography. *Proceedings of the National Academy of Sciences of the USA,* 93:321–325.

Schacter, D.L., Savage, C.R., Alpert, N.M., Rauch, S.L., and Albert, M.S. (1996b) The role of hippocampus and frontal cortex in age-related memory changes: A PET study. *NeuroReport,* 7:1165–1169.

Sereno, M.I., Dale, A.M., Reppas, J.B., Kwong, K.K., Belliveau, J.W., Brady, T.J., Rosen, B.R., and Tootell, R.B.H. (1995) Borders of multiple visual areas in humans revealed by functional magnetic resonance imaging. *Science,* 268:889–893.

Shulman, G.L., Ollinger, J.M., Petersen, S.E., Akbudak, E., Conturo, T.E., Snyder, A.Z., and Corbetta, M. (1998) Separation of cue and motion fMRI signals in a cued motion paradigm. *Society for Neuroscience Abstracts,* 24:506.

Squire, L.R., Ojemann, J.G., Miezin, F.M., Petersen, S.E., Videen, T.O., and Raichle, M.E. (1992) Activation of the hippocampus in normal humans: A functional anatomical study of memory. *Proceedings of the National Academy of Sciences of the USA,* 89:1837–1341.

Vallar, G. (1990) Hemispheric control of articulatory speech output in aphasia. In G. R. Hammond, (ed.), *Cerebral Control of Speech.* Amsterdam: North-Holland, pp. 387–416.

Vazquez, A.L., and Noll, D.C. (1998) Nonlinear aspects of the BOLD response in functional MRI. *NeuroImage,* 7:108–118.

Woods, R.P., Grafton, S.T., Holmes, C.J., Cherry, S.R., and Mazziotta, J.C. (1998) Automated image registration: I. General methods and intrasubject, intramodality validation. *Journal of Computer Assisted Tomography,* 22:139–152.

Zarahn, E., Aguirre, G., and D'Esposito, M. (1997). A trial-based experimental design for fMRI. *NeuroImage,* 6:122–138.

18

Computational Modeling of the Cortical Response to Focal Damage

JAMES A. REGGIA, SHARON GOODALL,
KEN REVETT, AND EYTAN RUPPIN

Efforts to understand the mechanisms of recovery following a stroke have traditionally been based on either clinical studies or animal models. In this chapter we will describe some initial steps in developing an alternative approach: computational models of the cerebral cortex and its reorganization following acute focal lesions. Ischemic stroke, where there is a loss of blood flow to a region of the brain, is a very complex multifactorial process. Acute and poststroke changes involve neural plasticity; metabolic and biochemical events; biophysical processes such as diffusion, mechanical displacement secondary to edema, altered autoregulation and metabolic regulation of blood flow; and other events. These events and their interactions are only partially understood; their complexity has led some investigators to suggest that novel ways of thinking about stroke are needed (Hallenback & Frerichs, 1993). Computational models provide a new approach that can be useful in furthering our understanding by supporting detailed examination of various hypotheses about stroke pathophysiology and recovery. In other words, the complexity of events in stroke suggests that computational models can be powerful tools for its investigation, much as they are in the analysis of other complex systems (e.g., climate prediction).

The work described in this chapter should be viewed in the broad context of other computational modeling studies of the effects of brain damage on neurological and cognitive functions. Research in this area has been growing rapidly during the last decade (Reggia et al., 1996). A sense of the scope of this computational research can be obtained by considering the range of disorders studied: Alzheimer's disease, amnesia, aphasia, depression, dyslexia, epilepsy, ischemic stroke, migraine, visual neglect, parkinsonism, schizophrenia, and others. Many of these models have included computational investigation of aspects of neuroplasticity, such as synaptic compensatory changes in Alzheimer's disease, cortical map reorganization following deafferentation, and changes in neural circuit efficacy after pharmacological therapy.

Our focus in this chapter is on developing a computer model of the pathophysiological events occurring in ischemic stroke. Ultimately, what is required is a sufficiently powerful model that can be used to understand better the acute poststroke changes in the ischemic penumbra, to determine which factors lead to worsening or recovery from stroke, and to suggest new pharmacological interventions and rehabilitative actions that could improve the outcome of stroke. However, the complexity of stroke pathophysiology, and the limitations of current neural modeling technology and neuroscientific knowledge, make it impractical to begin with a detailed, large-scale model of the brain and all the effects of a major stroke. In this chapter, we consider the more limited objective of creating computer models of circumscribed regions of cerebral cortex and of small, ischemic lesions. Magnetic resonance imaging (MRI) evidence suggests that small cortical and subcortical ischemic strokes are far more common and important than is generally recognized (Hougaku et al., 1994), and our models also relate to the small cortical infarcts that can be produced with contemporary animal models of stroke. The reason for focusing on small lesions in restricted cortical regions is the wealth of data on map organization in such regions and the fact that a model of this size provides the best match with the current state of the art in neural modeling technology.

Two specific computational models are described below to illustrate how focal brain damage can be modeled computationally. These models are explicitly intended to simulate map plasticity following small cortical ischemic strokes, i.e., to examine compensatory mechanisms in cortex immediately surrounding a site of focal brain damage. The first model uses a topographic map of the hand region of primary somatosensory cortex. Following a sudden focal cortical lesion, portions of the hand originally represented in the lesioned area reappear in the perilesion cortex, as has been observed experimentally in animal studies. The second model involves feature maps in proprioceptive and motor cortex regions that control a simulated arm moving in three-dimensional space. In this model, a sudden focal cortical lesion can produce a very different result: a perilesion zone of decreased cortical activity. These two models make testable predictions, among them that postlesion map reorganization occurs in two phases and that perilesion excitability is a critical factor in map reorganization. Current work is extending these studies to more realistic models incorporating biochemical and metabolic factors important in stroke and to models involving contralateral hemispheric changes as well. This chapter concludes with a summary and overview of this ongoing work.

Lesioning Topographic Sensory Maps

Cortical maps can conveniently be classified as *topographic maps* (Udin & Fawcett, 1988), which reflect the distribution and density of peripheral neurons over the

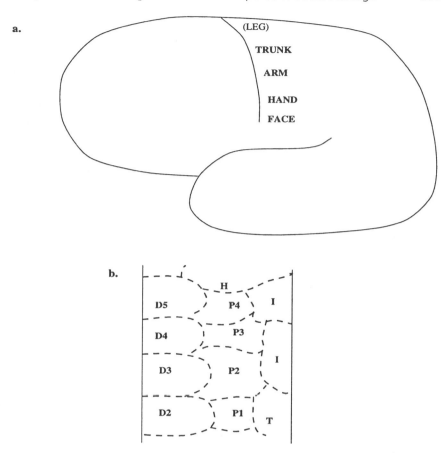

Figure 18-1. Primary somatosensory (SI) map. (a) The contralateral body surface is represented in the postcentral gyrus in a systematic, order-preserving fashion, forming a topographic map. (b) Simplified, enlarged caricature of the hand region shown in (a). Areas representing individual digits (D1–D5; only four pictured here), palmar surfaces (P1–P4), thenar eminence (T), are labeled.

body surface, or as *feature maps* (computational maps) (Knudsen et al., 1987), in which a computed feature varies across the cortical surface. For example, in primary visual cortex, line orientation and ocular dominance columns are organized into bands (a computational map) that are embedded in a topographic (retinotopic) map.

The Topographic Map in Primary Somatosensory Cortex

A familiar example of topographic map, which we deal with in this section occurs in primary somatosensory (SI) cortex, as illustrated in Figure 18-1a. In this lateral view of the left hemisphere, the opposite side of the body is systematically projected onto the postcentral gyrus. Electrophysiological studies in animals have carefully charted the details of this map; for example, the individual fingers and palmar areas of the hand can be identified (Fig. 18-1b) (Merzenich et al., 1983; Wall et al., 1993).

One of the most intriguing experimental observations in recent years is that maps in the sensory and motor cortices of adult animals are highly plastic (adaptable). For example, if a single finger of the hand is repeatedly stimulated over time, the area representing that finger in the SI cortical map increases substantially at the expense of areas of neighboring regions (Jenkins et al., 1990). If a cortical finger region is deafferented, say by peripheral nerve sectioning, then that region of the cortical map becomes initially unresponsive to skin stimuli. Within a few weeks, however, the representations of surrounding hand regions expand into the deafferented cortical region, which is once again responsive to peripheral stimuli (Kaas, 1991; Merzenich et al., 1983).

Studies in humans following deafferentation indicate that map reorganization similar to that seen in animals occurs, often associated with increased cortical excitability (Brasil-Neto et al., 1993; Cohen et al., 1991; Pascual-Leone & Torres, 1993). The extent to which such changes are due to neocortical plasticity, unmasking of normally silent subcortical pathways, or other mechanisms is unclear (Calford, 1991; Killackey, 1989). Only limited animal data are available on the effects of cortical lesions on map reorganization. These data indicate that following small focal lesions in SI cortex, the body surface represented in the lesioned area eventually reappears in the perilesion region (Jenkins & Merzenich, 1987). Movements originally represented in a primary motor cortical area reappear outside that area when it is lesioned (Glees & Cole, 1950), perhaps even in the somatosensory cortex (Sasaki & Gema, 1984) or contralaterally (Chollet et al., 1991), although there is some conflicting evidence (Boyeson et al., 1994).

During the last few years, several efforts have been made to develop computational models of cortical map self-organization and map refinement (Ritter et al., 1992). These models typically take the form of a two-layer network and use an unsupervised Hebbian learning method (often competitive learning). Such computational models of the hand region of the SI cortex have demonstrated map refinement and map reorganization in response to localized repetitive stimulation and deafferentation (Grajski & Merzenich, 1990; Pearson et al., 1987).

These and related computational studies provide an impressive demonstration that fairly simple but plausible assumptions about network architecture and synaptic modifiability can account qualitatively for several fundamental facts about cortical map self-organization and reorganization. These studies have been less successful, however, in accounting for some map reorganization effects, particularly those of direct relevance here. For example, in the only previous computational model we know of that simulated a focal cortical lesion, map reorganization did not occur unless relatively implausible steps were taken (complete re-randomization of weights following a simulated focal lesion) (Grajski & Merzenich, 1990). Map reorganization following a cortical lesion is fundamentally different from that involving deafferentation or focal repetitive stimulation. In both of the latter situations, there is a change in the probability distribution of input patterns seen by the

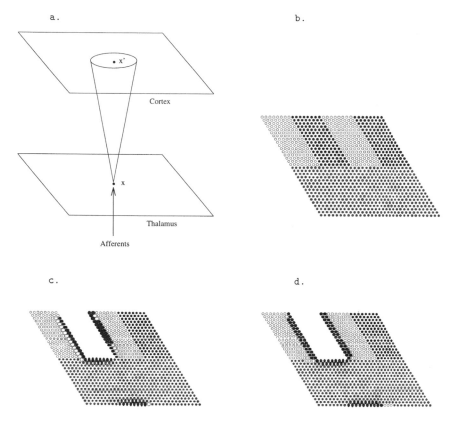

Figure 18-2. The SI model: (a) network architecture; (b) cortical map of the hand surface after training; (c) immediately after the lesion; (d) after further training.

intact cortex. This change has long been recognized to result in map alterations. In contrast, a focal cortical lesion does not affect the probability distribution of input patterns, so some other factors must be responsible for map reorganization.

A Model of Map Formation in Primary Somatosensory Cortex

To examine issues related to map plasticity, we created and studied a computational model of the hand region of primary somatosensory cortex that we refer to as the *SI model.* In our model, cortex and thalamus are viewed as two-dimensional sheets of small-volume elements (Fig. 18-2a). Each cortical element represents a small patch of cortex containing on the order of 100 neurons, i.e., roughly a microcolumn. As indicated in Figure 18-2a, each thalamic element x sends divergent excitatory connections to a set of cortical elements (circular region) centered on the corresponding cortical element x'. Each cortical element sends excitatory connections to nearby elements in cortex. In the simulations described here, each layer is a hexagonally tessellated grid of 32×32 nodes. Thalamic elements project into a radius four hexagonal region of cortex, resulting in 61 connections per thalamic node. Accordingly, there are 62,464 thalamocortical connections and 6144 cortico-cortical connections. To avoid possible edge effects, the front and back edges of each layer are connected, as are the right and left edges, so that conceptually the two layers form tori. Inputs are presented directly to the thalamic layer that implicitly defines a skin surface with direct thalamic connections.

Neural activity and synaptic changes are modeled mathematically (a full description is given in Sutton et al. [1994]). A Mexican Hat pattern of lateral interactions in cortex is present: Each cortical element tends to excite/activate its immediately adjacent elements but to inhibit more distant surrounding cortical elements. This is brought about in two different ways in variations of our model: by using *standard intracortical connectivity* (lateral/horizontal inhibitory connections) and by allowing cortical elements to *distribute their activity competitively*. Elsewhere, we have presented arguments that both forms of peristimulus inhibition are present in the cerebral cortex (Reggia et al., 1992). Simulations have demonstrated that both mechanisms produce qualitatively similar mapping results as long as an appropriate Mexican Hat pattern of lateral interactions is supported (Armentrout et al., 1994; Cho & Reggia, 1994; Goodall et al., 1994; Reggia et al., 1992; Sutton et al., 1994).

An unsupervised, Hebbian synaptic weight change rule is used to simulate map formation in SI cortex (area 3b). In other words, the synaptic strength between two connected neural elements tends to increase when both elements are active simultaneously and to decrease otherwise. Learning occurs only on thalamocortical connections. Initially, thalamocortical weights are random, so a precise cortical map of the hand surface does not exist. The model undergoes a developmental training period during which synaptic changes occur as random input stimuli (hexagonal patches) are applied to the hand. Because of the competitive Hebbian rule, synaptic strengths increase when presynaptic and postsynaptic activities are correlated; otherwise, they decrease.

The coarse topographic map that existed before training due to the initially random weights and network structure was transformed by training into a finely tuned, uniform topographic map (Armentrout et al., 1994; Sutton et al., 1994). Receptive fields decreased in size and changed from irregular to circular in shape (incoming weight vectors for cortical elements became roughly bell-shaped). These results were relatively insensitive to variations in input stimuli and the learning rule, i.e., the model was robust. Figure 18-2b (right) shows receptive fields of cortical elements plotted across the cortical surface after training. Each ellipse in this figure provides a rough measure of receptive field size. The general location of the receptive fields is shown by shading to indicate four finger regions (upper half) and the palm (lower half) of the cortical map representing the hand surface. A number of effects seen in animal studies were observed in the SI model. For example, if the relative frequency of input stimuli to a finger was increased, its cortical representation increased dramatically, Conversely, if the same cortical finger region was deafferented, some of the cortical elements originally in that finger region developed new receptive fields in adjacent fingers, also as observed in animals.

Lesioning the Model

We hypothesized that a version of our model based on competitive distribution of activation would demonstrate spontaneous map reorganization following a cortical lesion. To test this hypothesis, a contiguous portion of the trained cortical layer (elements representing the second finger from the left in Fig. 18-2b) was deactivated after training. After this lesioning, the topographic map showed a two-phase reorganization process (Armentrout et al., 1994; Sutton et al., 1994). Immediately after lesioning and before any retraining, the receptive fields of cortical elements adjoining the lesioned area shifted spontaneously toward the second finger and increased in size. As Figure 18-2c, shows, parts of the finger region originally represented in the now lesioned cortical area (solid black ovals) have shifted substantially into the surrounding intact cortex. This immediate shift was due to the competitive redistribution of thalamic output from lesioned to unlesioned cortical elements, which resulted in increased perilesion excitability. The second phase of map reorganization occurred more slowly with continued training and was due to synaptic weight changes. It resulted in further reappearance of the second finger in perilesion cortex (Fig. 18-2d). Receptive fields in perilesion cortex increased in size, consistent with the inverse magnification rule. This spontaneous map reorganization is consistent with that seen experimentally following small cortical lesions (Jenkins & Merzenich, 1987).

Having demonstrated for the first time that spontaneous map reorganization can occur in a computational model of focal cortical damage, we examined how a number of factors influence the extent and nature of the reorganization process (Armentrout et al., 1994). First, with either thalamocortical competitive distribution alone or intracortical competitive distribution alone (as opposed to both in the initial model), postlesion map reorganization still occurred but was reduced. Second, as lesion size increased, the mean distance that perilesion map representations moved increased at first but then leveled off; mean shift of the receptive field location was always highest close to the lesion and diminished with increasing distance. Third, allowing learning on intracortical connections in addition to thalamocortical connections produced few differences in map reorganization. Fourth, only minor improvements in map reorganization occurred when increased plasticity was present on connections to cortex from thalamic elements originally represented in the lesioned area.

Variation in the postlesion training stimuli also influenced map reorganization. As the input stimulus size was increased from radius 1 to radius 4, the speed of reorganization increased. Further, if the frequency of training stimulation to the region of sensory surface originally represented in the lesioned cortex was increased relative to other locations, there was a dramatic increase in the extent to which the lost sensory surface reappeared in the postlesion cortical maps. Moreover, the receptive fields obtained were smaller (Weinrich et al., 1994). Such results represent testable predictions that could be used to guide controlled clinical trials in stroke rehabilitation.

Finally, we simulated analogous lesions to a version of the SI model based on the use of lateral inhibitory connections rather than competitive distribution of activity. We found that, in general, map reorganization was more difficult to elicit and less marked than with the competitive SI model. However, with a suitable choice of parameters derived through a trial-and-error process, we were able to create a version of the standard SI model that demonstrated substantial, if irregular, reorganization. Like the competitive SI model, this reorganization could be enhanced by increased frequency of stimulation of the sensory surface in the region previously represented in the area of the cortical lesion.

Analysis of the factors that influence map reorganization in both types of models, and of the reasons why past efforts to demonstrate spontaneous map reorganization were unsuccessful, suggested that increased perilesion excitability is a critical factor in map reorganization (Armentrout et al., 1994). Our results thus lead to the hypothesis that the increased perilesion excitability observed in some animal models of stroke, in addition to contributing to neurological impairment, as some have suggested (Domann et al., 1993), may actually be an important aspect of brain recovery from focal injury.

In summary, the competitive SI model exhibits topographic map formation, and reorganization following both deafferentation and repetitive stimulation, that are qualitatively similar to experimental findings reported in the literature (Jenkins & Merzenich, 1987; Kaas, 1991). More important, our model exhibits spontaneous map reorganization in response to a focal cortical lesion. Sensory regions originally represented in the lesioned cortex reappeared spontaneously in cortex outside the lesion area as long as synaptic plasticity was continued after the lesion. This spontaneous map reorganization seen when competitive distribution of activity is present is consistent with that seen experimentally in adult primates following small cortical lesions (Jenkins & Merzenich, 1987). Further, receptive fields increased in size in perilesion cortex, as has also been described experimentally (inverse magnification rule) (Jenkins & Merzenich, 1987).

Most intriguing is how and why map reorganization occurred following a cortical lesion in our model. Map reorganization involved a two-phase process in which each phase, rapid and slow, was due to a different mechanism. Immediately after a cortical lesion, there was a dramatic change in map organization associated with increased excitability in the perilesion cortex: Some finger regions originally represented by the lesioned area of cortex "shifted outward" and now appeared in adjacent regions of intact cortex. This first, or rapid, phase of map reorganization was due to the competitive distribution of thalamic activity to cortex (see Reggia et al., 1992 for further explanation). This result provides a specific testable prediction: Significant shifts of sensory representation out of a lesioned cortical area should be observed immediately after a cortical lesion. While no definitive experimental data are available on this issue regarding SI cortex, a recent experimental study, motivated in part by our results, has found acute postlesion receptive field changes consistent with this prediction (Sober et al., 1997).

This first, rapid phase of map reorganization due to the competitive dynamics is followed by a second, slower phase due to synaptic plasticity. More of the hand region initially represented by the lesioned cortex appeared in the surrounding cortex. This second phase due to synaptic changes, like the first phase, occurred in spite of the fact that there was no change in the input stimuli. Increased perilesion excitability during the first phase of map reorganization appeared to be essential for jump-starting the second phase. The extent of reorganization in the SI model following a cortical lesion increased dramatically with the use of focal repetitive stimulation. Extrapolating this result to the clinical rehabilitation setting indicates some potentially practical implications of this research and represents another testable prediction of the model.

Lesioning Sensorimotor Feature Maps

The results described above and others (Ruppin & Reggia, 1995; Xing & Gerstein, 1996) indicate the important role of intracortical interactions in postlesion brain reorganization. Sometimes, unlike the SI model, a *structural lesion* that simulates a region of damage and neuronal death can result in a secondary *functional lesion* in surrounding cortex. This is due to loss of synaptic connections from the damaged area to surrounding intact cortex. In the following discussion, we use the term *functional lesion* in this limited sense and not to indicate the ischemic penumbra.

We have recently examined the generality of the results obtained with the SI model through simulations with a different cortical model. This more complex model represents the portion of cortex that controls the positioning of a simulated arm in three-dimensional space (Chen & Reggia, 1996). This model involves both proprioceptive input and motor output in a "closed-loop" network. Maps initially form in the two cortical regions represented in the model: proprioceptive sensory cortex and primary motor (MI) cortex. Unlike the SI model described in the previous section, the maps involved here are feature maps rather than topographic maps and involve motor output as well as sensory input information.

Model Description

The computational model used in this study consists of two parts: a simulated arm that moves in three-dimensional space and a closed loop of neural elements that controls and senses arm positions (Fig. 18-3). Each neural element in the model again represents a population of real neurons, not a single neuron. The transformation of activity in lower motor neurons to proprioceptive sensory neural activity is generated using a simulated arm (bottom of Fig. 18-3). This model arm is a significant simplification of biological reality, and is described in detail elsewhere (Cho & Reggia, 1994, Chen & Reggia, 1996). It consists of upper and lower arm segments connected at the elbow. It has six generic muscle groups, each of which corresponds to multiple muscles in a real arm. There are four muscle groups that control the upper arm and two that control the lower arm. Abductor and adductor muscles move the upper arm up and down through 180°, respectively, while flexor and extensor muscles move it forward and backward through 180°, respectively. The lower arm flexes and extends as much as 180°, controlled by the lower arm flexor and extensor muscles. Activation of the lower motor neuron elements places

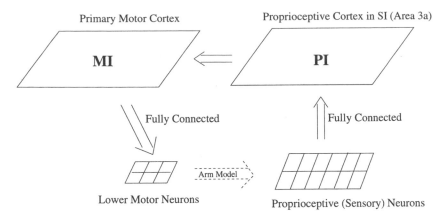

Figure 18-3. Structure of the motor control model: 12 proprioceptive receptor elements (lower right) form the proprioceptive input layer and are fully connected to the proprioceptive cortex layer (PI). The PI layer and the primary motor cortex layer (MI) are two-dimensional arrays of neural elements with lateral (horizontal) intracortical connections. The projection from PI to MI is partial, with a coarse topographic ordering. Each MI element is connected to the six lower motor neuron elements. Activity in lower motor neurons is transformed into proprioceptive input by a simulated arm.

the model arm in a specific spatial position. The simulated arm then generates input signals to the cortex via the proprioceptive neuron elements that indicate the length and stretch of each individual muscle group (Fig. 18-3). The biologically oriented proprioceptive input in this model, based on muscle stretch and tension, distinguishes it from previous robotically oriented neural models of arm control in which input is derived from a camera (e.g., Ritter et al., 1992).

Activation flows in a closed loop through the four sets of neural elements: MI cortex, lower motor neurons, proprioceptive neurons, proprioceptive cortex, and back to MI (Fig. 18-3). We use the nonstandard abbreviation PI to designate primary somatosensory cortex receiving proprioceptive input from the upper extremity (roughly Brodmann area 3a). The 12 receptor elements in the proprioceptive input layer are fully connected to PI; they provide 6 muscle length and 6 muscle tension measures. A length element becomes active when the corresponding muscle is stretched, while a tension element activates when the corresponding muscle is under increased tension. Similar to the SI model, the PI and MI layers are both two-dimensional, hexagonally tessellated arrays of elements with lateral (horizontal) intracortical connections. Each element of these layers represents a cortical column and is connected to its immediately neighboring elements. Each element of PI sends synaptic connections to its corresponding element in MI and to the surrounding elements in MI within a radius 4, providing a coarse topographic ordering for the connections from PI to MI. Each MI element is fully connected to the lower motor neuron layer.

Each neural element in the model has an associated activation level, representing the mean firing rate of neurons in that element. The activation and learning rules are similar to those used in the SI model discussed in the preceding section; a full description is given in Chen and Reggia (1996). During simulations, the only weights modified are those on interlayer connections.

Map Formation in the Intact Model

The model is initialized with small, random weights so that well-formed feature maps are not present initially in the cortical regions. The model is then trained as follows. A patch of external input is repeatedly provided at randomly selected positions in MI. This stimulus is applied as external *input* to the MI elements, i.e., none of the activation levels are clamped to a fixed value. Two thousand random stimuli to MI, covering the cortical space, are applied to the network during training, after which further training does not produce qualitative changes in the trained weights or the cortical feature maps that appear. To examine the resultant *proprioceptive maps* in the cortical layers, these two layers are analyzed to determine to which muscle length and tension input each cortical element responds most strongly. A cortical element is taken to be "maximally tuned" to an arm input element if the cortical element's activation corresponding to that input is largest and above a certain threshold.

The prelesion maps are described in detail in Cho and Reggia (1994) and in Chen and Reggia (1996) and are briefly summarized here. Figure 18-4 shows which PI and MI cortical elements are maximally responsive to stretch of specific muscles after training. For example, the third element to the right from the upper left corner of Figure 18-4a is maximally responsive to stretch of the lower arm extensor (O). The proprioceptive map in Figure 18-4a is for all six muscle groups for the PI cortical layer; the map in Figure 18-4c is the corresponding map for MI. Prior to training, elements maximally responsive to the same muscle group's stretch or tension were irregularly scattered across the map.

Although it is difficult to see in Figure 18-4a and 18-4c, the maps form clusters of adjacent elements that respond to the same input. This can be better seen in Figure 18-4b and 18-4d, which show only those elements that are maximally activated for the stretch of the lower arm extensor (O) and lower arm flexor (C) in PI and MI, respectively. Figure 18-4b illustrates the regular size and arrangement of the clusters across the PI layer. In both PI and MI the clusters responsive to antagonist muscle pairs tend to be separated, reflecting the constraint that simultaneous shortening of antagonist muscle pairs is not physically possible. For example, after training, the clusters of O's and C's are generally pushed apart (Fig. 18-4b). The PI and MI maps of responsiveness to muscle tension inputs often exhibit uniformity in size and spacing of clusters responsive to the same muscle group. When the length map for PI is compared with the tension map, the length map of a particular muscle has been found to match closely the tension map of its antagonist muscle (Chen & Reggia, 1996). The maps thus capture the correlated features of input patterns, reflecting the mechanical constraints imposed by the model arm.

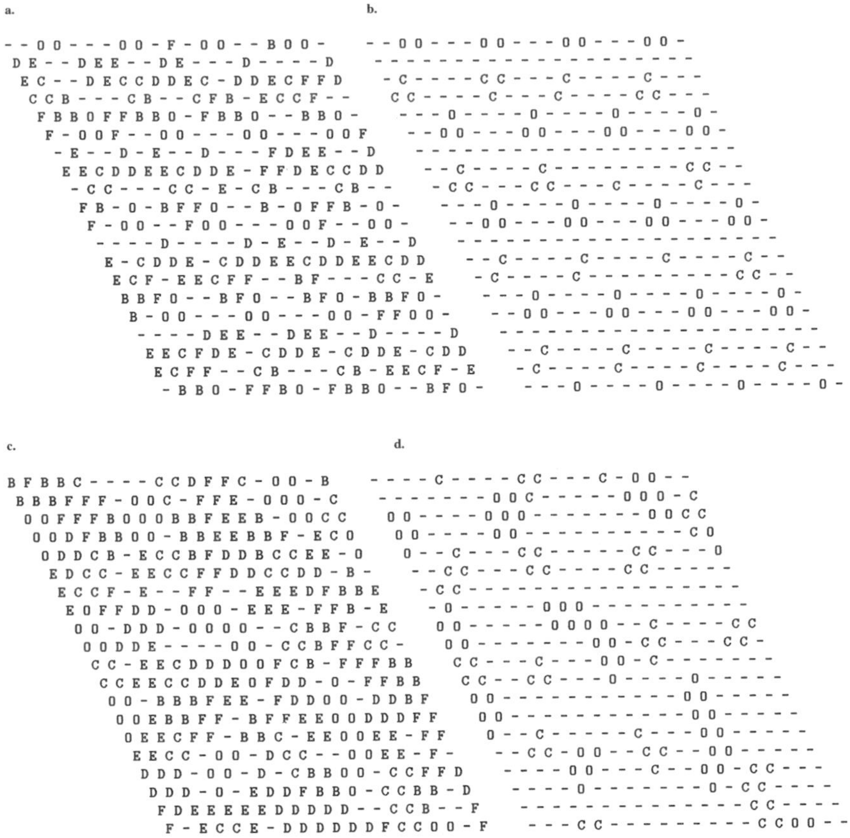

a.

```
- - O O - - - O O - F - O O - - B O O -      - - O O - - - O O - - - O O - - - O O -
D E - - D E E - - D E - - - D - - - - D      - - - - - - - - - - - - - - - - - - - -
E C - - D E C C D D E C - D D E C F F D      - C - - - - C C - - - C - - - - C - - -
C C B - - - C B - - C F B - E C C F - -      C C - - - C - - - C - - - - C C - - -
F B B O F F B B O - F B B O - - B B O -      - - - O - - - - O - - - - O - - - - O -
F - O O F - - O O - - - O O - - - O O F      - - O O - - - O O - - - O O - - - O O -
- E - - D - E - - D - - - F D E E - - D      - - - - - - - - - - - - - - - - - - - -
E E C D D E E C D D E - F F D E C C D D      - - C - - - - C - - - - - - - - C C - -
- C C - - - C C - E - C B - - - C B - -      - C C - - - C C - - - C - - - - C - - -
F B - O - B F F O - - B - O F F B - O -      - - - O - - - - O - - - - O - - - - O -
F - O O - - F O O - - - O O F - - O O -      - - O O - - - O O - - - O O - - - O O -
- - - - D - - - - D - E - - D - E - - D      - - - - - - - - - - - - - - - - - - - -
E - C D D E - C D D E E C D D E E C D D      - - C - - - - C - - - - C - - - - C - -
E C F - E E C F F - - B F - - - C C - E      - C - - - - C - - - - - - - - - - C C - -
B B F O - - B F O - - - B F O - B B F O -    - - - O - - - - O - - - - O - - - - O -
B - O O - - - O O - - - O O - F F O O -      - - O O - - - O O - - - O O - - - O O -
- - - - D E E - - D E E - - D - - - - D      - - - - - - - - - - - - - - - - - - - -
E E C F D E - C D D E - C D D E - C D D      - - C - - - - C - - - - C - - - - C - -
E C F F - - C B - - - C B - E E C F - E      - C - - - - C - - - - C - - - - C - - -
- B B O - F F B O - F B B O - - B F O -      - - - O - - - - O - - - - O - - - - O -
```

b.

c.

```
B F B B C - - - - C C D F F C - O O - B      - - - - C - - - - C C - - - C - O O - -
B B B F F F - O O C - F F E - O O O - C      - - - - - - - O O C - - - - - O O O - C
O O F F F B O O O B B F E E B - O O C C      O O - - - O O O - - - - - - - - - O O C C
O O D F B B O O - B B E E B B F - E C O      O O - - - - O O - - - - - - - - - - C O
O D D C B - E C C B F D D B C C E E - O      O - - C - - - C C - - - - - C C - - - O
E D C C - E E C C F F D D C C D D - B -      - - C C - - - C C - - - - C C - - - - -
E C C F - E - - F F - - E E E D F B B E      - C C - - - - - - - - - - - - - - - - -
E O F F D D - O O O - E E E - F F B - E      - O - - - - - O O O - - - - - - - - - -
O O - D D D - O O O O - - C B B F - C C      O O - - - - - O O O O - - - C - - - - C C
O O D D E - - - - O O - C C B F F C C -      O O - - - - - - - O O - C C - - - C C -
C C - E E C D D D O O F C B - F F F B B      C C - - - C - - - O O - C - - - - - - - -
C C E E C C D D E O F D D - O - F F B B      C C - - C C - - - O - - - - O - - - - -
O O - B B B F E E - F D D O O - - D D B F    O O - - - - - - - - - - - - - - O O - - - -
O O E B B F F - B F F E E O O D D D F F      O O - - - - - - - - - - - - - - O O - - - -
O E E C F F - B B C - E E O O E E - F F      O - - C - - - - - C - - - - - - O O - - - -
E E C C - O O - D C C - - O O E E - F -      - - C C - O O - - C C - - O O - - - - -
D D D - O O - D - C B B O O - C C F F D      - - - - O O - - - C - - O O - - C C - -
D D D - O - E D D F B B O - C C B B - D      - - - - O - - - - - - - - - - - O - C C - -
F D E E E E E D D D D D - - C C B - - F      - - - - - - - - - - - - - - - - - C C - - -
F - E C C E - D D D D D D F C C O O - F      - - - C C - - - - - - - - - - C C O O - -
```

d.

Figure 18-4. Maps of the intact proprioceptive cortex layer (a and b) and the motor cortex layer (c and d) showing which cortical elements respond most strongly to stretch of specific muscles after training. Each cortical element is labeled by a letter indicating the muscle whose stretch (increased length) maximally activates that element. The labels are E for upper arm extensor, F for upper arm flexor, B for upper arm abductor, D for upper arm adductor, O for lower arm extensor ("opener"), and C for lower arm flexor ("closer"). Cortex elements marked "-" were found not to be responsive to stretching of any muscle above an activation threshold of 0.4. Maps (a) and (c) indicate the cortical elements in PI and MI responding most strongly to stretch of all six muscle groups. Maps (b) and (d) show the same information but only for forearm extensor (O) and flexor (C) muscle groups, illustrating the clustering of cortical elements responsive to stretch for just these two antagonist muscles.

After training, the MI *motor output map* develops clusters of elements activating the same muscle group. The MI input map of a particular muscle's length closely matches the MI output map of its antagonist muscle, while the MI input map of a particular muscle's tension closely matches the MI output map of its corresponding muscle (Chen & Reggia, 1996). The motor output map in MI (not pictured here) thus resembles the proprioceptive input map in Figure 18-4d very closely, except that the C's and O's are reversed. The model's maps thus capture the proprioceptive feedback of an activated muscle from the increased stretch of its antagonist muscles and the increased tension of itself.

Figure 18-5a shows the model arm in four of six test positions for the intact prelesion model, corresponding to requests to contract the upper arm extensor, flexor, abductor, and adductor muscles. The four arm positions corresponding to these motor cortex stimuli are in the anticipated directions.

Lesioning the Model

Structural lesions of varying sizes were applied to the cortex ("simulated ischemic strokes") in which an area of focal damage was suddenly imposed on a previously trained network (Goodall et al., 1997). A focal lesion was simulated by clamping the activation levels of a contiguous set of "lesioned" cortical elements permanently at zero. In addition, connections to and from lesioned cortical elements were severed. The effect of each lesion on the trained, intact cortex was examined twice: immediately after the lesion and after continually training the network with 2000 additional random input stimuli in MI. Random stimuli were used as we were modeling the natural evolution of postlesion changes. Changes in the position of the model arm following cortical stimuli were also analyzed, both immediately after lesioning and after further training. All lesion effects were compared with the prelesion network, as well as with an unlesioned control network that continued to receive input stimuli.

Focal Lesions in Proprioceptive Cortex. Changes to the feature maps in PI were observable immediately after a structural lesion occurred in this layer, again as the first phase of a two-phase reorganization process. Following the primary structural lesion in PI, the activity of surrounding elements was *decreased,* forming a secondary functional lesion. For example, Figure 18-6a shows a perilesion zone of relatively inactive cortical elements (marked by dashes) seen immediately following an 8×8 focal structural lesion; these elements do not respond to the stretch of any of the muscles above a threshold of 0.4. A second phase of reorganization occurred more slowly with continued synaptic changes during the postlesion period. With time, as the map reorganized in the context of continued proprioceptive input and synaptic changes, the functional lesion gradually enlarged. For example, with an 8×8 structural lesion, there was a 77% increase in perilesion inactivity at distances 1 and 2 from the lesion edge over the long term (see Fig. 18-6b, in comparison with Fig. 18-6a). Similar changes were observed with the proprioceptive map of muscle tension. Over time, clusters of elements responsive to the stretch of a particular muscle also shifted position in the feature map.

The functional lesion effects described above occurred largely independently of the size of the structural lesion in PI. They are representative of the effects observed with lesions that varied incrementally in size from 2×2 to 8×8. There was an essentially uniform prelesion mean activation of the PI elements, averaged over all of the test input patterns, of roughly 0.12. Immediately following the structural

a.

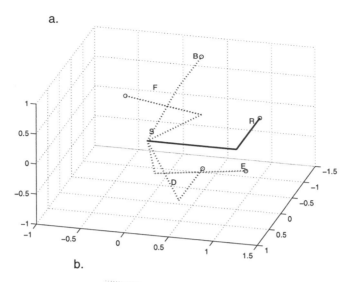

b.

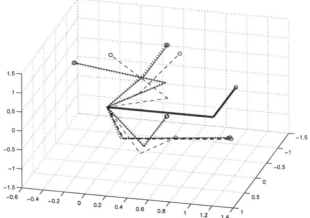

c.

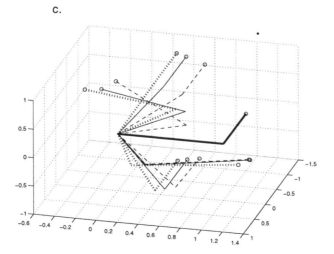

344

lesion, the mean activation level of cortical elements directly adjacent to the lesion site dropped to 0.08, about 70% of its prelesion value. With additional synaptic modifications following the lesion, these perilesion effects in the PI layer were intensified (about 25% of the prelesion value) and shifted outward. Perilesion cortical elements were activated essentially by the same amount for all input stimuli, in contrast to the prelesion cortex, where elements were activated selectively for some input stimuli but not for others. This uniformity occurred as a result of the loss of excitatory support from cortical elements in the structural lesion via intracortical connections. As the map reorganized following the lesion, the weights to these perilesion cortical elements tended to become uniform.

We attempted to prevent the spread of the perilesion functional deficit by providing a small, uniform external input to elements at a distance 1 from the lesion during the postlesion period of continued synaptic modifications. We did this to confirm that it is the low activation level in the perilesion elements that leads to the spread of the functional deficit. This change arrested the spread of the perilesion functional deficit; but when synaptic modifications were subsequently allowed to continue even further without the increased external input, all gains made in arresting the spread of the functional deficit were lost.

Immediately following larger structural lesions (5×5 and larger) in PI, an irregularly shaped area of inactive motor cortex elements appeared in the center of the sensory maps of the MI layer and did not resolve with further training. Given the coarsely topographic projections from PI to MI (projections from PI to MI elements within a radius 4), the observed inactive zone in the center of the motor cortex sensory map is expected and can be viewed as an example of diaschisis. In addition to these effects on the sensory maps of the MI layer, larger PI lesions produced a central region in the motor output map that did not activate any muscle groups in the lower motor neuron layer. This was due to the loss of excitatory input to this region from the corresponding lesioned area in PI. The percentage of MI elements activating one or more muscle group(s) in the motor output maps was 77%

Figure 18-5. (a) Position assumed by the model arm at rest in the absence of external stimuli (R, thick solid line) and in response to four of six cortical test stimuli. The arm is on the right side of the body and is viewed from the back (S, right shoulder; small circles, hand positions). Each test stimulus provides external input to cortical elements in MI that are most strongly connected to a specific muscle group (here, upper arm extensor E, flexor F, abductor B, and adductor D). For example, activating upper arm abductor elements in MI elevates the arm to position B. The positions assumed by the arm in response to cortical stimuli are appropriate and are indistinguishable for the trained prelesion (dotted lines) and control (crosshatched) states of the model. Similar results are found for the lower arm flexor and extensor (not shown). (b) Arm positions for an 8×8 focal lesion of PI shown prelesion (dotted line; largely obscured by overlapping solid lines), immediately postlesion (dashed line), and after 2000 further random input stimuli in MI (solid line). (c) Arm positions for a 16×16 lesion of MI, prelesion (dotted line), immediately postlesion (dashed line), and after 2000 further random input stimuli in motor cortex layer MI (solid line).

```
a.                                          b.

- - O O F F E O O - F B O O - - B O O -     F F O O D F - E - - - - - O - - - O O -
D E - F D E E - - D D - - - - - - - - D     D E E - D D E E O - - - - - - - - - - D
E C C - D E C C - D E C F D D E C - - D     C E B - - C C O O D E C F D D E C - D D
C C B - - C C B O E C C F O E C C F - -     C B B - - C B F D E C B F D E C B - - -
F B B O - F F - O - - B - O - - B B O -     - F F O - - F F - - - - O - - B F O - -
F - O O - - - - - - - - - - - - O O F       D F O O - - - - - - - - - - F O - -
D E - - D E * * * * * * * * - D E E - D     D - E E D - * * * * * * * * - D D E - D
E E C D E E * * * * * * * * - D E C - D     - - E D - - * * * * * * * * - D E C - -
- C C F E - * * * * * * * * - C C B - -     - C C F - - * * * * * * * * - C B - -
- B B O - - * * * * * * * * - F B O O -     - B B O - - * * * * * * * * - - F O O -
- B O O - - * * * * * * * * - - O O F F     - - O O - - * * * * * * * * - - O O D -
- - - - D - * * * * * * * * - D E - F D     - - E D - - * * * * * * * * - - E D D -
E - C D E - * * * * * * * * D E E C D D     - E C C - - * * * * * * * * - - C C - -
E F F E E - * * * * * * * * - - C C - E     - - F B - - * * * * * * * * - C C F - -
- B B O - B B - - - - - B O - F B - O -     - - B O O - - - - - - - - - - - B B O O
- B O O - B - O O F - B B O - F F O O -     - - - O E F - - - F - - E E - - - - O -
- - - F D E E O F D E E - - D - - - - D     - C - D D C B E E D C B E D D - C - D D
E - C F D E - C C D E - C D D E - C D D     C C - - - C B O D C C B F D D E C - D -
E - B - - - B B - - - C C - E E C F F E     E B - - - - - - - C B F F - E E B F - E
- B B O - - B - O - F B B O - - B F O -     B F - O - F F - - - - - - O O B F - O O
```

```
c.                                          d.

F - D D B B F - - O B B F - D O O B - F     F - D - B B F - D - B B F F O O O B B F
F D D D B F F F O O B B - - O O B B - F     F D D - B F F - O O C - E - O O B B F F
C D D - C F F O O - E E E O O B B - F F     C D D C C F F O O O E E E O O O B - F C
E E - C C C O O E E E E D O F F D - F C     - - - C C - O O O E E D D - F F D D F C
E O O C C O O - E E E D D F F D D F F E     E O - - E E - F F B B D C C F D D F F E
O O - B B - F F B B B D C C E E O B - E     O O B E E C F F F B B C C C E E O - E E
O - B B - F * * * * * * * * E O B B E E     O O B B C C * * * * * * * E O O B E E
D D - C C D * * * * * * * * E C B B E E     - B B C C D * * * * * * * * C C B B - D
D - - C D D * * * * * * * * C C B - E D     - O O D D D * * * * * * * * C F B B D D
F F - E E O * * * * * * * * F O O - D D     - O - D D O * * * * * * * * F F B C D -
F - E E O O * * * * * * * * O O B C C F     F - E E O O * * * * * * * * F O C C C F
F B E E O F * * * * * * * * O B B C C F     F B E E O C * * * * * * * * O O C C F F
B B E E C C * * * * * * * O F D D - F     B B E E C C * * * * * * * * O D D - F F
B O D D C E * * * * * * * * E D D - F F     B O O D B B * * * * * * * * D D - - F -
F F D D O O D D F F D E E E E O O - F F     O O D D B O D D F F E E E E O O - - -
F F - O O C F F F C C F B B O O O C C -     F F D B O O D F F F E E E E O O - C C C
F F - O C C F B B C C B B B O C C C C -     F F B B C C - B B C C - - B B C C C C C
B B - - C O E E C C D B B - C C D E E -     F B B C C O B B C C C - B B C C D D E -
B B E E O O E E D D D - F F C D D E E C     B - E E O O E E D D D B B F F D D E E -
- E E - O B E E D D - - F F D D O E C C     - E E O O E E E D D - B F F F - - E B B
```

Figure 18-6. Muscle length map of proprioceptive cortex layer PI (above threshold 0.4) for an 8 × 8 focal lesion of PI (a) immediately postlesion and (b) following 2000 further random input stimuli in motor cortex layer MI. Muscle stretch map of MI following an 8 × 8 lesion (c) immediately postlesion and (d) after 2000 further input stimuli in MI. The labels are the same as those in Figure 18-4. Asterisks indicate the imposed structural lesion.

before lesioning. This decreased with larger PI lesions (5 × 5 and larger); for example, with an 8 × 8 PI lesion, the percentage dropped to 68% over time.

The decrease in motor output map responsiveness with lesions of increasing size led to "weakness" of the model arm following a lesion in PI. Figure 18-5b shows the arm position for the same four test inputs to MI as in Figure 18-5a, for an 8 × 8 focal lesion in PI. Immediately after the lesion, a measurable shift was observed in the arm away from their prelesion position and toward the neutral, resting position. For example, the elbow immediately after the lesion for the upper arm flexor test was 20° away from its prelesion position, revealing a weakened flexor response. Similar weakened responses were seen with the contraction tests of the abductor, adductor, and lower arm flexor immediately after the lesion. This occurred due to functional loss of MI elements that activated each muscle group. However, over time with continued cortical plasticity, the arm positions for all test inputs realigned with their prelesion positions, representing essentially complete "recovery." With larger PI lesions, e.g., 16 × 16, recovery was incomplete.

Focal Lesions in Motor Cortex. A separate set of simulations was performed to study reorganization of the MI maps following focal structural lesions of varying sizes in MI (2 × 2 to 8 × 8). For sufficiently large lesions, reorganization after a structural lesion in MI was seen in both the MI sensory and motor output maps. Immediately after such large focal lesions to MI, both the stretch and tension sensory maps for MI adjusted so that there was an increase in the number of responsive elements in normal cortex near the lesion edge (Fig. 18-6c). In contrast to PI lesions, no perilesion zone of decreased activation was present. At distances 1 and 2 from the lesion edge there was an increase in the number of responsive elements over prelesion levels, from 91% before this 8 × 8 lesion to 96% immediately afterward. Although the change in the absolute number of responsive elements is small, it accurately reflects a substantial increase in the mean activation levels of all elements averaged over all inputs in this perilesion zone (from 0.14 before the lesion to 0.21 afterward). Over time, the distance 1 and 2 responsiveness stabilized at 99%, as is seen in Figure 18-6d. Overall rates of responsiveness for the MI sensory maps increased slightly immediately following the onset of the lesion but dropped back to prelesion levels with continued postlesion synaptic modifications. This postlesion reorganization result is similar to the results observed with the topographically ordered SI maps. In this context, it is important to note that the topographically ordered connections between PI and MI in the current model are similar to those between thalamus and sensory cortex in the earlier SI model.

Like the MI sensory maps described above, the MI output map in residual intact cortex experienced an increase in relative activity. The number of MI elements activating one or more muscle group(s) increased following an MI lesion of sufficient size (4 × 4 or larger). For an 8 × 8 lesion, the percentage of remaining MI elements activating one or more muscle group(s) increased from 77% to 86% of intact elements. This affected the positioning of the model arm as well when tested with six external inputs to MI. As seen in Figure 18-5c, with a 16 × 16 focal lesion in MI, the arm position revealed a weakened response immediately after the lesion. For example, the elbow position immediately after the lesion for the upper arm flexor test was 15° away from its prelesion position, roughly in the direction of the resting position. Further postlesion synaptic modifications in the presence of the MI lesion did not produce a complete realignment of the arm positions with their prelesion location, although complete recovery did occur with smaller MI lesions (e.g., 8 × 8).

The lack of any significant postlesion reorganization with small MI lesions (2 × 2 and 3 × 3) can be attributed to the coarseness of the topographic projections from PI to MI. Each MI element receives input from 61 PI elements, so with such small

MI lesions the distribution of output from PI elements was only minimally perturbed, and perilesion elements continued to experience a distribution of input patterns similar to that before lesioning. As a result their receptive fields, and thus the MI map, remained largely unchanged due to the correlational nature of the synaptic modification rule. Examination of the feature maps for PI (both after lesioning and with further training) did not reveal any qualitative reorganization following MI lesions.

Discussion

It is not well understood how the cerebral cortex adjusts to an ischemic stroke. In the work described in this chapter, we induced acute focal lesions in computational models of primary sensory and sensorimotor cortex to examine the resultant map reorganization in surrounding cortex. While our models involve substantial simplifications of reality, they are based on generally accepted concepts of cortical structure, activity dynamics, and synaptic plasticity. Postlesion effects in these models concerning cortical map reorganization represent testable predictions of the models. To our knowledge, they are the first demonstration that nontrivial computational models of ischemic strokes are possible.

In our simulations, it was observed that focal lesions resulted in a two-phase map reorganization process in the intact perilesion cortical region. The first, very rapid phase was due to changes in activation dynamics; the second, slow phase was due to synaptic plasticity. Thus, our models predict that biological perilesion map changes are demonstrable within a few minutes of a cortical lesion. To our knowledge, while there are a few experimental animal studies that have examined postlesion cortical map reorganization (see below), none of these have measured maps immediately following the lesion. Experimental studies in animals have repeatedly shown map reorganization within minutes following focal deafferentation of cortex (Gilbert & Wiesel, 1992; Metzler & Marks, 1979). Our model predicts that map reorganization occurs following cortical lesions as well and provides some details about their nature.

The second prediction of our model is that increased perilesion excitability is necessary for effective map reorganization in cortex surrounding an acute focal lesion. When increased perilesion excitability was present during the first phase of map reorganization, the cortex surrounding the lesion consistently participated in the map reorganization process, even achieving a higher-density feature map than in the prelesion cortex. Presumably such effective use of surrounding intact cortex following a lesion could contribute to behavioral recovery following an ischemic stroke. On the other hand, when there was decreased excitation in perilesion cortex, this intact cortex consistently did *not* participate in map reorganization, and the amount of perilesion cortex that "dropped out" of the map actually expanded with time due to the normal modifications of synaptic strengths. These very different findings, observed for pure feature maps (PI) and for feature maps involving topographically arranged inputs (to MI from PI) in the sensorimotor model, are consistent with similar results obtained in the SI model involving pure topographic maps.

The notion that perilesion excitability is an important factor may prove useful in interpreting animal studies of postlesion map reorganization. Under some conditions in these studies, functions originally represented in the infarct zone of sensorimotor cortex reappeared or expanded in nearby intact cortex (Castro-Alamancos & Borrel, 1995; Jenkins & Merzenich, 1987; Nudo & Milliken, 1996), while under other conditions they did not (Nudo et al., 1996). Our model suggests that assessing perilesion excitability under these differing conditions may shed light on why the different results occur.

The dependence of map reorganization on perilesion excitability in the model can be explained by examining the synaptic modification rule that produces map formation originally. Informally, this rule causes changes to a cortical element's receptive field (1) at a rate proportional to the activity of that element and (2) such that the receptive field shifts to become more like the pattern of input elements that activate that cortical element. Thus, when perilesion activity is low, its receptive field changes very slowly and little reorganization occurs. When perilesion activity is high, the receptive field changes quickly and substantial reorganization occurs. In this context, the differences in the input connections to PI and MI account for the differences in the way these two regions reorganize in the sensorimotor model. In PI, the diffuse afferent inputs have little influence on, and therefore little correlation with, the perilesion elements following a lesion. Thus, intact cortical elements adjacent to the original postlesion functional deficit lose correlated activity from neighbors, become less correlated with specific input patterns, and tend to drop out of the map. In contrast, the coarsely topographic connections from PI to MI that originally supply the outer region of lesioned cortex have an increased influence on, and become more correlated with, perilesion elements, causing the latter's receptive fields to shift and thus substantial map reorganization to occur.

In the context of these modeling results, it is interesting to note that there is direct experimental evidence of increased excitability in intact cortex following a small focal lesion (Domann et al., 1993; Eysel & Schmidt-Kastner, 1991; Mittmann et al., 1994). Such increased excitability has generally been viewed as detrimental, although this conclusion is controversial (Hossmann, 1994). Our computational models suggest that, in addition, increased excitability may play an important and previously unrecognized role in recovery from stroke. At the very least, the models indicate that further experimental investigation of this issue is warranted and will be useful in obtaining a better understanding of recovery after stroke. In our sensorimotor model, the primary factors determining whether perilesion activity increased or decreased were the extent of divergence of afferents to the cortical region and the ratio of intracortical lateral excitation to inhibition. In other words, in both PI and MI, the cortex immediately around the lesion lost excitatory input from the lesioned region. However, the widely divergent inputs to PI were insufficiently powerful to compensate for this loss of perilesion excitation from lateral connections arising in the lesion area, while the much more focused afferents to MI were powerful enough to provide compensation.

At present, we are extending our models in two ways. One issue currently under study involves adding to our models some biochemical and metabolic alterations occurring in the ischemic penumbra. In particular, we are interested in transient chemical and metabolic disturbances reminiscent of cortical spreading depression in the ischemic penumbra, a region of viable but nonfunctioning tissue that surrounds an infarction. This region is generally thought to be due to decreased blood flow that compromises neuronal functionality but does not immediately kill penumbra tissue (Heiss et al., 1993). The secondary biochemical changes and depolarizations seen with cortical ischemia are remarkably similar to those of cortical spreading depression (do Carmo, 1992; Lauritzen, 1994). Initially we undertook a series of computer simulations using an enhanced model of normal cortex that incorporates just a few biochemical factors. These simulations produce a traveling wave of markedly elevated potassium that slowly propagates in an expanding annular region, exhibiting several key features of cortical spreading depression. The patterns of cortical activity at the leading edge of spreading depression in the model, when projected onto the visual fields, resemble the visual hallucinations reported by patients with classic migraine (Reggia & Montgomery, 1995). Most recently, we have examined the effects of focal ischemia in a more complex version of the model involving metabolic supply, structural state variables, blood flow, and several biochemical factors (Revett et al., 1998).

The second new focus of our work is on the effects of focal cortical lesions on intact, contralateral hemispheric regions. We have recently implemented models of hemispheric regions, both left and right, interacting via a simulated corpus callosum. These models have been used to study the emergence of function lateralization during tasks such as learning to pronounce words (Reggia et al., 1998), learning to recognize letters (Shevstova & Reggia, 1999), and during self-organizing sensory map formation (Levitan & Reggia, 1999). Studies examining the effects of lesions of varying sizes on the acute and postrecovery performance of the nonlesioned hemispheric region are currently underway.

Finally, the results of our work raise more global issues about the role of computational models in neuroplasticity research in general. Computational modeling represents a truly novel approach to the study of neuroplasticity that complements traditional methods and may provide useful guidance for future empirical studies. The findings reported here, as well as recent modeling work involving a wide range of other brain and cognitive disorders (Reggia et al., 1996), are very encouraging in this respect. Ultimately, the utility of such computational models may prove to be their heuristic value in suggesting novel experimental investigations and new approaches to therapeutic and rehabilitative intervention.

ACKNOWLEDGMENT

This work was supported by NINDS Awards NS29414 and NS35460.

References

Armentrout, S., Reggia, J., and Weinrich, M. (1994) A neural model of cortical map reorganization following a focal lesion. *Artificial Intelligence and Medicine,* 6:383–400.

Boyeson, M., Jones, J., and Harmon, R. (1994) Sparing of motor function after cortical injury, *Archieves of Neurology,* 51:405–414.

Brasil-Neto, J., Valls-Sole, J., Pascual-Leone, A., Eracco, J., Hallett, M., and Cohen, L. (1993) Rapid modulation of human cortical motor outputs following ischemic nerve block. *Brain,* 116:511–525.

Calford, M. (1991) Curious cortical change. *Nature,* 352:759–760.

Castro-Alamancos, M., and Borrel, J. (1995) Functional recovery of forelimb response capacity after forelimb primary motor cortex damage. *Neuroscience,* 68:793–805.

Chen, Y., and Reggia, J. (1996) Alignment of coexisting cortical maps in a motor control model. *Neural Computation,* 8:731–755.

Cho, S. and Reggia, J. (1994) Map formation in proprioceptive cortex. *International Journal of Neural Systems,* 5:87–101.

Chollet, F., Di Piero, V., Wise, R., Brooks, D., Dolan, R., and Frackowiak, R. (1991) Functional anatomy of motor recovery after stroke in humans. *Annals of Neurology,* 29: 63–71.

Cohen, L., Bandinelli, S., Findley, T., and Hallett, M. (1991) Motor reorganization after upper limb amputation in man. *Brain,* 114:615–627.

do Carmo, R. ed. (1992) *Spreading Depression.* New York: Springer-Verlag.

Domann, R., Hagermann, G., Kraemer, M., Freund, H., and Witte, O. (1993) Electrophysiological changes in surrounding brain tissue of photochemically induced cortical infarcts in the rat. *Neuroscience Letters,* 155:69–72.

Eysel, U., and Schmidt-Kastner, R. (1991) Neuronal dysfunction at the border of focal lesions in cat visual cortex. *Neuroscience Letters,* 131:45–48.

Gilbert, C., and Wiesel, T. (1992) Receptive field dynamics in adult primary visual cortex. *Nature,* 356:150–152.

Glees, P., and Cole, J. (1950) Recovery of skilled motor function after small lesions of motor cortex. *Journal of Neurophysiology,* 13:137–148.

Goodall, S., Reggia, J., and Cho, S. (1994) Modeling brain adaptation to focal damage. *Proceedings of the 18th Symposium on Computer Applications in Medical Care* 860–864.

Goodall, S., Reggia, J., Chen, Y., Ruppin, E., and Whitney, C. et al. Acute focal cortical lesions. *Stroke,* 28:101–109.

Grajski, K., and Merzenich, M. (1990) Hebb-type dynamics is sufficient to account for the inverse magnification rule. *Neural Computation,* 2:71–84.

Hallenback, J., and Frerichs, K. (1993) Stroke therapy: Time for an integrated approach. *Archives of Neurology,* 50:768–770.

Heiss, W., Fink, G., Huber, M., and Herholz, K. (1993) Positron emission tomography imaging and the therapeutic window. *Stroke,* 24:150–153.

Hossmann, K. (1994) Glutamate-mediated injury in focal cerebral ischemia. *Brain Pathology,* 4:23–36.

Hougaku, H., Matsumoto, M., Handa, N., Macda, H., Itoh, T., Tsukamoto, Y., and Kamada, T. (1994) Asymptomatic carotid lesions and silent cerebral infarction. *Stroke,* 25:566–570.

Jenkins, W., and Merzenich, M. (1987) Reorganization of neocortical representation after brain injury. In F. Seil, *Progress in Brain Research,* Vol. 71. Elsevier, pp. 249–266.

Jenkins, W., Merzenich, M., Ochs, M., Allard, T., and Guic-Robles, E. (1990) Functional reorganization of primary somatosensory cortex in adult owl monkey after tactile stimulation. *Journal of Neurophysiology,* 63:82–104.

Kaas, J. (1991) Plasticity of sensory and motor maps in adult mammals. *Annual Review of Neuroscience,* 14:137.

Killackey, H. (1989) Static and dynamic aspects of cortical somatotopy. *Journal of Cognitive Neuroscience,* 1:3–11.

Knudsen, E., du Lac, S., and Esterly, S. (1987) Computational maps in the Brain. *Annual Review of Neuroscience,* 10:41–65.

Lauritzen, M. (1994) Pathophysiology of migraine aura. *Brain,* 117:199–210.

Levitan, S., and Reggia, J. (1999) Interhemispheric Effects on Map Organization Following Simulated Cortical Lesions, *Artificial Intelligence in Medicine,* 17:59–85.

Merzenich, M., Kaas, J., Wall, J., Nelson, R., Sur, M., and Felleman, D. (1983) Topographic reorganization of somatosensory cortical areas following deafferentation. *Neuroscience,* 8:33–55.

Metzler, J., and Marks, P. (1979) Functional changes in cat sensory-motor cortex during short-term reversible epidural blocks. *Brain Research,* 177:379–383.

Mittmann, T., Luhmann, H., Schmidt-Kastner, R., Eysel, U., and Heinemann, U. (1994) Lesion-induced transient suppression of inhibitory function in rat neocortex. *Neuroscience,* 60:891–906.

Nudo, R., and Milliken, G. (1996) Reorganization of movement representations in primary motor cortex following focal ischemic infarcts in adult squirrel monkeys. *Journal of Neurophysiology,* 75:2144–2149.

Nudo, R., Wise, B., SiFuentes, F., and Milliken, G. (1996) Neural substrates for the effects of rehabilitative training on motor recovery after ischemic infarct. *Science,* 272:1791–1794.

Pascual-Leone, A., and Torres, F. (1993) Plasticity of sensorimotor cortex representation of the reading finger in Braille readers. *Brain,* 116:39–52.

Pearson, J., Finkel, L., and Edelman, G. (1987) Plasticity in the organization of adult cerebral cortical maps: A computer simulation. *Journal of Neuroscience,* 7:4209–4223.

Reggia, J., D'Autrechy, C., Sutton, G., and Weinrich, M. (1992) A competitive distribution theory of neocortical dynamics. *Neural Computation,* 4:287–317.

Reggia, J., Goodall, S., and Shkuro, Y. (1998) Computational studies of lateralization of phoneme sequence generation. *Neural Computation,* 10:1277–1297.

Reggia, J., and Montgomery, D. (1995) A computational model of visual hallucinations in migraine. *Computers in Biology and Medicine,* 26:133–141.

Reggia, J., Ruppin, E., and Berndt, R. eds. (1996) *Neural Modeling of Brain and Cognitive Disorders.* World Scientific.

Revett, K., Ruppin, E., Goodall, S., and Reggia, J. (1998) Spreading depression in focal ischemia: A computational study. *Journal of Cerebral Blood Flow and Metabolism,* 18: 998–1007.

Ritter, H., Martinetz T., and Schulten, K. (1992) *Neural Computation and Self-Organizing Maps.* Reading, MA: Addison-Wesley.

Ruppin, E., and Reggia, J. (1995) Patterns of functional damage in neural network models of associative memory. *Neural Computation,* 7:1105–1127.

Sasaki, K., and Gema, H. (1984) Compensatory motor function of the somatosensory cortex for motor cortex temporarily impaired by cooling. *Experimental Brain Research,* 55:60–68.

Shevtsova, N., and Reggia, J. (1999) A neural network model of lateralization during letter identification. *Journal of Cognitive Neuroscience,* 11:167–181.

Sober, S., Stark, J., Yamasaki, D., and Lytton, W. (1997) Receptive field changes after strokelike cortical ablation: A role for activation dynamics. *Journal of Neurophysiology,* 78:3438–3443.

Sutton, G., Reggia, J., Armentrout, S., and D'Autrechy C. (1994) Map reorganization as a competitive process. *Neural Computation,* 6:1–13.

Udin, S., and Fawcett, J. (1988) Formation of topograhic maps. *Annual Review of Neuro-science,* 11:289–327.

Weinrich, M., Armentrout, S., and Reggia, J., (1994) A neural model of recovery from lesions in the somatosensory system. *Journal of Neurological Rehabilitation,* 9:25–32.

Wall, J., Nepomuceno, V., and Rascy, S. (1993) Nerve innervation of the hand and associated nerve dominance aggregates in somatosensory cortex. *Journal of Comparative Neurology,* 337:191–207.

Xing, J., and Gerstein, G. (1996) Networks with lateral connectivity. *Journal of Neurophysiology,* 75:184–232.

IV

Synthesis and Implications
for Rehabilitation

19

Conceptual Issues Relevant to Present and Future Neurologic Rehabilitation

PAUL BACH-Y-RITA

Major questions running through much of the substance of this book are: What changes can be obtained with appropriate rehabilitation? How is the work each of us is engaged in relevant to recovery of function for persons with brain damage? What does this scientific information suggest to clinicians developing rehabilitation programs?

In this chapter, I will comment on conceptual issues relating to neuroplasticity and reorganization of function following brain injury. Pertinent parts of the chapters of this book will be integrated with those comments and interpreted in regard to the relevance to clinical neurologic rehabilitation.

The Rediscovery of Plasticity

This book presents a modern vision of brain plasticity and reorganization of function after brain damage. This reflects the emergence over the last 30 years from the "dark ages" of brain plasticity: the 100 years that followed Broca's cerebral localization study of 1861. That pioneering study ushered in a century of domination by cerebral localizationists, whose excellent studies emphasized synaptic connectivity. The result for clinicians was that a concept of a hardwired brain with strict localization of function leaves no room for plasticity. Thus, there was little expectation of reorganization following brain damage, and the clinician's intervention was centered on obtaining maximum functional compensation (Bach-y-Rita, 1995).

Benton and Tranel (Chapter 1) present an insightful historical review of plasticity, reorganization of function, and the origins of rehabilitation, including data and comments from many centuries ago, which should be required reading for researchers entering the field.

Brain plasticity and reorganization have now been established experimentally and are part of the "conceptual substance" of the neurosciences. New mechanisms of plasticity continue to appear; the most recent one is the demonstration that neurogenesis can occur (at least in the hippocampus), which has been shown in both adult (Gould et al., 1999; Kemperman et al., 1998a) and senescent (Kemperman et al., 1998b) animals and adult humans (Erickson et al., 1998). While plasticity often produces functional improvement after brain injury, it may also produce unwanted effects, such as spasticity, and the kindling effect in the development of certain forms of epilepsy. The findings of Schallert and colleagues (Chapter 8) that overuse after cortical injury can cause dysfunctional alterations in cortical morphology may be another example of unwanted effects of plasticity. Furthermore, plasticity by itself is not enough to reestablish function. In an experimental model of paraplegia (but in the absence of rehabilitation), Guizar-Sahagún and collaborators (1999) noted that while sprouting at the lesion area was moderate following the lesion, and was abundant following the implantation of peripheral nerve tissue at the lesion area, function was less than the increased function obtained with methylprednisolone—which, however, inhibited sprouting.

Experimental Rehabilitation Studies

Experimental rehabilitation studies are now in the mainstream of the neurosciences, as is reflected in the majority of the chapters of this book. The results of such studies will have an increasing influence on clinical neurologic rehabilitation.

Information Transmission

Following brain damage, brain plasticity mechanisms offer the possibility of functional recovery. How is that task accomplished? To explore the role of plasticity in recovery, knowledge of the normal, prelesion mechanisms is essential. Much has been learned in recent years about neurotransmitters and about the extracellular space. Both synaptic and nonsynaptic mechanisms are altered by brain damage. How these mechanisms may play a role in the reorganization of the brain and in functional recovery, and how these are influenced by medications and rehabilitation, will be an active area of research in the coming years. Confirmation of the importance of these mechanisms will reveal their enormous flexibility, which may play roles in brain plasticity. As an example, the existence of a large number of recptor subtypes offers the possibility of selective neurotransmission at a distance by nonsynaptic diffusion neurotransmission (NDN), which may contribute to the survival of partially denervated neurons and to brain reorganization after brain damage by selective up- and downregulation of receptors. These issues have been discussed elsewhere (e.g., Bach-y-Rita, 1993, 1995, 1998), most recently in regard to spinal cord injury (Bach-y-Rita, 1999).

The effects of brain damage in the various neurotransmitter systems are not uniform. In a rat model, Westerberg et al. (1989) studied the effects of transient cerebral ischemia in the rat hippocampal subfields on excitatory amino acid receptor ligand binding. They noted that their results demonstrate a lack of correlation between receptor changes in the early recovery period following ischemia and the development of neuronal necrosis in different hippocampal regions. They also noted long-lasting receptor changes in areas considered resistant to an ischemic insult. Some receptors are downgregulated, while others appear to be upregulated on the surviving cells.

Hamm and colleagues (Chapter 3) pointed out that microdialysis studies have documented increased glutamate and acetylcholine levels after traumatic brain injury (TBI). The effects of brain damage on neurotransmitter mechanisms differ, depending on the time after injury. In a series of physiologic processes, there is a reversal in the measured variable between the acute and chronic phases. Moreover, the alterations are consistent with an acute phase characterized by excessive neuronal activation (which ends after an interval ranging from a few minutes to a few hours) and a chronic phase (the degree and duration of which depend on the severity of the lesion) typified by a state of neuronal depression or hypofunction. This suggests that the interventions during the chronic phase should be directed toward increasing neuronal activity. This conclusion has been borne out by a series of drug studies demonstrating cognitive improvement.

Kolb and Whishaw (Chapter 6) reported that nerve growth factor (NGF) administered intraventricularly reduced the behavioral deficits produced by a brain lesion. It is likely that the NGF diffused through the extracellular fluid to neural sites. The authors also noted that neuromodulatory catecholamines such as norepinephrine (which function largely extrasynaptically) are related to recovery of function.

Diffusion neurotransmission may play a role in the widespread connectivity of some systems in the brain. Up to recently, studies demonstrating such connectivity have been interpreted strictly within the synaptic model of neurotransmission. The studies of Barbas (Chapter 5) may offer the opportunity to reinterpret excellent experimental data within a conceptual framework that includes both synaptic and nonsynaptic neurotransmission. Barbas has presented evidence of widespread connectivity of the limbic system. Some of the plasticity exhibited by this system may be due to unmasking; Barbas (Chapter 5) states that the limbic cortex system behaves like a feedback system when it communicates with the rest of the neocortex. Prefrontal cortex receives projections from occipital, parietal, and temporal sensory cortex association areas. The prefrontal cortices have distributed connections. Although thalamocortical projections are generally ipsilateral, neurons from the contralateral thalamus project preferentially to the prefrontal limbic areas, while other projections are bilateral.

Development-related proteins (Gap-43) are denser in limbic associative areas that have a role in learning and memory than in other cortical areas in the adult. Barbas (Chapter 5) believes that the structural and neurochemical differences between limbic and eulaminate (lateral prefrontal) areas may provide clues for understanding why limbic areas are so vulnerable in neurologic and psychiatric diseases.

She also believes that the properties that render prefrontal limbic cortices plastic may also contribute to their preferential vulnerability in several neurologic and psychiatric disorders. She suggests that when the nervous system is damaged by injury or disease, it may revert to a more chaotic pattern of synaptic connections, perhaps comparable to what is seen in development, but may eventually settle into a more orderly pattern of local circuits, which may account for recovery after brain injury.

These studies of widespread connectivity may have escaped general knowledge because, as Barbas (Chapter 5) notes, traditional experimental studies all generally related to the more hardwired sensory and motor functions.

Multiplexing

Multiplexing in the brain consists of multiple uses of neurons and fibers so that they participate in various functions. A number of studies have demonstrated multiple sensory (e.g., Anton et al., 1996; Bach-y-Rita, 1964; Murata et al. 1965; cf. Nudo et al., Chapter 9, and motor (e.g., Leyton & Sherrington, 1917; cf. Nudo et al., Chapter 9) representations of a single brain region and overlap of representation. This may provide the neural substrates for plastic changes with training; examples include the greatly increased cortical representation of a fingertip area in monkeys following training in haptic exploration (Jenkins et al., 1990) and the expanded finger motor cortex representation in piano players as well as in the sensorimotor cortex in Braille readers, reported by Pascual-Leone and Torres (1993). Human functional magnetic resonance imaging (fMRI) studies (Anton et al., 1996) have strongly suggested that in the primary hand region around the central sulcus, the same neuronal population is active in the three tasks studied (active finger apposition, texture on fingers, and haptic exploration).

Lesions or temporary suppression of a sensory input can unmask multiple sensory inputs to a cell (Merzenich et al., 1983; Wall, 1980) that may be mobilized in motor and sensory recovery following peripheral nerve or brain damage. The nonvisual (auditory and tactile) sensory representation demonstrated in primary visual cortex (Murata et al., 1965) has been shown to be very active in the visual cortex of adult congenitally blind persons (Wanet-Defalque et al., 1988). This may represent the unmasking of previously weak tactile and auditory inputs to the primary visual cortex demonstrated by Murata and colleagues (1965). Almost half of the primary visual cortex cells that responded to visual stimuli also responded to tactile and auditory stimuli, but with longer latencies, and those nonvisual inputs were more easily blocked.

The nonvisual pathways to the visual cortex may also be unmasked in Braille readers. The positron emission tomography (PET) scan studies of Sadato et al. (1998) demonstrated rerouting of processing pathways: "tactile processing pathways usually linked in the second somatosensory area are re-rerouted in blind [Braille readers] . . . to the ventral occipital cortical regions originally reserved for visual shape discrimination" p. 121. Furthermore, transcranial magnetic stimulation (TMS) has shown a robust tactile representation in the visual cortex one of the important findings regarding brain plasticity that has emerged f. application of this noninvasive brain imaging technique (Wasserman et al., ter 15). Magnetic stimulation, which tends to activate cortical interneurons ra than output cells, reveals that changes in cortical maps can occur very quick after lesions or reversible blocks of sensory input to the brain, and that following hemispherectomy, the ipsilateral representations of the surviving hemisphere (ipsilateral representations are more anterior and lateral) are involved in functional recovery.

In Chapter 9, Nudo and colleagues present evidence that supports the concept of multiplexing. They report that individual somatosensory neurons in the cortex have the potential to respond to a wide array of inputs from widespread surfaces on the skin. They note the suggestion that the rapidly occurring changes in the functional topography of the cortex are mediated by unmasking of the latent excitatory connections via inhibition of local inhibitory synapses.

Reorganization of the brain after damage can occur over long distances. Erzenzinger and Pons (Chapter 4) discuss the evidence of reorganization over 5 mm or more. They believe that massive reorganization cannot be explained by unmasking. However, the results of Murata, and colleagues (1965), discussed above, suggest that inputs to the primary visual cortex from systems whose principal representation in the uninjured state is distant from the visual cortex may be unmasked following the loss of vision.

Erzenzinger and Pons (Chapter 4) suggest that in large-scale reorganization, a combination of initial unmasking and growth of new connections, may underlie the plastic reorganization. Changes in glutamate immunoreactivity and glial proliferation may be related to the initial process of reorganization, which may include growth of new connections. Indirect evidence of such growth has emerged from GAP-43 immunostaining studies, as noted by Erzenzinger and Pons.

Wasserman and colleagues (Chapter 15) suggest that it is possible that latent bilateral representation can become functional under certain circumstances. In patients with internal capsule infarcts, bilateral motor-evoked potentials (MEPs) to electrical and magnetic stimuli were recorded, which may have been conducted by corticoreticulospinal pathways unmasked by the lesion. The changes following a reversible nerve lesion become detectable within minutes, while more gradual and profound reorganization in the somatotopic map in M1 follows a peripheral nerve cross.

The studies reported in Chapter 7 by Xu and Wall have also demonstrated central reorganization following peripheral nerve lesions. The authors suggest that injury initiates rapid, concurrent, consistent, and reiterative changes in brain stem and cortical maps. They also suggest that changes in thalamic maps may occur. The authors consider the concurrent changes to represent "en masse" patterns of central reorganization, in contrast to purely intracortical reorganization. They show that the discontinuous, patch-like representation of radial nerve dorsal inputs becomes more continuous and increased in size, from a normal mean area of 12% of the hand map to a mean area of 37% after ulnar and median nerve injury. Their evidence suggests that nerve injury results in reorganization at both brain stem and cortical levels. Rapid spinal mechanisms operate in neuropil with convergences from C- and A-fiber inputs. In normal cats and primates, nociceptive and innocuous inputs clearly converge on sizable populations of dorsal column nuclei cells. Injury-triggered changes may "upmodulate" sensitization and disinhibition, thus making weak or subthreshold connections stronger.

Multiplexing of sensory convergent cells was demonstrated in the pontine brain stem (Bach-y-Rita, 1964); diffusion (NDN) mechanisms were considered to play a role in the inhibition of the sensory responses. A comparable inhibitory diffusion mechanism has been demonstrated in the hippocampus: dynorphin, which is stored together with glutamate in mossy fibers, can cause a long-lasting inhibition of mossy fiber synaptic responses by decreasing glutamate release (Weisskopf et al., 1993). The authors consider the distant heterosynaptic effects to be mediated by dynorphin diffusing in the extracellular fluid.

Extracellular Space Volume Fraction

The extracellular space (ECS) in the brain plays a role in many functions, including nonsynaptic diffusion neurotransmission. In an assembly of cells in the brain, the distance between neurons can be reduced by 50% with neuron activity that causes them to swell. This affects the excitability and metabolism of the cells by changing the distance between the neurons, producing, among other things, changes in ionic concentrations and dynamics (Aiello & Bach-y-Rita, 1997).

Changes in the size of the extracellular compartment (volume fraction, or VF) may play a role in membrane excitability in pathologic brain states such as brain damage, and in the survival of partially denervated neurons during the postinjury period of receptor upregulation that can lead to reorganization of brain function by unmasking and other mechanisms. Under pathologic conditions such as anoxia, the extracellular volume fraction (EVF) is reduced (Harreveld & Khallab, 1967; Lipton, 1973; McBain et al., 1990). It is also reduced (by up to 50%) in hyperexcitability, by changes in the concentration of potassium, and with epileptiform discharges (Dietzel & Heinemann, 1986; Dietzel et al., 1980).

Brain cell swelling due to anoxia and brain trauma, leading to a decreased EVF, may promote the survival of partially denervated neurons during the postinjury period of receptor upregulation [which has been shown to follow damage to the brain in animal models (e.g., Westerberg et al, 1989) as well in humans (De Keyser et al., 1989)]. Those cells may respond to previously subthreshold stimuli, either synaptically or by NDN, which generally involves activation of membrane surface receptors (cf.) Bach-y-Rita, 1995).

However, it is also possible that hyperexcitability due to a volume fraction decrease, either independently or in combination with excitotoxic activity, may increase secondary cell death following brain damage (Aiello & Bach-y-Rita, 1997). Computational neuroscience models comparable to those used by Reggia et al. (Chapter 18) may aid in the study of that possibility.

The computational models of Reggia and colleagues suggest that increased excitability may play an important and previously unrecognized role in recovery from stroke. In one of their models, portions of the hand originally represented in the lesioned area reappear in the perilesion cortex, as has been observed experimentally in some animal studies. In another model, a sudden focal cortical lesion produces a different result; a perilesion zone of reduced cortical activity.

Modeling studies are dependent on the type of connectivity built into the model. Thus, if connectivity is not purely synaptic, as discussed in the section "Information Transmission" (above), the accuracy of the computer model is limited. To predict the functional outcome of a lesion and the possible changes with different types of rehabilitation, future models will also have to reflect the physiological properties of the individual neurons, as well as the brain neuronal assemblies. Reggia and colleagues (Chapter 18) have provided exciting preliminary data from a partially charted sea.

Temporal Factors

The effects of brain lesions early in life differ from the effects of lesions that occur in adulthood. Functional results can be either better or worse, depending on the age at injury and on the area injured. Furthermore, the age at which the lesion occurs may influence motor as well as behavior lesion effects. Bachevalier and Malkova (Chapter 2) show that damage in infancy produces more profound socioemotional effects than does damage in adulthood. Compensatory mechanisms do not always operate to ensure recovery of functions after early brain damage.

Carlsson and Hugdahl (Chapter 12) discuss evidence supporting the conclusion that early lesions (such as in persons with congenital hemispherectomy), resulting in acquisition of language in the right hemisphere, may interfere with right hemisphere nonverbal functions due to the "crowding effect." The authors believe that functional plasticity seems to have a limited advantage with regard to total cognitive capacities.

It has been shown that tactile stimulation of premature babies leads to faster growth. Kolb and Whishaw (Chapter 6) found that tactile stimulation of lesioned laboratory rats also led to unexpectedly large attenuation of the behavioral deficits, correlated with reversal of atrophy of the cortical neurons normally associated with these lesions. Both premature infants and laboratory rats live in impoverished environments. Thus, the positive responses with tactile stimulation can be considered to be related to movement in the direction of a normal environment.

Carr (Chapter 13) concluded from her studies that reorganization of corticospinal projections may be demonstrated after early unilateral central nervous system damage. She noted that transcortical magnetic stimulation (TCMS) can evoke abnormal coactivation in both soleus and gastrocnemius muscles in persons with congenital spastic diplegia, and showed that children with infantile hemiplegia have a high incidence of persistent mirror movements. Some of her subjects developed a novel ipsilateral tract, which in some subjects had fibers that branched and were distributed bilaterally to the motoneuronal pools of the upper limbs. Carr cites human and animal evidence showing that for motor function, the earlier (including prenatal) the lesion, the better the outcome: lesions in early gestation resulted in a better outcome than perinatal lesions.

Filipek (Chapter 14) states that none of the developmental disorders are believed to have characteristic discrete focal lesions. Since there is no distinct "insult onset" in the developmental disorders, the effects of plasticity are little understood. Brain imaging studies have not identified conclusively the characteristics of each type of developmental disorder. However, Fillipek's studies have now demonstrated that in attention deficit/hyperactivity disorder (ADHD), frontostriatal developmental anomalies can be detected.

Reorganization and recovery of function do not cease at any arbitrary time, such as 6 months; the potential can exist for many years after injury (cf. Bach-y-Rita, 1995), and late changes (over a period of 33 months) in functional representation has been discussed by Wasserman and colleagues (Chapter 15). This is becoming an important area in the field of neurologic rehabilitation, since it appears that, in humans, specific late (after acute injury) rehabilitation programs are necessary to exploit that potential (Bach-y-Rita, 1995).

Environmental Factors

The most important functional gains noted by Hamm and colleagues (Chapter 3) in animal models of TBI were obtained with an enriched environment. Most animal studies are undertaken with environmentally deprived laboratory animals (Bach-y-Rita and de Pedro 1991), which may distort the experimental results. As an example, in beam-walking studies (e.g., Bjelke et al., 1992), laboratory rats had some difficulty crossing a gap on a 2 cm wide strip of wood, while rats in the wild can scamper across much narrower strips. The studies of Hamm et al. (Chapter 3) emphasize the importance of the environment both in animal studies and in the development of effective rehabilitation programs.

In addition to the physical environment for rehabilitation, and the content and timing of the rehabilitation programs, psychosocial factors and fitness level can affect the outcome of rehabilitation programs. Dustman and colleagues (1990) demonstrated that in older men, fitness affects a number of functional measures. The physically active men they studied had shorter event-related cortical potentials, stronger central inhibition, better neurocognitive performance, and better visual sensitivity.

The excellent functional recovery noted in some unusual cases of recovery from brain damage with home rehabilitation programs may be related not only to neuroplasticity factors, but also to psychosocial factors (Bach-y-Rita & Wicab-Bach-y-Rita, 1990a, 1990b), environmental considerations, and the functionality of the rehabilitation program. Recent studies discussed by Schallert and colleagues (Chapter 8) regarding the deleterious effects of excessively intense rehabilitation may also be relevant, with home rehabilitation being less intensive (at least in our Stockholm studies; see below).

Brain Changes with Rehabilitation

Rehabilitation can produce changes in brain function. However, Nudo and colleagues (Chapter 9) have noted that, with few exceptions, experimenters before Glees did not train their animals. They state that in their research model, spontaneous recovery (i.e., in the absence of postinfarct training) results in degenerative changes in the physiology of the remaining hand area, while with rehabilitation those degenerative changes do not occur.

Thus, studies describing the findings of lesion studies that do not include rehabilitation do not contribute valuable information concerning the *ability* of the brain to reorganize and the attainment of functional recovery.

Liepert et al. (1998) showed that with constraint-induced movement therapy for persons with chronic upper extremity dysfunction following stroke, functional recovery was accompanied by an increase in both the size of the motor output area and the amplitudes of the MEPs, which they believed to be evidence of enhanced neuronal excitability in the damaged hemisphere. There was also evidence of re-cruitment of motor areas adjacent to the original location.

Kolb and Whishaw (Chapter 6) state that since it seems unlikely that a localized structure like the cerebral cortex could undergo wholesale reorganization of cortical connectivity in the adult, they assume that recovery from cortical damage most likely results from a change in the intrinsic organization of local cortical circuits in regions directly or indirectly disturbed by the injury. They assume that the best place to look for evidence of cortical reorganization is the output (i.e., pyramidal) cells.

Kolb and Whishaw note that the adult mammalian brain maintains a quiescent population of stem cells in the subventricular zone, and state that it may be possible to induce these cells to divide after cerebral injury. Rats with large midline frontal lesions show severe deficits on various tests of spatial navigation followed by slow improvement. Following lesioning there is initially dendritic atrophy, but over time there is (in animals with an improved behavioral outcome) a net gain in dendritic arborization in regions adjacent to the lesion that is temporally correlated with recovery of performance on cognitive tasks.

The stem cells that are of interest to Kolb and Whishaw offer a possible morphologic basis for recovery from brain damage. If they are induced to divide, they must then be connected synaptically and/or by NDN to the rest of the brain. This creates intriguing possibilities about how they would be recruited into functional cell assemblies by rehabilitation procedures.

Brain Imaging Correlates

An important question in regard to scientifically based rehabilitation regimens is, how can brain imaging studies facilitate their development? Various chapters in this book offer relevant information. In Chapter 17, Buckner and Petersen evaluate various brain imaging methods in regard to the support they could provide for the study of the mechanisms of recovery. Each of these methods has advantages and disadvantages, notably in regard to temporal and spatial resolution, but they can help us to understand how remaining (intact) brain regions support compensation capabilities. Buckner and Petersen provide evidence from neuroimaging studies that the right frontal cortex may compensate, in certain instances, for damaged left frontal regions. They are interested in how rehabilitation may be influenced by observations from neuroimiging, and they believe that the characterization of various brain imaging activation patterns "may have clinical worth by contributing a variable that will help predict which patients can benefit from specific rehabilitative strategies."

Information important for the interpretation of fMRI studies is discussed by Rickard (Chapter 16), who pointed out that the spatial resolution of fMRI studies is 0.50 cc^3 and that effective resolution is decreased by the variability in normal brains. Cognitive studies pose the most technical challenges in controlling for various potentially confounding factors. Rickard suggested that combined MEG, MRI, and TMS are advisable. Each of these methods has spatial resolution limitations that may mask small amounts of brain plasticity.

Relevance to Clinical Rehabilitation and Recovery of Function

The chapters in this book have described a variety of studies on brain plasticity and recovery of function. A major purpose of this book is to help provide the infrastructure for the development of rehabilitation strategies for brain-damaged persons. A thorough understanding of the factors influencing brain reorganization and recovery of function is the foundation of modern neurologic rehabilitation. There are also social, philosophical, and financial issues that affect the transfer of data from the laboratory to the clinic. Moreover, while important, these issues are not included in this book.

Areas critical to clinical rehabilitation that could have received more attention in this book are those related to what are often considered to be the "soft" sciences. These include psychosocial factors, environmental factors, and learning. They will be discussed briefly in this section, together with an analysis of the relevance of the studies presented in the previous chapters to clinical rehabilitation.

Historical Considerations

The capacity for early and late brain reorganization is no longer in doubt. The chapters in this book provide evidence of interventions and mechanisms by which reorganization is achieved. Behavioral interventions (rehabilitation), growth factors, pharmacological agents, and sex hormones are some of the interventions explored. The results obtained by the authors of these chapter and by other researchers must now be applied to clinical procedures to obtain optimal recovery of function in persons with damage to the brain.

In a previous search of the experimental literature for relevance to rehabilitation, many physiology studies on the role of environments on the development of rat brains and recovery from lesions were interpreted in terms of their potential relevance to neurologic rehabilitation of brain-damaged humans by Rosenzweig (1980).

The prevailing conceptual framework affects the therapy for specific disease entities. The conclusions of Hubel and Wiesel (1970; Dews & Wiesel, 1970) (made at a time when plasticity was not generally accepted) regarding the permanence of amblyopia following lid suturing were not likely to have inspired plasticity-based rehabilitation approaches to brain dysfunction due to developmentally induced abnormalities. However, just a short time later, Chow and Stewart (1972) challenged that interpretation within the conceptual framework of plasticity; they provided "rehabilitation" and obtained functional, physiologic, and morphologic evidence of at least partial recovery. I consider their study to be a seminal one in the field of rehabilitation. Although it was an animal study, it also offered evidence of the importance of psychosocial factors: no recovery was obtained unless the experimentor established an affective bond with the cats and "gentled" them.

Franz and colleagues (1915; their work is further interpreted by Nudo et al. in Chapter 9) demonstrated recovery from brain damage with appropriate rehabilitation in both animals and humans and published their results in the *Journal of the American Medical Association* more than 80 years ago. (In that article, they suggested that we should not speak of permanent paralysis in hemiplegic patients, but rather of untreated paresis.) However, their study did not influence the clinical management of stroke patients; plasticity was out of favor at that time. Furthermore, cerebral ablation experiments leading to the conclusion of permanent loss of function have contributed to the long-dominant clinical concept of permanent loss of function following stroke or traumatic brain damage; little recovery was expected within that conceptual framework, and [consistent with Merton's (1968) ideas on the "self-fulfilling prophesy"] little recovery was obtained (Bach-y-Rita & Wicab-Bach-y-Rita, 1990b).

Absent a conceptual framework of plasticity, even most practitioners in the field of neurologic rehabilitation have sought functional adaptation to the disability resulting from a brain lesion rather than reorganization of function. Yet in other parts of the world, plasticity has been part of the conceptual framework for many decades. In Russia, Pavlov stated in 1932 (cf. Luria, 1963) that plasticity had not yet been accorded its true place in physiology. Luria, in his book, published in 1948 (English edition in 1963), noted that automatic and instinctive reorganizations after a lesion simply exclude the dysfunctional part of the body, and that with appropriate rehabilitation, including conscious effort, function is reorganized to include the motorically dysfunctional parts of the body, resulting (within certain limits) in functional recovery.

Rehabilitation and Learning

Rehabilitation resembles the developmental learning process. Both include important elements of inhibition in regard to selective function and precisely coordinated movements. For example, a child learning to write initially demonstrates electromyographic activity in virtually all the muscles related to the hand. As ability increases, muscle activity decreases progressively until it becomes minimal and is coordinated precisely to produce just the muscle action necessary for writing. It then becomes virtually fatigue-free (Paillard, 1960). Following brain damage, coordinated movements often are disturbed. Patients become fatigued when attempting controlled movements; rehabilitation is then oriented toward the restoration of precise, fatigue-free movements, using a minimum of muscle activity to achieve the desired movement. Comparably, reflexes that are normal shortly after birth (e.g., Babinski's) are inhibited during maturation and can reappear following brain damage.

There are many other similarities to the learning process. Rehabilitation cannot be injected; passive procedures have little value except to prevent complications such as contractures or bed sores. The patient has to cooperate actively for rehabilitation to be successful. Therefore, the psychosocial factors (e.g., social support, motivation, supportive and optimistic rehabilitation therapists, a positive rehabilitation environment) that are discussed elsewhere (Bach-y-Rita, 1995; Bach-y-Rita & Wicab-Bach-y-Rita, 1990a, 1990b) are critical to the effectiveness of rehabilitation programs.

Scientifically Based Rehabilitation

Clinical rehabilitation has developed in an ad hoc fashion. The first formal stroke rehabilitation method, published by Frenkel in the mid-nineteenth century, emerged from a program that a nonprofessional woman had developed to rehabilitate her husband successfully (Licht, 1975). Rehabilitation clinicians still rely on nontheory-related methodologies. This is hard to understand, since there is a considerable literature in experimental psychology, behavioral psychology, neurophysiology, and other disciplines (much of it discussed in the chapters in this book) that could and should be brought to bear on the development of clinical rehabilitation programs.

Taub and Wolf (1997) noted that, except for a paper by Andrews and Stewart (1979), little has been written about the fact that rehabilitation as presently practiced has meager carryover to real-life activities and even little carryover from one session to another. Taub and Wolf noted that this situation reinforces the "widespread impression in the physical rehabilitation field that once a patient reaches a plateau, usually 6–12 months after a stroke, further administration of rehabilitation therapy does not have useful results" (p. 39). Andrews and Stewart (1979) found that there was a difference between what stroke patients did in the hospital stroke unit and what they did at home. Each activity of daily living was less well performed in the home situation in 25%–45% of the cases, and in 52% of the cases the chief carer claimed that the patient did not do two or more activities at home that were performed in the hospital.

In several publications, Taub and collaborators (Taub & Crago, 1995) make a strong case for basing therapy on experimental findings. Taub is particularly interested in the results of different means of training. Taub and Crago (1995) have evaluated theoretical issues, drawn from Taub's extensive animal and more recent human studies, and have noted that carryover to real-life activities requires programs specifically developed to do so. They have examined issues such as the nature of the interaction between behavioral and neural plasticity and the nature of rehabilitation programs that produce functional carryover. Programs based on conditioned responses have no carryover, while those based on shaping and on constraint-induced facilitation have excellent carryover to real-life tasks. Taub and Crago (1995) noted that motor status improves no more in developmentally disabled children given well-executed traditional physical therapy than in either untreated or attention-placebo-treated control subjects.

There are a number of excellent recent studies on the scientific basis of recovery of function with rehabilitation, including those reported by Nudo and his associates (Chapter 9), who note the following:

1. Rehabilitation must be varied and must not be repetitive. They state, "If physiologic plasticity in cortical maps is critical for functional recovery, then it follows that tasks requiring progressively increasing motor skills are more important than tasks that simply require the patient to move the limb repetitively in the absence of skill acquisition."
2. Changes in the motor cortex are driven by the acquisition of new motor skills, not simply by motor use. (I consider this to be evidence that the repetitive, boring activities of standard rehabilitation programs are virtually useless and that functional rehabilitation with motivating activities may avoid this pitfall.)
3. Functional plasticity is accompanied by structural plasticity.
4. Unmasking, multiplexing, synaptic plasticity, sprouting, and inhibition are mechanisms of functional reorganization following brain damage.
5. Functional plasticity in intact cortex begins immediately after injury.
6. Activity (rehabilitation) results in an increase in the neuropil, in dendritic arborization, in the number of synapses, and in the separation between neurons, resulting in the reduction of the number of neurons per cubic millimeter.
7. Spontaneous motor recovery cannot be explained by substitution of function in the spared motor cortex immediately adjacent to the lesion. The retention of functional representation in tissue adjacent to the lesion requires motor training (rehabilitation), which appears to have a modulatory effect on plasticity in the surrounding tissue.

Of equal relevance to clinical rehabilitation is Chapter 8 by Schallert et al. Some of their relevant findings are as follows:

1. Mechanisms of both neuroplasticity and neurodegeneration, including behavioral, anatomy, and neurochemistry, can be influenced by manipulations of motor behavior.
2. Blocking the N-methyl-D-aspartate (NMDA) receptors may be neuroprotective in the early postinjury period, but blocking them later on may reinstate deficits. (This is another finding in the complicated field of the effect of neuroactive substances in recovery of function. Many have powerful effects, and much work is needed to develop effective pharmacologic therapy.)

3. Immobilizing the good limb too soon after brain damage in a rat model can have "extremely deleterious effects," both in behavioral responses and in causing a "dramatic expansion of the original lesion." (It appears that either too much or too little activity can have profoundly negative consequences.)
4. In rats, forced disuse for 1 week has a number of measurable negative effects. (What is the negative effect of forced bed rest in brain-damaged humans?)
5. In rats, minimal forelimb use may initiate at least partial plasticity and afford protection against later "aggressive" rehabilitation, while early immobilization extends the period of vulnerability to forced overuse.
6. Mild rehabilitation may improve the functional outcome, while early moderate rehabilitation can have negative effects including an increase in the size of the infarct.
7. Human stroke patients had a worse outcome with forced speech therapy for several weeks than with brief (15 minute) conversations.

Chapters 8 and 9 challenge several dogmas of rehabilitation. Intensive (how much?) rehabilitation is not good for the eventual recovery of function. Immobilization and forced use, although shown to be positive in late rehabilitation (see Taub, above) has extremely negative effects early on. Mild rehabilitation, and conversations rather than intensive speech therapy may be indicated. Some time ago, I discussed the timing and organization of rehabilitation (Bach-y-Rita, 1990) and proposed a much more extended and gradual rehabilitation program than is usually the goal of inpatient rehabilitation. Mild rehabilitation, home programs, and late rehabilitation may produce the best outcome. However, as Schallert et al. (Chapter 8) note, "the optimal program of rehabilitation has not yet been established."

In clinical neurologic rehabilitation, there have been few randomized prospective studies (De Pedro-Cuesta et al., 1992). We discovered how difficult such studies are to carry out. In 1989 we explored the feasibility of early home rehabilitation for stroke at the Karolinska-Huddinge Hospital in Sweden, with home visits by a physical or occupational therapist. A pilot study was completed that suggested its feasibility and cost effectiveness (Bach-y-Rita & de Pedro-Cuesta, 1991; De Pedro-Cuesta et al., 1992, 1993; Widén-Holmqvist et al., 1993, 1994, 1995, 1998).

A model for logistic regression was used to evaluate the impact of different factors on functional recovery and was adjusted for potential confounding. The adjusted odds ratio with 95% for high level of motor capacity (2.77, 0.75–10.15), Bartel activities of daily life (ADL) (2.19, 0.63–7.62), extended Katz ADL (1.80, 0.68–4.74), and social activity (2.54, 0.71–9.09) indicated a trend toward a better outcome in the home rehabilitation group. The mean duration of the hospital stay for the home rehabilitation group was 13 days, and the patients received on average nine home visits after discharge. In contrast, the mean hospital stay for the routine rehabilitation group was 28 days, and 50% of the patients visited therapists or used day care after discharge. Patients preferred home rehabilitation (Widén-Holmqvist, 1996).

Rehabilitation in the Future

Prospective, randomized clinical studies, such as the stroke study described above, offer the opportunity to obtain scientifically valid evidence by which rehabilitation methods can be evaluated. Such clinical trials, together with the objective, quantified studies to be discussed below, should lead to scientifically validated rehabilitation.

I take the optimistic view that greater attention to theory and research will lead to radical changes in the delivery of rehabilitation services that will virtually eliminate rehabilitation as practiced today. Traditional neurologic rehabilitation is costly, inefficient, labor intensive, and artificially fractionated into multiple specialties. There is little rationale for the timing and intensity of presently practiced rehabilitation therapy.

Shorter hospital stays, often with sicker patients than in the past, have already forced many hospitals to reorganize their rehabilitation services, although these services are still based on traditional ineffective models. The absence of objective, quantitative data on most procedures is leading to reimbursement difficulties, so the changes will be driven by economic considerations, hastened by the changes affecting the organization and financing of medicine.

Those programs that can be demonstrated, with hard evidence, to provide cost-effective, measurable recovery of function will dominate rehabilitation. This means that objective, quantified data on recovery are essential and that randomized, prospective clinical trials of theory-based rehabilitation are needed now more than ever.

Demands for demonstrated efficacy at a reasonable cost will bring to the fore approaches such as the constraint-induced (CI) movement therapy developed by Taub for late rehabilitation (Taub & Crago, 1995) and the interesting and motivating real-life activity therapy that we have been emphasizing over the last 20 years (Bach-y-Rita, 1995).

Taub has been a pioneer in the development of a scientifically validated rehabilitation procedure (Taub & Crago, 1995; replicated in another country: Miltner et al., 1999). He and his colleagues have completed a series of brain imaging studies (e.g., Liepert et al., 1998) correlating brain changes with functional changes.

Since the 1960s, we have explored functional changes obtainable with rehabilitation in persons with known lesions. The first model was designed to demonstrate that adults who were blind since infancy (and therefore had major changes in visual pathways and central representation), and had acquired the capacity to perceive visual images through a tactile sensory system, had to reorganize their brain mechanisms to do so. Positron emission tomography scan data support that conclusion (Wanet-Defalgue et al., 1988). Thus, sensory substitution systems offer the possibility of demonstrating human brain plasticity.

The tactile vision substitution systems (TVSS) deliver visual information to the brain via arrays of stimulators in contact with the skin of one of several parts of the body, including the abdomen, back, thigh, fingertip, and tongue (Bach-y-Rita, 1972, 1995, 1999; Bach-y-Rita et al., 1969, 1998). Optical images picked up by a TV camera are transduced into a form of energy (vibratory or direct electrical stimulation) that can be mediated by the skin receptors. The visual information reaches the perceptual levels for analysis and interpretation via somatosensory pathways and structures.

After sufficient training with the TVSS, blind subjects reported experiencing the images in space instead of on the skin. They learned to make perceptual judgments using visual means of analysis, such as perspective, parallax, looming and zooming, and depth judgments. Our studies with the TVSS have been extensively described.

The sensory substitution systems for sensory losses other than blindness (technically, blindness from retinal damage is due to brain damage, since the retina is part of the brain) also require major adaptations, which apparently include brain reorganization (Bach-y-Rita, 1995). The brain plasticity mechanisms that are involved in sensory substitution may be similar to those related to recovery from brain damage.

Another postacute program has been developed for persons with long-standing facial paralysis due to facial nerve damage during the removal of an acoustic neuroma, who had undergone a VII–XII cranial nerve anastomosis (connecting part of the tongue nerve to innervate the facial muscles). In this model, it is clear that the facial muscles are now innervated by nerve fibers from structures genetically programmed to move tongue muscles. Yet with appropriate rehabilitation, persons recover spontaneous and voluntary bilateral facial symmetrical movements and learn to inhibit dyskinetic movements. We have developed prototypes of objective, quantified computer image analysis–based evaluation of progress (Bach-y-Rita, 1995). Like the studies of the Taub group discussed above, the image analysis studies are designed to provide objective, quantitative evidence of recovery with a specific rehabilitation method. More than a comparison of rehabilitation methods, this study was designed to evaluate brain plasticity in a human model in which the extent of the lesion is definitely known and in which, due to the complete loss of connectivity from the brain regions genetically programmed to control facial movements, another system (in this case, the brain regions that had previously controlled tongue movements) could be demonstrated to have reorganized to obtain functional recovery.

These studies, as well as the studies reported in the chapters of this book and in the cited research reports, as well as future studies along these lines, will be the basis for major changes in the organization of rehabilitation services. I predict that among the major changes that will occur, the rehabilitation team will virtually disappear. In any case, there is no evidence that it is better than other forms of delivery of rehabilitation services (Keith, 1991), and it is very expensive in terms of cost, time, and efficiency. In a preliminary study (never completed because of his fatal illness) of the efficiency of dividing rehabilitation therapy into numerous subdisciplines such as physical Occupational therapy, recreational speech psychology, and others, B. Berenson, a distinguished architect, followed patients leaving their hospital rooms in the morning to go to the various special rehabilitation services. He held a stopwatch and recorded the number of minutes of actual therapy; they were surprisingly few. Most of the time was spent transporting the patient, waiting for the therapist, and having the therapist determine the readiness and general state of the patient that day in the initial stage of each session.

What will replace the rehabilitation team? If intense therapy is appropriate, a single cross-trained therapist, who can spend more hours with a patient than several separate therapists, may provide therapy more efficiently. Thus, I predict that a neurologic rehabilitation therapist, combining aspects of each of the present therapies, will emerge in the reorganization of rehabilitation services. For home rehabilitation, which I predict will be the norm for those patient for whom it is appropriate, a single therapist is practical and efficient, as demonstrated in our Stockholm studies (see above). Inpatient rehabilitation will still be required for many patients, and for parts of the programs (in some cases, several short hospital stays) of even those patients rehabilitated principally at home. My experience over the years, and the results of our Stockholm project, suggest that stroke patients and their families are least stressed, and happier in general, when rehabilitation can be provided at home in a familiar and supportive environment for patients who have such support systems. Furthermore, outside of the hospital, patients are less likely to acquire hospital infections. Many home rehabilitation tasks can be related to real-life activities, such as washing the dishes or sweeping the floor. Carryover is less difficult when the rehabilitation is already based on functional real-life activities.

Other forms of therapy (some already in use) and other approaches to the timing of rehabilitation (Bach-y-Rita, 1990) will become more common. At present, rehabilitation has a plethora of named therapies (e.g., Brunstrom, Bobath) for which scientific validation is insufficient; reported therapeutic successes may have more to do with the attitudes toward the patient resulting from the conviction that the particular therapy is the most effective than with the specific merits of the therapy itself. But certainly, attitude alone has a dramatic effect (e.g., Bach-y-Rita, 1995; Bach-y-Rita & Wicab-Bach-y-Rita, 1990a, 1990b), and the environment and psychological factors are of enormous importance.

For neurologic rehabilitation, cost-effective rehabilitation programs that are well documented and validated should include the packaging of programs, possibly on compact disks or on the Internet. These could be provided as a library of programs from which not only specialists (physiatrists and neurologists) but also primary care physicians could select to prescribe the rehabilitation of their patients and monitor their progress.

At present, medical students have little exposure to rehabilitation and little understanding of the issues related to long-term care. I predict that including rehabilitation in family practice training programs will help to counteract the acute care mentality that develops in medical school and persists in our delivery-of-care systems.

Rehabilitation in nursing homes (in the true sense of the word—not final repositories, as is now generally the case), outpatient facilities, and other organizational modes will develop. In the best cases, programs outside of the hospital can be more motivating in more friendly environments, as well as being cost-effective. Social aides will help patients living at home.

Neuropharmacology offers the possibility of major advances, not only for specific problems such as agitation, motivation, and spasticity, but also for correcting lesion-induced neurotransmitter imbalances and for facilitating pathways of the various sorts discussed above (neural as well as those related to the microenvironment of the brain cells).

Motivating therapy will dominate. An example is the ingenious approach taken by Gauthier and his colleagues (1978) to obtaining eye movement control in children with cerebral palsy who had eye coordination deficits. They noted, as had others before them, that watching a pendulum aided in the training, but they found that the children refused to watch because they found it too boring. They developed a fascinating functional pendulum by projecting children's movies (*Snow White, Lassie*) at a galvanometer-controlled mirror that reflected the image to the back side of a projection screen. The children sat in front of the screen with their heads fixed, so that to follow the pendular movements of the image, they had to use eye movements. They had 6 hours a week of intense therapy (three movies) and within a month improved to the point where they could learn to read.

We had previously used a comparable approach when the early electronic pong games, which could be connected to home TV sets, appeared in the early 1970s (Cogan et al., 1977). We substituted for one of the joystick controls a device used in the clinic to train arm movements in hemiparetic persons. Instead of meaningless exercise, the effort to move the arm could then control a paddle (paddle size and ball speed were varied according to the capabilities of individual patients), allowing participation in a highly motivating game. A virtual reality version of this system is planned. Other forms of simple devices, game-based Internet therapy, and other technological advances will be widely used in both home and institutional rehabilitation, and the more general acceptance of both early and late plasticity will influence attitudes and produce a more supportive environment for the patient.

Finally, the timing of rehabilitation service delivery will change. No longer will intense therapy be forced on sick patients, many of whom are not ready for it. Various forms of rehabilitation therapy will be spread more judiciously across the full course of the disability.

Thus, a typical stroke patient in the future will have a short acute inpatient stay on a medical unit, where rehabilitation will begin from day 1 with passive range of motion and appropriate positioning; at this time, the physiatrist or neurologist will initiate pharmacological therapy and work with a cross-trained neurologic rehabilitation therapist, who will be the primary contact with the patient for the entire course (up to several years) of the rehabilitation. From this hospitalization, some patients will be released home and some will be transferred to an inpatient rehabilitation unit. In both hospital units, rehabilitation will take place in the patient's room and in therapy rooms, which will be mostly small, individual patient rooms primarily with electronic and computation-based rehabilitation. The patient interfaces will be simple, inexpensive mechanical devices, but some of the rehabilitation will occur in a gym setting with machines.

For patients who can undergo rehabilitation at home, close monitoring will occur over the Internet, and rehabilitation will be electronic and computation based, again with simple, inexpensive mechanical patient interfaces. The computer-based devices will also facilitate data collection. A new class of therapy aide will be developed for home visits. These aides will interact closely, personally, and electronically with the therapy staff, and will monitor both the rehabilitation program and the psychosocial factors, helping to create a positive, hopeful, and motivating environment. Equipment such as walkers and parallel bars will be simple and inexpensive, and wheelchairs will be plastic, easily assembled from molded parts. Motivating video game–based therapy appropriate for the age and interests of the patient will be available as a library of programs, so that the therapy staff will modify the rehabilitation, based on progress, by means of changes in the programs in the electronic library. The Internet and virtual reality rehabilitation will substitute for presently used expensive devices. There will be no separation of acute and postacute rehabilitation; rather, there will be a continuum, lasting as long as is needed—usually several years.

Stroke patients who live in rural areas or areas with difficult access to rehabilitation services will be more dependent on programs, largely electronically based, that will be monitored by their family practitioner (and staff), who will have received training in rehabilitation during residency training.

I began this chapter with a comment on the "dark ages" of brain plasticity, and throughout I have discussed what could be considered medieval neurologic rehabilitation. We are now ready to enter the modern age. It is up to all of us who have contributed chapters to this book, and all of our colleagues in the fascinating fields of neurological rehabilitation, neuroplasticity, and reorganization of function after brain injury, to continue to expand the knowledge contained in this book, which will lead to the development of modern, scientifically validated, effective rehabilitation procedures.

ACKNOWLEDGMENT

This chapter was completed during a sabbatical leave at the Facultad de Medicina, Universidad Autonoma del Estado de Morelos, Mexico, supported in part by a Cátedra Patrimonial of the Consejo Nacional de Ciencia y Tecnología (Mexico).

References

Aiello, G.L., and Bach-y-Rita, P. (1997) Brain cell microenvironment effects on neuron excitability and basal metabolism. *NeuroReport,* 8:1165–1168.

Anton, J.L., Benali, H., Guigon, E., Di Paola, M., Bittoun, J., Jolivet, O., and Burnod, Y. (1996) Functional MR imaging of the human sensorimotor cortex during haptic discrimination. *NeuroReport,* 7:2849–2852.

Andrews, K., and Stewart, J. (1979) Stroke recovery: He can but does he? *Rheumatology and Rehabilitation,* 18:43–48.

Bach-y-Rita, P. (1964) Convergent and long latency unit responses in the reticular formation of the cat. *Experimental Neurology,* 9:327–344.

Bach-y-Rita, P. (1972) *Brain Mechanisms in Sensory Substitution.* New York: Academic Press.

Bach-y-Rita, P. (1990) Timing and organization of neurorehabilitation. *Giornale Italiano di Medicina Riabilitativa*, 4:321–322.

Bach-y-Rita, P. (1993) Nonsynaptic diffusion neurotransmission (NDN) in the brain. *Neurochemistry International*, 23:297–318.

Bach-y-Rita, P. (1995) *Nonsynaptic Diffusion Neurotransmission and Late Brain Reorganization*. New York: Demos-Vermande.

Bach-y-Rita, P. (1998) Nonsynaptic diffusion neurotransmission and some other emerging concepts. *Proceedings of the Western Pharmacology Society*, 41:211–218.

Bach-y-Rita, P. (1999) Theoretical aspects of sensory substitution and of neurotransmitter-related reorganization in spinal cord injury. *Spinal Cord*, 37:465–474.

Bach-y-Rita, P., Collins, C.C., Saunders, F., White, B., and Scadden, L. (1969) Vision substitution by tactile image projection. *Nature*, 221:963–964.

Bach-y-Rita, P., and de Pedro-Cuesta, J. (1991) Neuroplasticity in the rehabilitation. In A. Molina, J. Parreño, J.S. Martin, E. Robles, and A. Moret (eds.), *Rehabilitation Medicine*. Amsterdam: 5–12

Bach-y-Rita, P., Kaczmarek, K., Tyler, M., and Garcia-Lara, J. (1998) Form perception with a 49-point electrotactile stimulus array on the tongue. *Journal of Rehabilitation Research and Development*, 35:427–430.

Bach-y-Rita, P., and Wicab-Bach-y-Rita, E. (1990a) Biological and psychosocial factors in recovery from brain damage in humans. *Canadian Journal of Psychology*, 44:148–165.

Bach-y-Rita, P., and Wicab-Bach-y-Rita, E. (1990b) Hope and active patient participation in the rehabilition environment. *Archives of Physical Medicine and Rehabilitation*, 71:1084–1085.

Bjelke, B., Bach-y-Rita, P., Anderson, C., and Fuxe, K. (1992) Changes in patterns of c-*fos* immunoreactive neurons in the rat tel- and diencephalon following *d*-amphetamine treatment. *Society for Neuroscience abstracts*, 18:871.

Broca, P. (1861) Nouvelle observation d'aphemie produite par une lesion de la motie posterieure des deuxieme et troisieme circonvolutions frontales. *Bulletin de la Societé Anatomie de Paris*, 6:398–407.

Chow, K.L., and Stewart, D.L. (1972) Reversal of structural and functional effects of long-term visual deprivation. *Experimental Neurology*, 34:409–433.

Cogan, A., Madey, J., Kaufman, W., Holmlund, G., and Bach-y-Rita, P. (1977) Pong game as a rehabilitation device. *Proceedings of the Fourth Annual Conference on Systems and Devices for the Disabled*. Seattle, WA: University of Washington pp. 187–188.

De Keyser, J.D., Ebinger, G., and Vauquelin, G. (1989) Evidence for a widespread dopaminergic innervation of the human cerebral cortex. *Neuroscience Letters*, 104:281–285.

de Pedro-Cuesta, J., Sanström, B., Holm, M., Stawiarz, L., Widen-Holqvist, L., and Bach-y-Rita, P. (1993) Stroke rehabilitation: Identification of target groups and planning data. *Scandinavian Journal of Rehabilitation Medicine*, 25:107–116.

de Pedro-Cuesta, J., Widen-Holmqvist, L., and Bach-y-Rita, P. (1992) Evaluation of stroke rehabilitation by randomized controlled studies: A review. *Acta Neurologica Scandinavica*, 86:433–439.

Dews, P.B., and Wiesel, T.N. (1970) Consequences of monocular deprivation on visual behavior in kittens. *Journal of Physiology*, 206:437–455.

Dietzel, M.A., and Heinemann, I. (1986) Dynamic variations of the brain cell microenvironment in relation to neuronal hyperactivity. *Annals of the New York Academy of Science*, 481:72–86.

Dietzel, M.A., Heinemann, I., Hofmeier, U., and Lux, H.D. (1980) Transient changes in the size of the extracellular space in the sensorimotor cortex of cats in relation to stimulus-

induced changes in potassium concentration. *Experimental Brain Research*, 40:432–439.

Dustman, R.E., Emmerson, R.Y., Ruhling, R.O., Shearer, D.E., Steinhaus, L.A., Johnson, S.C., Bonekat, H.W., and Shigeoka, J.W. (1990) Age and fitness effects on EEG, ERPs, visual sensitivity, and cognition. *Neurobiology and Aging*, 11:193–200.

Ericksson, P.S., Perfilieva, E., Björk-Eriksson, T., Alborn, A.M., Nordborg, C., Peterson, D.A., and Gage, F.H. (1998) Neurogenesis in the adult human hippocampus. *Nature and Medicine*, 4:1313–1317.

Franz, S., Sheetz, M., and Wilson, A. (1915) The possibility of recovery of motor function in long-standing hemiplegia. *Journal of the American Medical Association*, 65:2150–2154.

Gauthier, G.M., Hofferer, J.M., and Martin, B. (1978) Film projecting system as a diagnostic and training technique for eye movements of cerebral palsied children. *Electroencephalography and Clinical Neurophysiology*, 45:122–127.

Gould, E., Beylin, A., Tanapat, P., Reeves, A., and Shors, T.J. (1999) Learning enhances adult neurogenesis in the hippocampal formation. *Nature Neuroscience*, 2:260–265.

Guízar-Sahagún, G., Grijalva, I., Salgado-Ceballos, H., Espitia, A., Orozco, S., Ibarra, A., Franco-Bourland, R., Castañeda-Hernández, G., and Madrazo, I. (1999) Methylprednisolone limits plasticity at the lesion area following experimental paraplegia. Proceedings of the 45th Annual Conference, American Paraplegia Society, pp 46–47.

Harreveld, A.V., and Khallab, F.I. (1967) Changes in cortical extracellular space during spreading depression investigated with the electron microscope. *Journal of Neurophysiology*, 30:911–929.

Hubel, D.H., and Wiesel, T.N. (1970) The period of susceptibility to the physiological effects of unilateral eye closure in kittens. *Journal of Physiology (London)*, 206:419–436.

Jenkins, W.M., Merzenich, M.M., Ochs, M.T., Allard, T., and Guic-Robles, E. (1990) Functional reorganization of primary somatosensory cortex in adult owl monkeys after behaviorally controlled tactile stimulation. *Journal of Neurophysiology*, 63:82–104.

Keith, R.A. (1991) The comprehensive treatment team in rehabilitation. *Archives of Physical Medicine and Rehabilitation*, 72:269–274.

Kempermann, G., Brandon, E.P., and Gage, F.H. (1998a) Environmental stimulation of 129sv/J mice causes increasing cell proliferation and neurogenesis in the adult dentate gyrus. *Current Biology*, 8:939–942.

Kempermann, G., Kuhn, H.G., and Gage, F.H. (1998b) Experience-induced neurogenesis in the senescent aged dentate gyrus. *Journal of Neuroscience*, 18:3206–3212.

Leyton, A.S., and Sherrington, C.S. (1917) Observations on the excitable cortex of the chimpanzee, orangutan and gorilla. *Quarterly Journal of Experimental Physiology*, 11:135–222.

Licht, S. (1975) Brief history of stroke and its rehabilitation. In S. Licht (ed.), *Stroke and Its Rehabilitation*. Baltimore: Waverly Press, pp. 1–27.

Liepert, J., Miltner, W.H.R., Bauder, H., Sommer, M., Dettmers, C., Taub, E., and Weiller, C. (1998) Motor cortex plasticity during constraint-induced movement therapy in stroke patients. *Neuroscience Letters*, 250:5–8.

Lipton, P. (1973) Effects of membrane depolarization on light scattering by cerebral cortical slices. *Journal of Physiology*, 231:365–383.

Luria, A.R. (1963) *Restoration of Function After Brain Damage*. New York: Macmillan.

McBain, C.J., Traynelis, S.F., and Dingledine, R. (1990) Regional variation of extracellular space in the hippocampus. *Science*, 249:674–677.

Merton, R.K. (1968) The self-fulfilling prophecy. In R.K. Merton (ed.), *Social Theory and Social Structure.* New York: Free Press, pp. 475–490.

Merzenich, M.M., Kaas, J.H., Wall, J.T., Nelson, R.J., Sun, M., and Felleman, D. (1983) Topographic reorganization of somatosensory cortical areas 3b and 1 in adult monkeys following restricted deafferentation. *Neuroscience,* 8:33–55.

Miltner, W.A.R., Bauder, H., Sommer, M., Dettmers, C., and Taub, E. (1999). Effects of constraint-induced movement therapy on chronic stroke patients: A replication. *Stroke,* 30:586–592.

Murata, K., Cramer, H., and Bach-y-Rita, P. (1965) Neuronal convergence of noxious, acoustic and visual stimuli in the visual cortex of the cat. *Journal of Neurophysiology,* 28:1223–1239.

Paillard, J. (1960) The patterning of skilled movements. In J. Field (ed.), *Handbook of Physiology, American Physiological Society,* Section 1, Vol. 3. Baltimore: Williams & Wilkins, pp. 1679–1708.

Pascual-Leone, A., and Torres, F. (1993) Plasticity of the sensorimotor cortex representation of the reading finger in Braille. *Brain,* 116:39–52.

Rosenzweig, M. (1980) Animal models for the effects of brain lesions and for rehabilitation. In P. Bach-y-Rita (ed.), *Recovery of Function: Theoretical Considerations for Brain Injury Rehabilitation.* Bern, Switzerland: Hans Huber, pp. 127–172.

Sadato, N., Pascual-Leone, A., Grafman, J., Deiber, M.P., Ibañez, V., and Hallett, M. (1998) Neural networks for Braille reading by the blind. *Brain,* 121:1213–1229.

Taub, E., and Crago, J.E. (1995) Behavioral plasticity following central nervous system damage in monkeys and man. In B. Julesz and I. Kovacs (eds.), *Maturational Windows and Adult Cortical Plasticity.* Redwood City, CA: Addison-Wesley, pp. 201–215.

Taub, E., and Wolf, S.L. (1997) Constraint induced techniques to facilitate upper extremity use in stroke patients. *Topics in Rehabilitation,* 3:38–61.

Tononi, G., and Edelman, G.M. (1998) Consciousness and complexity. *Science,* 282:1846–1851.

Wall, P.D. (1980) Mechanisms of plasticity of connection following damage in adult mammalian nervous systems. In P. Bach-y-Rita (ed.), *Recovery of Function: Theoretical Considerations for Brain Injury Rehabilitation.* Bern, Switzerland: Hans Huber, pp. 91–105.

Wanet-Defalque, M.C., Veraart, C., DeVolder, A., Metz, R., Michel, C., Dooms, G., and Goffinet, A. (1988) High metabolic activity in the visual cortex of early blind human subjects. *Brain Research,* 446:369–373.

Weisskopf, G.P., Zalutski, R.A., and Nicoll, R.A. (1993) The opioid peptide dynorphin mediates heterosynaptic depression of hippocampal mossy fiber synapses and modulates long-term potentiation. *Nature,* 662:423–427.

Westerberg, E., Monaghan, D.T., Kalimo, H., Cotman, C.W., and Wieloch, T.W. (1989) Dynamic changes of excitatory amino acid receptors in the rat hippocampus. *Journal of Neuroscience,* 9:798–805.

Widén-Holmqvist, L. (1996) An interim data analysis of a randomized controlled trial of rehabilitation at home after stroke in South-West Stockholm. *European Journal of Neurology,* Supplement 3, 2:27.

Widén-Holmqvist, L., de-Pedro-Cuesta, J., Möller, G., Holm, M., and Sidén A. (1996) A pilot study of rehabilitation at home after stroke: A health-economic appraisal. *Scandinavian Journal of Rehabilitation Medicine,* 28:9–18.

Widén-Holqvist, L., de-Pedro-Cuesta, J., Holm, M., and Kostulas, V. (1995) Intervention design for rehabilitation at home after stroke; a pilot feasibility study. *Scandinavian Journal of Rehabilitation Medicine,* 27:43–50.

Widén-Holqvist, L., de-Pedro-Cuesta, J., Holm, M., Sandström, B., Hellblom, A., Stawiarz, L., and Bach-y-Rita, P. (1993) Stroke rehabilitation in Stockholm. Basis for intervention in patients living at home. *Scandinavian Journal of Rehabilitation Medicine,* 25:173–181.

Widén-Holmqvist, L., von Koch, L., Kostulas, V., Holm, M., Widsell, G., Tegle, R.H., Johansson, K., Almazan, J., and de Pedro Cuesta, J. (1998) A randomized controlled trial of rehabilitation at home after stroke in south-west Stockholm. *Stroke,* 29:591–597.

Index

Note: Page numbers in *italics* indicate figures; page numbers followed by t indicate tables.